Pharmacy Practice Research Methods

Zaheer-Ud-Din Babar
Editor

Pharmacy Practice Research Methods

Adis

Editor
Zaheer-Ud-Din Babar
Faculty of Medical and Health Sciences
University of Auckland
Auckland
New Zealand

ISBN 978-3-319-14671-3   ISBN 978-3-319-14672-0 (eBook)
DOI 10.1007/978-3-319-14672-0

Library of Congress Control Number: 2015936045

Springer Cham Heidelberg New York Dordrecht London
© Springer International Publishing Switzerland 2015
This work is subject to copyright. All rights are reserved by the Publisher, whether the whole or part of the material is concerned, specifically the rights of translation, reprinting, reuse of illustrations, recitation, broadcasting, reproduction on microfilms or in any other physical way, and transmission or information storage and retrieval, electronic adaptation, computer software, or by similar or dissimilar methodology now known or hereafter developed.
The use of general descriptive names, registered names, trademarks, service marks, etc. in this publication does not imply, even in the absence of a specific statement, that such names are exempt from the relevant protective laws and regulations and therefore free for general use.
The publisher, the authors and the editors are safe to assume that the advice and information in this book are believed to be true and accurate at the date of publication. Neither the publisher nor the authors or the editors give a warranty, express or implied, with respect to the material contained herein or for any errors or omissions that may have been made.

Printed on acid-free paper

Adis is a brand of Springer
Springer International Publishing AG Switzerland is part of Springer Science+Business Media (www.springer.com)

To Aneequa and Danyal

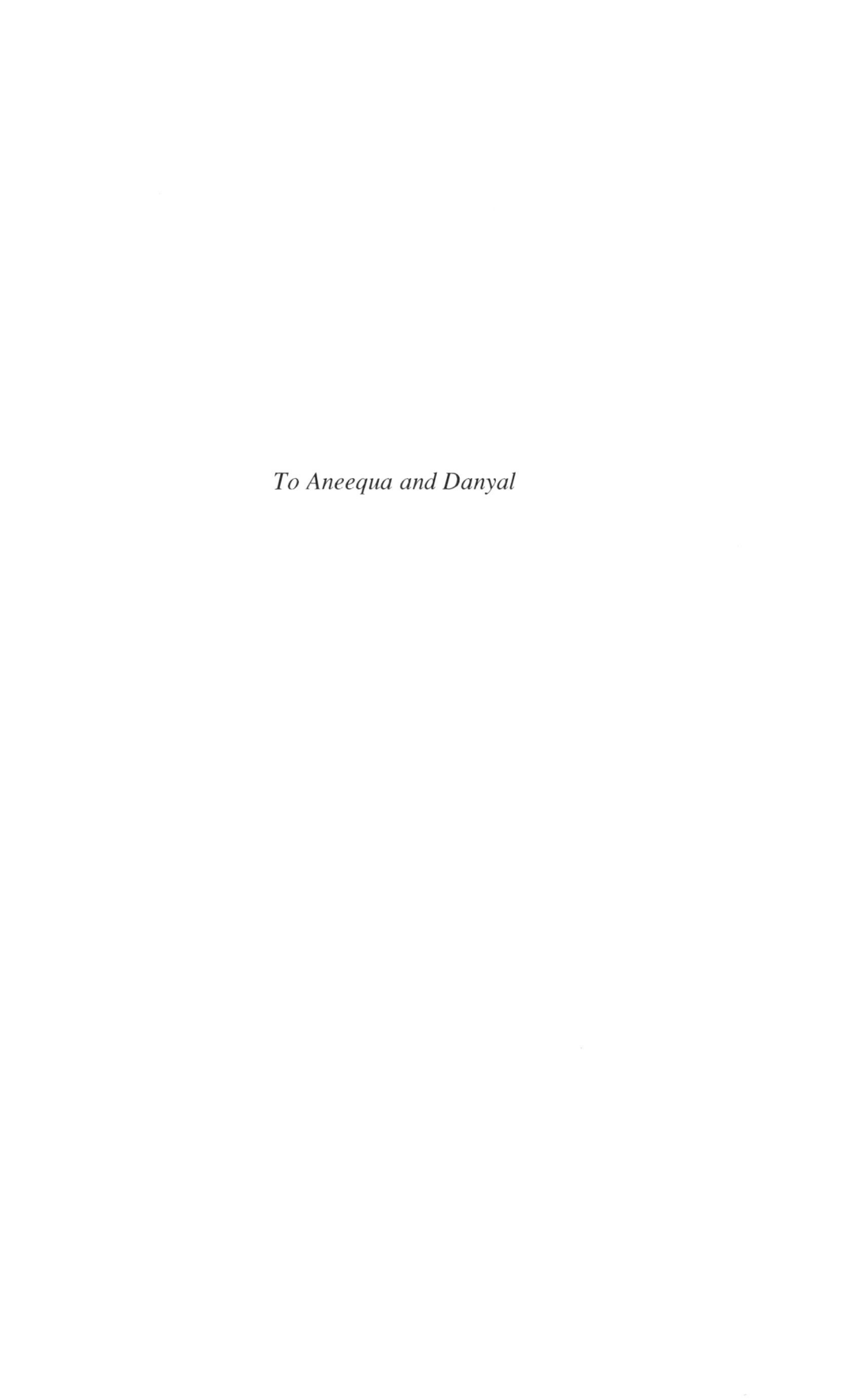

Foreword

The publication of this collection of methodologies and methods surely signals that Pharmacy Practice Research has come of age in providing an evidence base for the clinical effectiveness of pharmacy as an academic discipline and profession that places the person at the centre of care in medicine use.

Findings from gold standard research design and conduct must underpin pharmacy practice in the twenty-first century. The challenges of this century, including the discovery, delivery and use of medicines and therapeutic devices, revolve around the larger complex issues of climate change, border security, demographic changes, economic shifts, communications technology and resources sustainability all of which will impact the research in which pharmacists and their interdisciplinary colleagues engage. The role of the pharmacist will expand beyond medicines delivery, health education, public health, health promotion and policy development into areas that address health inequalities and their social determinants at the local level and on a global scale.

The various chapters in this edited volume provide a comprehensive but not exhaustive research toolkit for guiding the future practise of pharmacy in the technological age of the health literate patient requiring personalised pharmacotherapeutics for the chronic diseases of affluence and for understanding how to achieve equitable access to cost-effective medicines and culturally appropriate pharmaceutical care in developed and developing countries. Readers will find the descriptions helpful in building their own methodologies to address their diverse questions about the use of medicines, delivery of pharmaceutical services, pharmacists' employment and evidence-based policy to inform improvement in the quality and safety of pharmacy practice.

This book will be of interest to pharmacy students, academics, researchers and practising pharmacists. It provides general chapters on the broad paradigms of quantitative, qualitative and mixed methods research alongside chapters on specific research methods, including the application of methods from other disciplines, such as the social and behavioural sciences, economics and epidemiology, to the practice of pharmacy.

Melbourne, VIC, Australia									Kath Ryan
November 2014

Contents

1. **Pharmacy Practice Research: Evidence and Impact** 1
   Christine Bond

2. **Research Methodologies Related to Pharmacy Practice: An Overview** 25
   Parastou Donyai

3. **Quantitative Methods in Pharmacy Practice Research** 31
   James A. Green and Pauline Norris

4. **Qualitative Methods in Pharmacy Practice Research** 49
   Susanne Kaae and Janine Marie Traulsen

5. **Action Research in Pharmacy Practice** 69
   Lotte Stig Nørgaard and Ellen Westh Sørensen

6. **Participatory Action Research in Pharmacy Practice** 91
   Hazel Bradley

7. **Mixed Methods Research in Pharmacy Practice** 107
   Cristín Ryan, Cathal Cadogan, and Carmel Hughes

8. **Applying Organisational Theory in Pharmacy Practice Research** 123
   Shane Scahill

9. **Applying Pharmacoeconomics in Community and Hospital Pharmacy Research** 157
   Syed Tabish Razi Zaidi and Zaheer-Ud-Din Babar

10. **Concept Mapping and Pattern Matching in Pharmacy Practice Research** 175
    Shane L. Scahill

11	**Pharmacoepidemiological Approaches in Health Care** 197
	Christine Y. Lu
12	**The Future of Pharmacy Practice Research** 223
	Zaheer-Ud-Din Babar and Anna Birna Almarsdottir
13	**Pharmacists' Attitudes Towards Pharmacy Practice Research:**
	A Review 237
	Ahmed Awaisu, Nadir Kheir, Noor Alsalimy,
	and Zaheer-Ud-Din Babar

Chapter 1
Pharmacy Practice Research: Evidence and Impact

Christine Bond

Abstract This chapter summarises the current challenges that exist when matching increasing demand for health-care services to available capacity and funding. This has led to a drive to implement new services and redesign existing services in line with evidence of their clinical and cost-effectiveness. These principles are then translated into the context of pharmacy with consideration of the quality of the evidence available for pharmacy and related medicines services. Finally, there is an examination of the interplay between practice, policy and research, and examples are given of four different ways in which research can inform policy. The chapter concludes with a summary of the remaining challenges that need to be addressed to ensure that in pharmacy we can deliver an evidence-based service.

1.1 Evidence and Evidence-Based Health Care

It is important in 'health-care decision making' that both populations and individual patients are given a treatment that is likely to work and represents value for money. This is especially important at a time when in most of the countries in North America, Europe and Australasia (that is the majority of what is known as the developed world), the demand on health care is increasing. This is due largely to changing demographic profiles with a greater proportion of older people than previously. As age increases, there is an equivalent chance of poorer health and thereby requirement for treatment. This will therefore be a cost to countries, regardless of how their health-care systems are funded—i.e. whether they have a Beveridge-based approach such as in the taxation-funded universal health care offered under the NHS in the UK, or a Bismarck system, whereby health-care costs are covered by third party insurance systems, such as Germany or the USA.

To ensure limited budgets are used efficiently, the central question is which treatments are, and which treatments are not, both clinically- and cost-effective.

C. Bond (✉)
Centre of Academic Primary Care, University of Aberdeen, Aberdeen, UK
e-mail: c.m.bond@abdn.ac.uk

© Springer International Publishing Switzerland 2015
Z.-U.-D. Babar (ed.), *Pharmacy Practice Research Methods*,
DOI 10.1007/978-3-319-14672-0_1

This knowledge can inform decisions taken at both country wide level by policy makers and at individual patient level by the health-care professional in partnership with the patient. Indeed, the current drive towards more joint decision making at patient level is driven by research findings which suggest that this leads to better clinical outcomes and more satisfied patients who are likely to adhere to treatments.

1.1.1 Multiplicity of Research

There is already much research conducted to address questions about clinically-and cost-effective health care. Such studies range from pharmaceutical industry pre-licensing studies and post marketing surveillance, often not reported in peer reviewed journals, through to rigorous independently conducted substantive studies. However, these often only address the 'big' questions; a classic example would be the early studies demonstrating the value of reducing lipid levels in reducing morbidity and mortality from heart disease. Many conditions of lower prevalence remain under researched, although taken together, they represent a large proportion of the health care delivered.

However, there remains a challenge even when answering the big question. Is there a generic way of accessing, collating and interpreting results from the multiplicity of research reports in the peer-reviewed literature which can help 'answer' the question of finding the 'best treatment' for a particular population suffering a particular condition. Furthermore, whilst at a first glance the published literature may seem to offer some understanding, studies often report conflicting results and may not be conducted in the exact context for which information is required. For example, do results of a study conducted in North America with a largely Caucasian population aged averagely 50-years translate to a community in an area of Australia with a population of mixed ethnicity and ages over 65-years.

1.1.2 Quality of Research

The way research is conducted can also influence the bottom line as reported, potentially leading incorrect conclusions to be drawn. For example, a study conducted to explore whether taking an antidepressant relieves symptoms of depression, conducted without a control group could lead to a gross overestimation of the effect of the medication, because of the now well-documented size of the placebo effect. Randomised controlled studies, regarded as the best study design, cannot, however, automatically always be judged as rigorous. For example, it is important that all participants allocated to a treatment group are analysed in that group, and that those unable to be contacted for whatever reason at follow-up are classified as treatment failures. A good example of this would be smoking cessation studies, where those who are successful in stopping smoking are more likely to come back for follow-up assessment than those who have failed, leading to an overestimation of the effect of the smoking cessation intervention, be it a pharmacological or behavioural one. Therefore, in deciding to what extent a single piece of research can contribute to informing policy, the study design and conduct of the study must all be critically evaluated.

1.1.3 The Evidence-Based Medicines Movement

The conundrum, therefore, is how to develop techniques which allow the 'true' answer of what is the most clinically- and cost-effective choice to be distilled and synthesised from the literature, then to be understood, articulated and translated into practice at the front line of service delivery.

1.1.3.1 The Cochrane Collaboration

One of the first people to think through the above issues systematically was Archie Cochrane, founder of the Cochrane Collaboration[1] and one of the fathers of evidence-based medicine. In later parts of this chapter, we will talk more specifically about evidence-based pharmacy, but for now the principles of evidence-based medicine apply equally to evidence-based pharmacy.

The classic logo of the Cochrane Collaboration[2] illustrates the dilemma that people face when trying to understand what a multiplicity of research reports tell us about a specific question. The Cochrane Collaboration logo is itself a schematic representation of one of the first questions answered by the collaboration. This was to identify the right way to manage a woman with a history of repeated premature births, to prevent this happening in subsequent pregnancies. Each of the horizontal lines in the logo represents the outcome of a trial in which pregnant women were treated with varying doses of corticosteroid and the confidence limits around the estimated odds ratio of a successful outcome. The vertical line is the line through an odds ratio of 1, namely that there is no effect of treatment. Thus of the eight trials depicted, three show a benefit of using steroids. However, the diamond at the bottom shows the overall beneficial effect of this treatment in reducing premature births when all the studies are combined as if in one big trial. In this technique, now known as meta-analysis, all the individual studies are treated as one big study and one big population; increasing sample sizes in this way means the confidence interval around the estimated effect size is narrowed, and the robustness of the estimate is greater. Until this approach was understood, use of corticosteroids in

---

[1] www.cochrane.org/ accessed 27 Oct 2014.

[2] http://www.cochrane.org/about-us/history/our-logo accessed 16 Oct 2014.

pregnancy was only 20 %. It steadily rose thereafter reducing rates of premature births, preventing much human suffering and reducing NHS costs.

The Cochrane Collaboration itself is now an international group of health-service researchers, information scientists, statisticians and others who on a voluntary basis agree to conduct reviews of published literature to answer topical questions of relevance to health-care providers. There are Cochrane groups specific to different conditions, e.g. a Urology group, and those for more general topics such as what is the best way to encourage health-care professionals to change their behaviour—the Cochrane Effective Practice and Organisation of Care group.

1.1.3.2 Systematic Reviewing and Critical Appraisal

Accepting that meta-analysis is the solution to synthesising the literature and informing policy decisions about the best treatment, it becomes critical to ensure that prior to any meta-analysis, all eligible studies are identified. This has led to an understanding of the way to search the electronic databases of published research in the topic area. Gone are the days of manually searching journals until sufficient articles had been identified which made the required point. In a systematic review, the aspiration would be to find and include all relevant papers, regardless of their final conclusion, although the reality is often somewhat different. Even highly skilled information scientists cannot find everything, but if there are omissions, these should be by chance and not by intent. Once papers are identified, they also have to be critically appraised. One of the issues to consider is the extent to which it is valid to combine the individual studies into one big virtual study. Are the studies similar enough in terms of characteristics of the population, the health service in which they were delivered, the co-morbidities and risk factors of the participants, the outcomes used and the follow-up period. All of this has to be taken into account when looking at the value of the final figure and its applicability to any single setting. Furthermore, as mentioned earlier, what was the quality of the research that was done, were non-responders included in the follow-up, was an intention to treat analysis undertaken and were the assessors blind to group allocation. Perhaps of greatest importance is the study design. Ideally to compare two treatments, a randomised controlled trial design should be used, to allow for the multiple confounders that might spuriously suggest a treatment will work when assessed by a simple before and after analysis.

1.1.3.3 Grades of Evidence

The Cochrane Collaboration has devised a set of quality rules and standards which, as far as they can, allow for the limitations in published studies to be systematically examined and reported. There are Cochrane standards for the conduct of studies of different study designs, including most recently standards for assessing qualitative research and combining the results using meta-ethnography. There are even checklists for assessing systematic reviews of systematic reviews! These widely accepted quality tools therefore allow a review to be judged or graded, both on the rigour of the study designs and the quality of the studies. Amongst individual study designs, randomised controlled trials are the gold standard, followed by controlled trials, cohort studies, case studies and case reports. Both quality and study design can then be taken into account when assessing the importance which can be attributed to the bottom line finding.

1.1.4 Using Evidence to Influence Practice

Since the founding of the Cochrane Collaboration, the model of systematic reviewing and critical appraisal of the existing research have become the accepted approaches to inform health-care decision making, and 'an evidence-based service' has become the mantra. The Cochrane Collaboration is an international movement, and reviews are driven by researcher led groups. Therefore, in addition to Cochrane, individual countries have realised the need to develop their own organisations to undertake such reviews, answering questions driven by national priorities.

So, for example, in England and Wales, NICE (National Institute for Health and Care Excellence formally National Institute for Clinical Excellence)[3] was established in 1999. NICE undertakes and commissions reviews of the evidence, which are often directed at major issues such as whether or not a newly launched drug for a particular condition should be used. Initially, most interest was focussed on synthesising the evidence for choice of pharmacological agent. Given increasingly constrained budgets and demands on the health service, there has also been a steady move towards considering not only effectiveness but costs. In order to compare different treatments for cost, the concept of the quality-adjusted life year (QALY) was born. The QALY is a measure of disease burden, including both the quality and the quantity of life lived and provides a common standardised measure to allow comparisons between treatments, for example, between a new and an established treatment. It provides an objective measure of the additional cost of the new treatment and can demonstrate whether possibly marginal health gains come at an unaffordable cost. The synthesis of the evidence to support NICE decisions may need to be commissioned. One centre which often undertakes this synthesis is the NHS Centre for Reviews and Dissemination[4] based at the University of York.

Similarly, the Scottish Medicines Consortium[5] was established in Scotland in 2001, prompted by a need to remove replication of decision making across the then 15 individual Health Boards and to promote consistency in medicine use across

---

[3] www.nice.org.uk/ accessed 27 Oct 2014.
[4] www.york.ac.uk/inst/crd/ accessed 27 Oct 2014.
[5] https://www.scottishmedicines.org.uk/ accessed 27 Oct 2014.

Health Board boundaries. The SMC has been credited with providing more timely advice than NICE, but in practice the two groups work in tandem and complement each other's activities. In adopting evidence-based decision making in this way, the UK is reflecting practice in other countries such as Canada and Australia. For example, there is a pan-Canadian process [CADTH Common Drug Review (CDR)][6] which reviews the clinical effectiveness and cost-effectiveness of drugs and provides recommendations for Canada's publicly funded drug plans. In Australia, the Pharmaceutical Benefits Advisory Committee (PBAC)[7] recommends new medicines which can be provided under the Pharmaceutical Benefits Scheme (PBS) (medicines subsidised by the Australian Government). No new medicine can be listed unless the committee makes a positive recommendation. Reassuringly, a recent academic publication (Clement et al. 2009) demonstrated that conclusions about effectiveness and cost-effectiveness across the three countries were consistent, but that there was also variation in final recommendation because of differences in other contextual factors such as agency processes, ability for price negotiation and social values.

As well as high level use of evidence to inform policy, individual practitioners also need evidence-based guidance on managing individual patients with a particular condition, when they may be faced with a plethora of management and pharmacological treatment options. In Scotland, the Scottish Intercollegiate Guideline Group[8] undertakes wide ranging disease-based reviews, recognising that in some areas, the level of evidence is not as strong as in others and making this clear in the final recommendations. The development groups include clinicians, researchers and lay representatives, and findings are disseminated as guidelines to inform practice, with an accompanying quick reference guide for professionals and good practice points highlighted. Condition specific guidelines are also produced by specialist societies, e.g. for pain or hypertension.

1.2 Evidence-Based Pharmacy

1.2.1 From Drugs to Services

As noted above the original focus of evidence-based medicine was mostly about the choice of drug. There was an increasing recognition that similar techniques could also be applied to choices about different procedures or diagnostic tests and perhaps most recently about choice of personnel actually delivering the service. These developments and the need for appropriate methodologies to apply when moving from

---

[6] http://www.cadth.ca/ accessed 27 Oct 2014.

[7] http://www.health.gov.au/internet/main/publishing.nsf/Content/Pharmaceutical+Benefits+Advisory+Committee-1 accessed 27 Oct 2014.

[8] www.sign.ac.uk/ accessed 27 Oct 2014.

clinical research and studies of medicines contributed to the development of the discipline of Health Services Research (HSR).[9] HSR investigates 'how social factors, financing systems, organisational structures and processes, medical technology and personal behaviours affect access to health care, the quality and cost of health care and quantity and quality of life. Compared with medical research, HSR brings together social science perspectives with the contributions of individuals and institutions engaged in delivering health services'. It is a relatively new discipline whose methodologies are continually developing and becoming more sophisticated. Initially, HSR focussed more on the different ways of understanding and delivering patient care from the perspective of the effectiveness of the medical workforce, in both secondary and primary care. However, crucially it was not about whether a doctor could do something in a more effective or efficient way than another health-care professional but more about the optimal way a doctor should work. For example, should a surgeon use technique 'a' or technique 'b' or should stroke patients be cared for in specialist units or community units.

1.2.2 Pharmacy Practice Research

In applying an evidence-based approach to pharmacy, a sub-speciality within health services research has been developed known as pharmacy practice research. Its focus is on exploring how and why people access pharmacy services, the costs of pharmacy services and the outcomes for patients as a result of these services, and comparison of these costs and outcomes compared to the same or similar services delivered by other providers. Its aim is to support evidence-based policy and practice decisions where pharmacists are employed or medicines are prescribed or used.[10] Pharmacy practice research often challenges traditional professional boundaries, reflecting the shift in the balance of care currently observed in health-care delivery. For example, many conditions that were once primarily managed solely in a hospital setting are now managed in primary care settings, and many roles, particularly those delivered previously by doctors, are now being delivered by other health-care professionals including pharmacists. Pharmacy research aims to understand the clinical, humanistic and economic impact of these changes from the perspectives of pharmacists, patients and other health-care professionals.

1.2.2.1 Quality of Research

The approaches taken in pharmacy research can be summarised under the broad areas of understanding and describing the way care is accessed and delivered,

---

[9] http://en.wikipedia.org/wiki/Health_services_research accessed 25 Sept 14.

[10] http://en.wikipedia.org/w/index.php?title=Pharmacy_research&redirect=no accessed 25 Sept 2014.

identifying areas for improvement and evaluating new service models using rigorous research approaches. However, we should spend a moment now to reflect on the need, as in medicine, for rigorous approaches and to be critical of using research, to inform practice, which is not conducted to such standards.

As pharmacy practice research has developed, it has become inextricably linked to the move to change the whole paradigm of pharmacy from a technical supply function to a cognitive-based profession exploiting the unique expertise pharmacists have about medicines and their use, alongside the worldwide need to address the increasing demands on health care, financial constraints and predicted workforce shortages. Unfortunately, enthusiasm to demonstrate the contribution pharmacists can make to a wider role in health care has resulted in a multiplicity of small studies which were designed with the *a priori* assumption that a pharmacist could deliver a role effectively, for example, they could improve a patient's medication regime or increase their adherence, compared to current usual care. Critical also was the fact that with a few notable exceptions, much of the research was done by pharmacists themselves, generally with little insight into the increasingly sophisticated methodological approaches being used in HSR more generally. It is not surprising therefore that this body of research was widely criticised by the wider Health Services Research community and dismissed as not generating the necessary evidence for policy change. In response, in the UK, the Pharmacy Practice Research Resource Centre (based at the University of Manchester) commissioned a review of pharmacy practice research from Nicholas Mays, then Director of the Health and Health Care Research Unit at the Queens University Belfast. The results of the review were disseminated at a conference in 1994, but they made for uncomfortable reading for the majority of the pharmacy practice research community. The review concluded that the discipline of pharmacy practice research was largely immature, was limited to small descriptive and feasibility studies and most damningly that it was mostly designed and conducted by pharmacists with an apparent aim of demonstrating the value of pharmacy *per se*. The outcome was a plethora of studies interesting in that they could be used as proof of concept studies, but of little value in providing generalisable data, often only reporting intermediate process outcomes rather than clinical or humanistic patient outcomes and with health economic input extremely rare. In summary, in an evidence-based age, such research could not inform policy.

A core recommendation made in the review by Nicholas Mays referred to above was that as pharmacy practice research integrates several research paradigms and perspectives, it should be delivered by multidisciplinary groups including not only pharmacists and other members of the clinical team but also statisticians, health psychologists, social scientists, health economists and epidemiologists, among others.

1.2.2.2 Systematic Reviews of Pharmacy-Related Research

Just as in other areas of science, evidence from pharmacy practice research should be formally collated using a systematic review approach, involving comprehensive identification of all papers addressing a topic, selecting them against predefined inclusion and exclusion selection criteria, quality assessing them and reporting them. Ideally for quantitative studies, this should be in a meta-analysis. The critical quality review is really important for highlighting deficiencies in studies which may tend to favour more positive outcomes such as lack of an objective outcome measure, evaluation of the study by the same person who delivered the intervention, small numbers, failure to follow up non-responders or failure to use an intention to treat analysis. A relatively recent paper in Annals of Pharmacotherapy has emphasised the value of systematic reviews for pharmacy practice (Charrois et al. 2009) and gives good guidance on searching, evaluating, interpreting and disseminating the findings. Systematic reviews of pharmacy roles are increasing but readers need to critically consider the quality of the review method and the quality of the study inclusion criteria before quoting any conclusions. To take the profession forward, only the highest level of evidence should be cited.

Conducting a systematic review is a piece of research in its own right, often referred to as 'secondary' research. Just as primary studies can be done to differing levels of quality so can a systematic review. As noted earlier, there are quality criteria for assessing reviews, and even for reviews of reviews. Publishing a systematic review through the Cochrane Collaboration is beneficial on several counts. First, all Cochrane reviews have a certain status; they are also easily found by those searching for evidence as one of the first actions is always to search the Cochrane library. Second and linked to the above is the fact that there is knowledge that Cochrane reviews have been conducted to the highest standards; in order to publish a review under the Cochrane banner, a detailed protocol must first be submitted and approved through a peer review and editorial process. Finally, Cochrane reviews have a finite life and if not updated at regular predefined intervals, they are no longer considered valid.

There are already several systematic reviews relevant to pharmacy practice in the Cochrane library. Importantly, they often involve multidisciplinary teams of researchers and are therefore less likely to have any bias in favour of pharmacy in the interpretation and reporting.

One of the earliest was a review of the effect of outpatient pharmacists' non-dispensing roles on patient outcomes and prescribing patterns (Nkansah et al. 2010). Publication of the third update of this review is pending. In the most recent update in the public domain (2010), the authors comment that many of the studies show improvements but these are not statistically significant. The authors also comment that because of heterogeneity across the studies, no overall conclusion is possible.

In an evidence-based age, non-significant findings, however positive, cannot be claimed as evidence. Studies do not only need to be well designed but also to have included an appropriate sample size calculation to ensure they are not underpowered. Indeed the importance of undertaking an iterative approach to intervention design and testing is now well accepted[11] by the research community who follow the MRC guidance on developing and evaluating complex interventions. Pilot work to assess likely effect size and provide factual data to guide the power calculation for the definitive study is now *de rigueur*, and without this publication of studies in the leading journals is unlikely.

Similarly in 2012, a Cochrane review on polypharmacy and the elderly (Patterson et al. 2012) including a range of study designs showed a reduction in inappropriate prescribing and drug-related problems but conflicting results on hospital re-admissions,i.e. making a difference only to process rather than to a clinical outcome. The conclusion was, therefore, that it was unclear whether interventions to improve appropriate polypharmacy, such as pharmaceutical care, resulted in clinically significant improvements to patients.

Finally, a 2013 review (Alldred et al. 2013), again on improving prescribing but this time in care homes only, could not come to a definitive conclusion due to heterogeneity in design intervention and outcomes. This review could have had the potential to be considered a stronger more robust review, as it only included RCTs. However, individually few if any of these RCTs got high scores on the quality assessment. All of the eight studies, remaining after selection from 7,000 hits, included a pharmacist as the main deliverer of intervention.

Systematic reviews are of course published in many places, additional to the Cochrane library. They are printed by academic Journals, after going through appropriate peer review, and are prized by Editors as they get cited frequently. Holland et al undertook a review of papers evaluating the outcomes of pharmacist-led medication review in the elderly (Holland et al. 2008). Only RCTs were eligible for inclusion, and there was a meta-analysis for the main outcome of unscheduled hospital admissions. The authors comment on the steadily increasing quality of pharmacy practice research but once again were not able to provide a definite answer on changes if any in the 'clinical outcome of hospital re admission or mortality'. Some process improvements, e.g. patient knowledge and adherence were noted.

Finally, a review of the views of pharmacists, their staff and the public on a public health role for community pharmacy (Eades et al. 2011) concluded that overall whilst pharmacists were positive about providing public health services, these were secondary to medication-related and dispensing roles. Support staff were less confident and positive about providing a public health role, and whilst consumers were positive in principle about pharmacists providing such a service, they did not expect it and had rarely been offered it in practice. This review has identified descriptive studies such as surveys which are methodologically less challenging to conduct than an intervention studies, yet the authors of the review once again comment on the poor quality of the studies.

---

[11] http://www.mrc.ac.uk/documents/pdf/complex-interventions-guidance/ accessed 13 Oct 2014.

Small studies can of course be done to the highest quality, but to conduct a strong study eligible for any of the reviews cited above would require an experienced team and a substantive grant. Accessing such funds for pharmacy-related research is becoming easier, but it still represents a formidable challenge if pharmacy-related studies are being assessed for prioritisation against studies of, for example, a new surgical intervention. It is also sometimes difficult to get pharmacy colleagues in clinical practice to take part in research because they themselves are already very busy, and many funding arrangements do not pay for pharmacists' time. In Australia, there have been moves to integrate pharmacy practice and research, and the community pharmacy contract global sum includes money to fund pharmacy-related research. An excellent example of how this has been put to good effect follows in the next section.

1.2.3 Importance of Right Outcome

In their Cochrane review, Nkansah et al. commented on the heterogeneity of many components of the research including variation in the types, intensity and duration of interventions or differences in timing of follow-up measurements. They also comment on the lack of detail in the papers on the development processes of the interventions or how staff were trained to deliver the intervention or what constituted successful delivery of the intervention—what is sometimes referred to as fidelity. All of these are important things for any researcher to consider in designing, conducting and reporting a study.

The uncertainty around many of the aforementioned items could account for the conflicting results observed and also make it difficult to combine studies in a meta-analysis.

However, the main area of heterogeneity that the authors identify as requiring attention in the future is the need to select an appropriate outcome measure. At the study design stage, it should be possible to provide a theoretical reason for why the intervention in question is likely to change the selected primary outcome and whether the measure selected is likely to be sensitive enough to identify any changes. The gold standard choice of outcome to assess the clinical cost-effectiveness of intervention in general is a quality of life measure such as the SF36 or EQ5D which can be converted into QALY. Thus, NICE and equivalent organisation can compare diverse interventions on the basis of a common unit—the QALY, to which they can also attach a price.

However, in delivering pharmaceutical care we need to realistically ask ourselves the likelihood of changing these broad brush measures which have several domains. For example, the EQ5D, now the favoured measure in the UK, has five domains covering mobility, self-care, usual activities, pain/discomfort and anxiety/depression. Whilst there is a youth version there is no older people's version, and the scale itself has not been validated in every disease to which it has been applied. Nkansah et al. comment that in older people their likelihood of co-morbidities means that even improving outcomes in one of their conditions may not be sufficient to change the global assessment of overall quality of life and they call for a new universal, easily applied, valid and reliable outcome to be developed to use in these populations, who because of polypharmacy regimes often comprise the majority of participants in pharmaceutical care interventions.

In a study of community pharmacist-led medicine management for patients with coronary heart disease (The Community Pharmacy Medicines Management Project Evaluation Team (C. Bond Principal Investigator) 2007), there was no change in the primary outcome measure of patient quality of life as measured by the SF36 in the intervention group compared to the control. Yet there was significant increase in the patient satisfaction score for the care they received from the pharmacists. This leaves a conundrum of what is driving that increased satisfaction. Indeed, there is a general move to begin to consider the use of more patient-centred outcomes such as discrete choice experiments to value of what it is that the patient liked about the intervention. Early work has suggested that a DCE can be used to quantify and value the pharmacy input and reverse the take-home policy message to be more positive (Tinelli et al. 2010).

However, whilst the pharmacy profession and the research community all see the logic of this argument, the new pharmacy-delivered intervention is competing for funds with other new exciting developments, and the rationale for the EQ5D and SF36 QUALY were that they could bring a heterogeneous mix of interventions down to a single common unit of benefit. At this present time it is unclear how policy makers would view an alternative set of outcomes, and it remains unclear whether they would be prepared to pay for more satisfied patients.

1.3 The Policy, Practice and Research Triangle in Pharmacy

In 1986, the Nuffield report (Nuffield 1986) was the first to clearly identify in the UK that community pharmacists could play a more central role in health-care delivery. It was particularly important because it was seen to be an objective pronouncement by opinion leaders outwith the pharmacy profession who would have little, if any, vested professional interest in its recommendations.

The overall message of Nuffield was embraced in the context of health care in general. It was immediately adopted by policy makers in a succession of publications, which iteratively have been more ambitious in widening the scope of pharmacy practice and for changing a profession from having a predominantly technical medicine supply function to being a clinical profession with interfaces with both patients and other health-care professionals. The extent of change in the intervening years has been ground breaking. Whilst the UK has in many ways led the implementation of the extended role, this has also been happening elsewhere, most notably in Australia and Canada. In an evidence-based health-care system, it is interesting then to reflect on what has driven that change and to what extent it has been informed by research.

The reality is that to effect a change in role as significant as the one seen in pharmacy requires more than research evidence. For such a change to happen, it has to be acceptable to society—the public, fellow health-care professional and the pharmacy profession itself; it has to meet a policy need and there has to be some evidence of feasibility and benefit.

Applying these ideas specifically, and as noted earlier in this chapter, demographic changes will mean an inevitable increased future demand for health care. Furthermore, technological advances mean that many conditions previously treated surgically and requiring long stays in hospital can now be managed medically with pharmacotherapeutic approaches or as day cases. So there is a secondary care–primary care shift moving care out of hospitals. At the same time there are medical workforce shortages, a move to have longer consultation times reducing patient throughput, and a changing cultural expectation of the need to see a doctor for relatively minor symptoms, increasing demand although arguably not needed. The potential for other health-care professions including pharmacy to fill that capacity gap has been recognised, and the ambition for pharmacy to extend its role has actually coincided with a policy need. Furthermore, pharmacists have increasingly taken on new roles informally, for example, in hospitals advising medical staff of the best medicine regime for a patient, in the community issuing repeat prescriptions in advance of receipt of the formal form in the interest of continuity of supply for the patient, and pursuing the long-held traditional role of providing advice to patients on the management of minor ailments. Today it is a formal role in many countries for pharmacists to prescribe prescription only medicines; to prescribe on the NHS or equivalent pharmacy medicines rather than patients paying for them; to manage repeat dispensing; to advice on adherence; to provide a clinical medication review and make changes to drug regimens; to provide a multiplicity of public health roles including formal intensive advice to stop smoking, issuing emergency hormonal contraception, screening for chlamydia, giving brief interventions to address hazardous drinking and administering flu vaccinations to give but a few examples.

Practice research can be categorised under four broad areas with respect to its role in relation to policy. The first category is where **research has informed policy** and has been the trigger for innovation (e.g. smoking cessation, repeat dispensing, new medicines service) and where it was conducted before any service rollout. The second is again where the research was undertaken before service rollout but after a policy decision had been made, that is it was to **support a planned policy** (e.g. medicine management). Third is research that has been conducted after a new service had been introduced to **confirm the appropriateness of implemented policy**, (e.g. pharmacist prescribing). The final category is where it has been used to evaluate an innovation or service in order to **understand the processes in place**, identify good and less good aspects and make recommendations for the future (e.g. evaluation of the new English community pharmacy contractual framework). Each of these will be considered in turn, but it will be clear as the descriptions are read that there is some overlap between groups and in many ways it is a continuum. Because much of the professional change has been spearheaded in the UK, and because the author is UK based, there is no apology that the following examples are all from that country.

1.3.1 Research Informing Policy

1.3.1.1 Smoking Cessation

In 1991, as part of a progressive trend in many countries to widen safe and convenient access to medicines, the first nicotine replacement therapy (NRT) (nicotine gum 2 mg) was deregulated in the UK from a prescription-only medicine to a pharmacy medicine. Since then many other nicotine-replacement therapies at higher strength and in different formulations have been deregulated and many are now freely available as a General Sales List medicine. The wider availability of NRT made it possible for pharmacists to take on a very clear public health function of supporting smoking cessation. This led to the idea that pharmacists and their staff could be trained to provide a formal smoking cessation service. A randomised controlled trial was designed and funded to test whether the smoking cessation outcomes of people attending trained pharmacies were any different than those attending community pharmacies providing advice on smoking cessation as per usual practice. In other words, could the quality of the service provided by community pharmacists be enhanced by training. A 2-h training package was developed for pharmacists and their staff based on the theory of behavioural change. Smokers were followed up at 1 month, 4 months and 9 months after their first pharmacy visit. The study showed that smoking cessation rates at all three time points were better for those people attending trained compared to untrained pharmacies (Sinclair et al. 1998), and the cost of intensive pharmacist support was £300 per quitter and £83 per year of life gained (Sinclair et al. 1999). Despite this good evidence of benefit, endorsed by a Cochrane review (Sinclair et al. 2008), it was some time before smoking cessation advice became a core role for all community pharmacists in Scotland with appropriate recognition and a professional payment. First small local contractual arrangements were entered into, fighting professional turf wars on the way. Gradually, pharmacists demonstrated that as a profession they could deliver on smoking cessation, and in 2008, the service became embedded in the national contract. Today in Scotland, 70 % of all quit attempts go through community pharmacy, and thus community pharmacy is tackling one of the biggest public health problems of this, and the last, century. It is salutary to emphasise this long time line between the generation of the evidence and implementation into policy, and also to remember it was not just the research that led to the change. It also happened because society was ready to stop smoking and because smoking was suddenly identified as a priority public health policy issue.

1.3.1.2 Repeat Dispensing

With a similar time frame and in a similar way, a randomised controlled trial of pharmacists managing repeat dispensing conducted in the mid 1990s (Bond et al. 2000) led to repeat dispensing by pharmacists becoming embedded in both English and Scottish community pharmacy contractual frameworks. In the original RCT, when pharmacists managed repeat dispensing, they detected more medicine-related problems than were detected in the control group of usual care, they reduced the annual costs of drugs prescribed per patient in the system and GPs, managers and patients liked the service. Once again in the years following the academic publication, small pilot projects of the service were implemented widely in various local areas and ultimately the service became standard for all pharmacists.

1.3.1.3 New Medicines Service

The final example in this category is of the New Medicines Service recently introduced and evaluated in England. It is generally accepted that many people who are prescribed a new medicine do not necessarily take it for a range of reasons. Many people may even not take the first dose. A study published in 2006 (Clifford et al. 2006) showed that when patients prescribed a new medicine for a chronic condition were followed up by phone there was an improvement in their positive beliefs about taking the medicines, there was reduced non-adherence and reduced problems compared to a control group who did not receive the follow-up call. This research underpinned the New Medicines Service introduced into English community pharmacy contracts on a 1 year pilot basis in 2012 and now set to continue after an ongoing positive evaluation report. Thus, the New Medicines Service could also in fact fit into the next category of research confirming the appropriateness of a policy, especially as the way the service was implemented in practice was not through the centralised telephone service used in the trial but through individual pharmacists.

1.3.2 Research to Support a Planned Policy

In the early 2000s, new community pharmacy contracts were being developed in the home countries of the UK to reflect the aspirations of policy documents to move the pharmacy profession to a more cognitive role. Whilst most of the professionals believed at the time that this was the future for the profession, whilst contractual payments were driven by volumes of items dispensed, it was unlikely that the focus of community pharmacy services would change. Building on the success of the practice-based primary care pharmacists, it was believed that community pharmacists could deliver at least some of these roles from their community pharmacy base, by delivering a holistic pharmaceutical care service. In pharmaceutical care, pharmacists would take responsibility for the management of a patient's medicines and their associated drug-related needs. Research was commissioned by the Department of Health to derive evidence of the benefits of a community pharmacy-led pharmaceutical care service for patients with coronary heart disease. At the time there was evidence from published studies of the benefits of individual components of a pharmaceutical care or medicine management service (e.g. life style advice, blood pressure monitoring, adherence support), but there had been no studies of the whole service. A large definitive randomised controlled trial was conducted. This study has been previously referred to in this chapter as the one in which choice of outcome measure was critical. The study failed to show that there was an increase in appropriateness of treatment or patient quality of life although as noted earlier, there was increase in patient satisfaction and observed individual improvements in prescribing. However, whilst some community pharmacists identified many areas of improvement, others were less successful, so on average there was little change (Krska et al. 2007). When the new contract was implemented, it was emphasised that the Medicines Use Review component was about supporting the patient and not about improving appropriateness of care. This study also shows the challenges of generalising from small trials with self-selected participants to larger studies involving whole populations. The former are more likely to give positive results as the participants will be those who are more likely to have an interest in and commitment to the project. The larger whole population studies are more likely to reflect subsequent national implementation but may be more conservative in their estimate of benefit.

1.3.3 Research to Confirm the Appropriateness of Implemented Policy

Research defending policy is often commissioned as a formal evaluation after a service has been introduced. In the UK, this has been the case, for example, after the introduction of non-medical, including pharmacist prescribing.

1.3.3.1 Pharmacist Prescribing

Non-medical prescribing was introduced in the UK after the Crown review (Department of Health 1999), a group established to review the supply and administration of medicines, recognising that much current practice was operating on the edge of the current regulations and legal frameworks. The Review recommended the implementation first of non-medical supplementary prescribing in which trained nurses or pharmacists with the agreement of patients and medical staff could continue to prescribe specified drugs for a patient, altering them as necessary within an agreed clinical management plan. Supplementary prescribing, introduced in the UK in 2003 was quickly followed by independent prescribing (2007), which gave trained nurses and pharmacists the right to prescribe any drug they wanted within their areas of professional competence including controlled drugs. More recently other health-care professionals such as podiatrists and opticians have also been given some prescribing rights. Newly agreed accreditation criteria for undergraduate pharmacy degrees in the UK, to be introduced from 2015, will provide all pharmacy graduates with the requisite competencies to prescribe. These significant changes were introduced without prior research evidence of safety or benefit. The rationale might have been that the stepwise introduction starting with supplementary and then followed by independent prescribing allowed a staged opportunity to reflect on the rollout supported by commissioned evaluations (Department of Health 2011). These evaluations focussed mostly on experiences and safety aspects and did not include evidence of effectiveness or efficiency compared to traditional approaches. There is now a considerable body of subsequent research on non-medical prescribing, mostly focused on nurses and pharmacists. However, the bulk of this research has been descriptive exploring the extent of implementation and the medical specialities where most non-medical prescribing is delivered, the views and experiences of patients, medical doctors and the new prescribers themselves. A few studies have looked at the clinical outcomes of non-medical prescribing. One exploratory study (Bruhn et al. 2013) showed that in the field of chronic pain, pharmacist prescribing compared to traditional GP led care for patients with chronic pain led to significantly improved pain outcomes at 6 months (as measured using the validated Chronic Pain Grade) but interestingly only some effect on the mental health sub-scale of the SF36. This again reflects earlier discussion in this chapter on the importance of choosing the right outcome measure.

1.3.3.2 Primary Care Pharmacy

In the late 1990s and early 2000, the value of a pharmacist working closely with a general practitioner based in the practice became apparent. The role was purely advisory, and based on the clinical pharmacy role then well established in the hospital setting. It included for most early post holders reviewing practice prescribing and looking at a practice level at trends in prescribing, adherence to guidelines and formularies and making recommendations for changes to improve efficiency and effectiveness, at both practice and individual patient level. At individual patient level, some posts involved the pharmacist having face-to-face consultations with patients (McDermott et al. 2006), but until the advent of pharmacist prescribing (see previous example) any recommended changes had to be mediated by the medical prescriber.

The pharmacists working in general practice in the UK came to be known as primary care pharmacists, and over the course of approximately 10 years, the pharmacy profession evolved from being split into hospital and community pharmacists to having a third significant group of pharmacists delivering a clinical service. No large-scale definitive study was ever published of the added value that pharmacists brought to the practice team, although small uncontrolled studies and case reports appeared to confirm that the pharmacists saved money for practices and brought prescribing into line with current guidelines. This is a very interesting example of a sea change in the pharmacy profession which emerged on the basis of a slowly building body of descriptive evidence and local roll out rather than a big study and national implementation. However, reassuringly, a systematic review of practice-based pharmacy services (Fish et al. 2002) including studies from North America (7), the UK (5), Australia (2) and Sweden (1) showed that most published RCTs suggested benefits from the roles although studies were generally very small, not powered and did not include measures of cost-effectiveness.

1.3.4 Research to Inform Future Service Review

In this final category, the value of research in giving constructive feedback to providers and policy makers on how a service could be improved to support improved efficiency and effectiveness is illustrated. In 2005, a programme of work was commissioned to evaluate the introduction of the new Community Pharmacy Contractual Framework in England. As mentioned earlier, this new contract represented a significant change from earlier contracts as it was structured to formalise and recognise through remuneration professional advisory services alongside traditional dispensing roles. The emphasis of the evaluation[12] was to describe implementation processes and provide constructive recommendations on addressing identified barriers to optimal service delivery. So for example, one option introduced in the contract was for local organisations to commission advanced services from accredited community pharmacists. One such service was the Medicine Use Review (MUR) service. The research, which adopted a mixed methods approach, showed great variation in rate of uptake of the service in different local areas and by different pharmacists. The qualitative data revealed that there was a misunderstanding on the part of general practitioners, pharmacists, patients and commissioners about the purpose of the MUR. GPs either expected and pharmacists delivered a full clinical review rather than providing supportive communication with the patient. There was also concern about the record keeping, inability to assess quality and communication with the GPs. Thus the report could highlight these areas and allow local solutions to address these to be put in place. Subsequently small studies of MURS have been able to demonstrate the benefits

---

[12] http://www.pharmacyresearchuk.org/waterway/wp-content/uploads/2012/11/National_evaluation_of_the_new_community_pharamcy_contract.pdf accessed 14 Oct 2014.

they can confer,[13] and the service has continued to be delivered by increasing numbers of pharmacists.

1.3.5 An Integrated Example

In Australia, the introduction of Home Medicine Reviews provides an interesting comparator and an example of excellent integration between service provision and research. Since the mid-1990s, the global sum allocated to fund professional pharmacy services under the 5-yearly Community Pharmacy Agreements (CPA) has increased from $5 million in the second CPA (1995–2000) to $663 million in the fifth CPA (2010–2015). Several Commonwealth-funded research projects undertaken to evaluate the impact of pharmacist involvement in medication review for consumers living at home were conducted in the late 1990s, following a successful randomised controlled trial within the nursing home sector. This research subsequently informed negotiations within the third CPA to fund pharmacist and GP involvement in the Home Medicines Review (HMR) Programme. An HMR[14] involves a comprehensive medication review conducted by an accredited pharmacist. The process begins with a referral from the patients' GP to either their preferred pharmacy or pharmacist. The pharmacist then conducts an interview with the patient, usually in their own home, before writing a report to the referring GP, documenting specific medication review findings and recommendations. The GP then meets with the patient to develop a medication management plan based on the pharmacist's report. This successful programme has been developed and iteratively refined by research, much led by Professor Chen of the University of Sydney, Prof Gilbert from the University of South Australia and Prof Roberts from the University of Queensland. It is a real example of policy makers and researchers working together for the benefits of an improved service to patients.

1.4 Challenges

In the last decade the volume of good quality research on the cost effective and clinically effective prescribing, supply and use of medicines has increased exponentially. Nonetheless there remain challenges to bridging the policy research divide, and it is frustrating for researchers when policy is introduced for which there is no evidence, or where there is evidence that does not seem to have been

---

[13] http://www.pharmaceutical-journal.com/news-and-analysis/news/inhaler-technique-murs-sig nificantly-improve-outcomes/11107200.article

[14] http://5cpa.com.au/programs/medication-management-initiatives/home-medicines-review/

taken into account. Some of these challenges and reasons for them are considered briefly below.

1.4.1 Expertise, Time and Money!

A robust study that generates gold standard evidence requires an experienced team, appropriate iterative developmental and pilot work and substantive funding. All of these remain challenges for those working in the field of practice research. Capacity and expertise are being developed in Universities and in the workforce but it is a steep learning curve until a researcher would be judged 'a safe pair of hands' to lead a programme of work. Doctoral and post-doctorial experience are core to a research career as is the ability to network and link with those from relevant complementary disciplines. Commissioned research programmes addressing a national priority can often seem to have short deadlines between the initial call and its submission date, unrealistic objectives to be addressed within the funding envelope and tight timescales for when results should be available. It is better to argue the case to do part of the commission well than to spread efforts, expertise and resource too thinly.

1.4.2 Engaging Colleagues

Research of relevance to pharmacy frequently depends on peers in practice collecting data, recruiting participants or delivering a new service, often referred to as an intervention. It is important that in all these roles, adequate training and monitoring are in place to ensure accurate and consistent recording of data, non-biased recruitment or delivery of the new service in the planned way. This requires patience from those on the research team and commitment from colleagues for whom maintaining services represent an ever increasing workload to say nothing of the increased regulatory hurdles that are introduced.

1.4.3 Changing the Status Quo

Many new pharmacy roles are not new roles per se but are new to pharmacy. They will most likely have been delivered previously by medical colleagues, and there will be some resistance from those colleagues to another professional taking them on, especially if a transfer of funding would be implied. This attitude is slightly surprising, given that it is acknowledged by all, including the medical colleagues that they currently do not have the capacity to deliver all that is demanded and that new ways of working need to be identified. Further, there may initially be resistance from patients if they think that the move to transfer care is to 'save money' or that the new provider is not as well as qualified. Finally other non-medical colleagues may also be aspiring to take on the role that is being devolved, as in prescribing. The role of research therefore is to generate the evidence that shows that patients are not getting second best care, and to design the new service with stakeholder input so all concerns are addressed, and the new service is not seen to fail for the wrong reasons, for example, in the case of medication management that GPs are not referring patients to the service.

1.4.4 Negative Findings

Negative findings can be challenging to reveal especially if positive results had been central to implementation of a new service. This is where it is important at the design stage to think about incorporating a parallel strand of research which does not just focus on outcomes but is explanatory. For example, was the training sufficient to give the pharmacists the skills to deliver the new service, was the new service acceptable to patients, did the GPs implement the recommendations? Identify what, if anything, went wrong and provide recommendations for change. Most importantly, difficult though it might be, do not be persuaded to hide the negative findings, and ensure that at the project start the researchers have independence to publish findings.

1.4.5 Funding

Securing adequate funding is also a challenge. Whether applying to a dedicated call or applying for response mode funding (i.e. getting your own ideas funded) will always be within a competitive context. In general, pharmacy specific funds are modest so it is wise to try and access other funding streams and to collaborate with colleagues from other disciplines. Persuading grant giving bodies to prioritise funding on services such as aspects of medicine management (e.g. improving adherence or improving appropriateness of prescribing) or symptom management compared to developing a new cancer treatment may also appear challenging. However, at a time when patient safety is high on everyone's agenda, reducing prescribing errors is central, improving adherence is also a facet of medicines safety, and non-adherence leads to costs both in terms of medicines wastage and sub-optimal treatment. Finally, appropriate symptom management in the community pharmacy could lead to improved earlier diagnosis of serious diseases such as cancer and COPD, which when treated earlier have a better prognosis.

1.4.6 Duplication of Research

Finally, to what extent is it necessary to repeat research done in one country in another country? Will policy makers acknowledge the relevance of generalising from a different health-care setting, with different ethnic populations, different cultural attitudes? The answer to this is not simple, as it will depend on the exact intervention or development in question, but nonetheless it is important to learn from others and draw on their experiences. A good example of this is the interest in North America in the HMR service introduced in Australia. Whilst recognising that the evidence in the US about the value of extending pharmacists' roles in relation to medication management is increasing, authors of a recent paper have also explicitly drawn on evidence from elsewhere, namely Australia (Zagaria and Alderman 2013). The authors highlight that 'it is instructive to look at how similar practice models have been established and evolved in other countries'. This is an interesting example of where local research has been complemented by selected research from elsewhere generating a stronger body of evidence for the US than could have otherwise been achieved in the same timescale.

1.4.7 Communicating with Policy Makers

There is, as noted at the start of this chapter, a need to reconfigure health services if future need is to be managed within an affordable budget. Those interested in generating evidence that identifies a role for pharmacy in this service redesign must reflect not only the quality of their research but also on improving the way these findings are communicated to policy makers. This may not be just about recycling academic papers as policy briefings but is also about building real and virtual networks, and using the social media to promote awareness and disseminate findings widely.

1.5 Conclusion

Pharmacy has come a long way in the last three decades in becoming a truly clinical profession. A recent paper (Mossialos et al. 2013) has described the expanded role for pharmacy as 'policy making in the absence of policy relevant evidence' and claims further research is needed. We would not argue with this but also would assert that there is a building body of evidence confirming the value to patients of this paradigm shift. However, as we move forward more consideration need to be given to improving the quality of the evidence, ensuring that cost effectiveness as well as clinical effectiveness is considered, making sure the right outcomes are chosen, and finally opening up better lines of communication with policy makers to ensure greater partnership in planning a research strategy fit for the future.

References

Alldred DP, Raynor DK, Hughes C, Barber N, Chen TF, Spoor P (2013) Interventions to optimise prescribing for older people in care homes. The Cochrane Library 2. doi:10.1002/14651858. CD009095.pub2

Bond CM, Matheson C, Williams S, Williams P (2000) Repeat prescribing: an evaluation of the role of community pharmacists in controlling and monitoring repeat prescribing. Br J Gen Pract 50:271–275

Bruhn H, Bond CM, Elliott AM, et al (2013) Pharmacist led management of chronic pain in primary care: results from a randomised controlled exploratory trial. BMJ Open 3:e002361. doi:10.1136/bmjopen-2012

Charrois TL, Durec T, Tsuyuki RT (2009) Systematic reviews of pharmacy practice research: methodological issues in searching, evaluating, interpreting, and disseminating results. Ann Pharmacother 43(1):118–122

Clement FM, Harris A, Li JJ, Yong K, Lee KM, Manns BJ (2009) Using effectiveness and cost-effectiveness to make drug coverage decisions: a comparison of Britain, Australia, and Canada. JAMA 302(13):1437–1443. doi:10.1001/jama.2009.1409

Clifford S, Barber N, Elliott R, Hartley E, Horne R (2006) Patient-centred advice is effective in improving adherence to medicines. Pharm World Sci 28(3):165–170

Department of Health (1999) Review of prescribing, supply and administration of medicines. Final report. Department of Health, London

Department of Health (2011) Evaluation of nurse and pharmacist independent prescribing in England – key findings and executive summary. Final report. Department of Health, London

Eades CE, Ferguson JS, O'Carroll RE (2011) Public Health in community pharmacy: a systematic review of pharmacists and consumer views. BMC Public Health 11:582

Fish A, Watson MC, Bond CM (2002) Practice based pharmaceutical services: a systematic review. Int J Pharm Pract 10:225–233

Holland R, Desborough J, Goodyer L, Hall S, Wright D, Loke YK (2008) Does pharmacist-led medication review help to reduce hospital admissions and deaths in older people? A systematic review and meta-analysis. Br J Clin Pharmacol 65(3):303–316

Krska J, Avery AJ, on behalf of The Community Pharmacy Medicines Management Project Evaluation Team (including Jaffray M, Bond CM, Watson MC, Hannaford P, Tinelli M, Scott A, Lee A, Blenkinsopp A, Anderson C, Bissell P) (2007) Evaluation of medication reviews conducted by community pharmacists: a quantitative analysis of documented issues and recommendations. Br J Clin Pharmacol 65:386–396

McDermott E, Smith B, Elliott A, Bond CM, Hannaford PC, Chambers WA (2006) The use of medication for chronic pain in primary care, and the potential for intervention by a practice-based pharmacist. Fam Pract 23:46–52

Mossialos E, Naci H, Courtin E (2013) Expanding the role of community pharmacists: policy making in the absence of policy relevant evidence? Health Policy 111(2):135–148

Nkansah N, Mostovetsky O, Yu C, Chheng T, Beney J, Bond CM, Bero L (2010) Effect of outpatient pharmacists' non-dispensing roles on patient outcomes and prescribing patterns. Cochrane Database Syst Rev (7):CD000336. doi:10.1002/14651858.CD000336.pub2

Nuffield (1986) Pharmacy: a report to the Nuffield Foundation. Nuffield Foundation, London

Patterson SM, Hughes C, Kerse N, Cardwell CR, Bradley MC (2012) Interventions to improve the appropriate use of polypharmacy for older people (review). The Cochrane Library (5) Art. No.: CD008165. DOI: 10.1002/14651858.CD008165.pub2

Sinclair HK, Bond CM, Lennox AS, Silcock J, Winfield AJ, Donnan P (1998) Training Pharmacists and pharmacy assistants in the stage of change model of smoking cessation: a randomised controlled trial in Scotland. Tob Control 7:253–261

Sinclair HK, Silcock J, Bond CM, Lennox AS, Winfield AJ (1999) The cost effectiveness of intensive pharmaceutical intervention in assisting people to stop smoking. Int J Pharm Pract 7:107–112

Sinclair HK, Bond CM, Stead LF (2008) Community pharmacy personnel interventions for smoking cessation (review). The Cochrane Collaboration (2) doi/10.1002/14651858.CD003698.pub2/pdf

The Community Pharmacy Medicines Management Project Evaluation Team (C. Bond Principal Investigator) (2007) The MEDMAN study: a randomized controlled trial of community pharmacy-led medicines management for patients with coronary heart disease. Fam Pract 24(2):189–200

Tinelli M, Ryan M, Bond C (2010) Discrete choice experiments (DCE's) to inform pharmacy policy: going beyond quality-adjusted life years (QALYs). Int J Pharm Pract 18(S1):1

Zagaria MA, Alderman C (2013) Community based medication management in the US and Australia. US Pharmacist. http://www.uspharmacist.com/content//d/senior_care/c/38678/. Accessed 16 Oct 2014

Chapter 2
Research Methodologies Related to Pharmacy Practice: An Overview

Parastou Donyai

Abstract This chapter considers the research methodologies presented throughout the book in relation to their philosophical basis. Qualitative research is related to the interpretative perspective, and quantitative research to the empirical perspective. Thus, the *right* or *wrong* way of 'doing research' depends on the standpoint of the individuals conducting or judging the work. Viewed in this way, the very definition of pharmacy practice research can be brought into question, and the reader is nudged to think about their own acceptance of what is and what is not likely to lead to meaningful data within the context of the book's chapters.

The next chapter on the evidence and impact of pharmacy practice research paints a landscape nestled in the scientific paradigm, which by its very virtue asserts and values work that meets the positivist truth-seeking approach to knowledge creation and, less so, work that takes a more open-ended, interpretative approach. Interpretative researchers, those who view 'science' more as an ideology (one of many ideologies) than a singular truth, would argue that meaning is not necessarily to be derived from clear, testable outcomes of empirical research. Instead, to interpretative researchers, meaning can be just as validly derived from studying people and social structures in open systems to explore interactions and subjectivities. Although it can be a false dichotomy to divide researchers into empiricist (quantitative) versus interpretative (qualitative) investigators, it is important to highlight these vastly different philosophies that can underpin pharmacy practice research—if for no other reason than to demonstrate the relative validity and value of each. Pharmacy practice research and its methodologies are 'situated knowledge'. There is no inherently 'truthful' way of conducting research, but what is deemed acceptable, and by whom, depends on the temporal and spatial continuum along which research is being conducted, as well as the prevailing norms and expectations.

In this chapter, I provide an overview of research methodologies used in pharmacy practice research, detailed throughout this book, not as duplication of this material but by way of positioning the chapters within different research paradigms. It is important to articulate early on that pharmacy practice researchers

P. Donyai (✉)
University of Reading, Whiteknights, 226, Reading, Berkshire RG6 6AP, UK
e-mail: p.donyai@reading.ac.uk

do not in the main choose their research methods to suit the circumstances, but rather they conduct research based on their beliefs about what does and what does not constitute valid research. Of course, it is likely that researchers will have also developed expertise in their preferred methodology, and so to them, the right way of reflecting the reality of the 'researched' will be a result of their expertise as well as beliefs and perceived norms. Beliefs about what represents appropriate research are routed in different philosophical perspectives about how we create knowledge and, in effect, *how we know what we know*. Different epistemologies (theories about knowledge) dictate what should count as knowledge, the validity of knowledge, what distinguishes belief from knowledge, the kinds of things that are to be known, and indeed whether anything can be known for certain (Donyai 2012). Epistemology thus drives research methodology and ultimately results in the type of data generated through research.

In pharmacy practice research, those who subscribe to the empiricist tradition believe that science can (and should) provide an objective, value-free picture of the world—through the notion that people and social structures can be studied 'scientifically' within closed systems of research—that somehow, akin to laboratory research, a limited number of variables relating to people can be identified, their behaviour and interrelationship observed, while accounting for or avoiding interference from external (confounding) variables, to generate causal laws. In this way, scientific 'truth' can emerge through empirical evidence. If the 'truth' *ascertained* in this way returns unexpected results, empiricists may defend the findings by highlighting the superiority of the scientific method or contest them by identifying methodological deviations in the work conducted that invalidated the resulting 'truth'. However, people and social structures are too complex, according to interpretivists, for study in simple closed systems. This is because social objects, with their intrinsic properties and inherent complexities, can interfere with the assumptions made by empiricist researchers in countless ways, so that outcomes cannot ever be predicted and ascertained with any degree of certainty. Ideas about what it means to be human (ontology) are closely linked with epistemology and methodological approaches. Interpretivist researchers, not accepting reductionist ideas, stress the importance of language and communication in creating knowledge and thus explore and examine people's thoughts and experiences in detail for their qualitative meanings without the need for creating value-free, generalisable knowledge.

One of the 'interesting' consequences of the existence of different philosophical and methodological standpoints within pharmacy practice research is the resulting interplay of power and control in relation to what is deemed acceptable research and what is not by the dominant research community. This 'power play' has many effects—which research should be funded, published, applauded, taught, and taken up by policy makers? These outcomes depend clearly on the arbiters of such decisions. But to what extent are the decision-makers (publishers, peer reviewers, funders, academics) influenced by their own philosophical perspectives and what do they stand to gain from sanctioning research of one type and not another? If we define pharmacy practice research, as in the previous chapter (evidence and impact), as having a focus on 'exploring how and why people access pharmacy services, the costs of pharmacy services, and the outcomes for patients as a result of these services, and comparison of these costs and outcomes compared to the same or similar services delivered by other providers' (a 'hard' definition), then we stand potentially to invalidate or exclude certain other types of research that do not set out to measure and make comparisons through empirical research.

The chapter on qualitative methods provides a much broader definition of pharmacy practice research including the identification, improvement, and development of pharmacy practice, 'for example to explore various types of existing practices and beliefs in order to understand attitudes, values, and perspectives underlying these practices'. Thus, the emphasis here is not on hard outcome measures and a study of research variables but on much broader questions relating to human beliefs and interpretations. Research that uses qualitative methods captures the subjective nature of phenomena for assigned meanings and explanations, often through the analysis of language. Thus, the mechanism of qualitative research enables the researchers to relate with the field of study to uncover how the people being studied are creating, and being created by, their understanding of the world. An important element of qualitative research is that it need not follow distinct, predetermined stages, but can allow researchers instead to move back and forth between research questions, collecting and analysing data in an iterative process. As well as creating an understanding of people's inner experiences, researchers who study subjectivities and meanings can compare their results between different groups of people. Qualitative research involves a range of data-collection methods and approaches to data analysis. The chapter authors describe interviews, observations, documentary analysis, and the use of online communities ('netnography') as research methods, providing recommendations for the conduct and analyses of data generated through each technique. Importantly, the authors discuss validity, reliability, and transferability in qualitative studies.

Returning to the hard definition of pharmacy practice research, the chapter on action research is a good example of a pharmacy practice methodology, which by its very nature also cannot set out to measure and make comparisons with the same or similar services elsewhere (and therefore lacks generalisability). Instead, action research focusses on transformatory action at a local level and a recording of the outcomes of these changes as well as accompanying learning. As the chapter authors acknowledge, action research has local significance which cannot (and should not) be generalisable, but this does not invalidate such research. After all, instead of a scientifically valid experiment which is potentially unworkable in wider real-life settings, action research actually involves the development of everyday practices with potential for direct impact on patients involved. In the UK at least, propelled by the language of the 'research excellence framework', which assesses the quality of research within universities, 'impact' from research is a contemporary buzzword, and certainly action research viewed in this way delivers on this measure of quality. In addition, the chapter authors highlight a number of quality criteria that can guide researchers to demonstrate the validity of the processes followed within their own action research. As well as numerous examples of different action research projects, the authors provide a list of recommendations for conducting action research in pharmacy practice. As a methodology, action research certainly has value in engaging researchers with practitioners to collectively bring about practicable, transformative changes for improving patient care.

The situation is different with quantitative methods, seated in the empirical paradigm, where the primary aims are to establish general laws or statements that apply across different participants at different times. With quantitative methods, the entire mechanism of research including the study design, the nature of the data and the manner in which they are to be collected all should lend themselves to objectivity. The researchers collect the data in an impartial manner to exclude their own and others' personal values and biases. They establish the research hypothesis at the outset of the study and maintain consistency in data collection, for example, through the use of standardised instruments. The aim is to produce generalisable data, 'universal truths', where such studies can be repeated with another sample at a different time to produce similar results. The chapter on quantitative methods thus outlines firstly a variety of data-gathering methods in pharmacy practice research, which includes the collection of existing data and direct observation, as well as self-reports. Sources of bias are then identified as response bias (e.g. from self-reports to overt observation) as well as low response rates. Finally, the authors examine future trends through a discussion of reliability measures, implicit measures, and statistical norms. The concluding comments are apt, highlighting the importance of understanding what the data are being collected for, and what the limits are.

This recognition of the limitations of quantitative measures has resulted in the advent of mixed-methods research, which is another appropriate chapter in this book. This type of methodology uses a mix of empirical and interpretivist approaches within the same study or research programme to create contextual understanding as well as to validate the findings. The chapter authors discuss the advantages of mixed-methods research through the use of examples that demonstrate the added meanings gained through qualitative research, which are otherwise absent from quantitative measurements. The disadvantages of this type of research rests with the added burden of work created through the use of additional methods. The authors use the example of the UK's Medical Research Council's (MRC) guidance on the development of complex interventions to validate the place of mixed methods within pharmacy practice research. There is also a focus on outlining the typology of mixed-methods research in some detail, as well as a case study example detailing the application of a protocol for triangulation (for validating, enriching, and completing the knowledge gained). Mixed-methods research presents an interesting idea to interpretative researchers because it demonstrates an acknowledgement (by empiricists) that the quality and nature of experiences must also be a part of research in order to produce valid and meaningful data.

This is interesting, because the chapter on organisational theories and pharmacy practice research in fact begins with a clear acknowledgement that the positivist, empiricist 'stronghold' on pharmacy practice research can hinder the subjective, interpretative approach. The focus of this chapter is on management science as it applies to pharmacy practice research. The framework used examines micro-, meso-, and macro-level theories in relation to organisational research. The micro-level theories focus on individuals within their organisation, the meso-level theories focus on individual organisations, and the macro-level theories encompass larger communities such as 'community pharmacy organisations'. Yet the chapter has a wider reach than is portrayed by its title of organisational research. This is because there is also a very useful consideration of the empiricist ('positivist/objectivist/functionalist') versus the interpretative ('interpretative/subjectivist/naturalistic') perspectives with a detailed focus on ontology and epistemology, referred to earlier in the current chapter. There is also a focus on developing and testing theory, again with sufficient detail to be a very useful reference for those newer to research as well as experienced researchers from other fields. The chapter concludes with a consideration of rigour and how it might be ensured within organisational research.

The same author then focusses the next chapter on explaining the application of concept mapping and pattern matching techniques to pharmacy practice research. A methodology related to organisational research, this is again another accessible chapter that is of interest to both novice and experienced researchers. The idea of concept mapping is described as 'any process which helps to represent ideas as pictures or maps'. The chapter author sets out to explain the relevance of this methodology to community pharmacy research, specifically organisational culture and effectiveness. It is argued that concept mapping is helpful for 'structured thought about complex issues and action required to remediate these'. The technique is describes as a mixed method, using interpretative as well as statistical (quantitative) methods. This is because in addition to concept mapping, the author talks about pattern matching, which allows comparison of rating scales. There is a helpful step-by-step guide to concept mapping and also pattern matching, as well as two specific examples. The chapter ends with a brief consideration of the limitations as well as future applications. It serves as a useful entry-level explanation of this subject and provides ample references for those interested to pursue further reading and perhaps even make an attempt at applying the method.

The chapter on pharmacoeconomics and pharmacy practice research is strictly positioned in the empiricist paradigm, relying on hard-science analysis of health economics to enable comparison of pharmaceutical agents/services/programmes with one another. A number of pharmacoeconomic analyses are outlined. Where health resources are scarce and pharmaceutical expenditure has to be controlled, pharmacoeconomic evaluations are meant to enable prioritisation of spending through objective means. The authors rightly highlight that apart from cost-effectiveness studies involving medicines, it is rare to see pharmacoeconomic analyses as a part of pharmacy practice papers. Perhaps this is avoided because of a bias on the part of researchers, whose starting position is that pharmacy services are justified. According to the authors, the main area where pharmacoeconomic evaluations have been conducted relates to pharmacist interventions and some disease management activities. The chapter also provides some guidance for designing pharmacoeconomic analysis in pharmacy practice research. Sufficient examples and material are referenced to enable readers to look elsewhere for the additional detail needed to start a pharmacoeconomic analysis by one's self.

So what can someone unacquainted with pharmacy practice research methods conclude from reading this interesting set of chapters that make up the current book? Certainly, this is a field that is developing and growing as research ideas from other disciplines diffuse in and morph pharmacy practice research into a larger, more all-encompassing approach. While certain elements of the discipline are gaining credibility, there is still the power play that means one method is promoted and considered more credible than another. Apart from that, the authors of the last chapter consider drivers for change to include population demographics; technology; pharmacy as institution and as profession; consumer expectations; and finally new research capabilities. In the latter section of this chapter, the authors consider areas of focus for the future, working collaboratively, and moving towards large-scale initiatives. The authors highlight the demarcation between pharmacy practice research and other related fields—even inviting other fields to join the family of practice research. There is also the issue of capacity-building and making sure that we are training future generations of pharmacy practice researchers. Certainly this book is a step in the right direction in terms of defining the breadth of pharmacy practice research and providing some very useful descriptions, examples, and references for the reader.

Reference

Donyai P (2012) Social and cognitive pharmacy: theory and case studies. Pharmaceutical Press, London

Chapter 3
Quantitative Methods in Pharmacy Practice Research

James A. Green and Pauline Norris

Abstract Quantitative research methods in pharmacy practice complement qualitative research methods by providing estimates of frequency, commonness and size. Researchers use existing data or collect their own via observation or self-report. Challenges facing the use of quantitative methods include increasing levels of non-response and dealing with social desirability effects. We finish with a brief outline of how to start a quantitative research project.

3.1 What Are Quantitative Research Methods?

A simple definition of quantitative research is "research in which things are counted". The "things" might be people, medicines, opinions, behaviours, etc. While qualitative research is very useful for describing phenomena in depth (particularly motivations, feelings, understandings), quantitative research can tell us how common and widespread phenomena are. So, for example, qualitative research might show us that some people do not take their medicines because they worry about side effects, and quantitative research might tell us how common this is in the population.

J.A. Green (✉) • P. Norris
School of Pharmacy, Te Kura Mātauraka Wai-whakaora, University of Otago, P.O. Box 56, Dunedin, New Zealand
e-mail: james.green@otago.ac.nz; pauline.norris@otago.ac.nz

3.2 What Quantitative Methods Are Used in Pharmacy Practice?

A wide range of quantitative methods are commonly used in pharmacy practice research. Many projects explore medicines use, appropriateness of prescribing and medicines safety, by **analysing existing datasets**. There are a variety of sources of such data (discussed in the section below). These projects can provide valuable insights into important questions about how medicines are used and how to maximise the benefits and minimise the harms of medicines (see Box 3.1 for an example).

> **Box 3.1**
> Dr. I. A. Dhalla and others carried out a study of opioid prescribing amongst family doctors in Ontario, Canada, and also looked at opioid-related deaths amongst patients, using existing data from prescription records and data from the Office of the Chief Coroner. Many studies over several decades have found a high level of variation in prescribing habits (often unexplained) between prescribers. In this study, the authors found that the fifth of doctors (quintile) who prescribed the most opioids prescribed 55 times as much as the fifth of doctors who prescribed the least. The number of opioid-related deaths increased between each quintile according to the volume of opioids prescribed. The authors suggest that attempts to reduce opioid prescribing and therefore opioid-related deaths should be targeted at doctors who prescribe high volumes of opioids (Dhalla et al. 2011).

Another quantitative research strategy is **direct observation** (see Box 3.2 for an example). This has many advantages as a way to find out how things work in the real world of pharmacy practice, without the self-report bias (discussed in a later section) of methods like surveys.

> **Box 3.2**
> Abushanab and colleagues investigated how many and what kind of medicines were kept in Jordanian households, and how and where these were stored. They found many medicines were stored inappropriately, for example, within the reach of young children. Many were not in original containers and many were expired or had no clear expiry date. They recommended increasing public awareness of how to store medicines appropriately and also improving prescribing practices to prevent medicines wastage. (Abushanab et al. 2013)

Surveys or self-report data are also commonly reported in published pharmacy practice literature (see Box 3.3) and provide valuable information about the opinions, knowledge and practices of pharmacists, pharmacy staff, customers, the general population and other health professionals. Student projects often involve surveys of pharmacy staff or customers and explore a wide range of topics (see Box 3.4). Even unpublished student reports can often inform professional practice and policy.

> **Box 3.3**
> Claire Anderson and Tracey Thornley explored why some people in the UK choose to pay for influenza vaccinations in pharmacies when they are eligible for free vaccinations in general practices. As part of their study, they surveyed 921 patients who paid for vaccinations in pharmacies. Twenty two percent of these were eligible to get their flu vaccination for free. The results suggest that community pharmacies are convenient and easy to access and some patients prefer to receive their vaccination in a community pharmacy. (Anderson and Thornley 2014)

> **Box 3.4**
> In New Zealand, pharmacists who have undergone a training course can now sell trimethoprim to women with uncomplicated urinary tract infections, without a prescription. Fourth year students at the University of Otago, supervised by Associate Professor Rhiannon Braund and Natalie Gauld, designed and administered a simple survey to explore pharmacists' satisfaction with the training provided to them, the impact of selling trimethoprim on their practice and their views about how the service was perceived by others. They found that pharmacists were pleased to be able to provide the service, but the demand for it varied substantially between pharmacies. The participants thought that women really appreciated being able to get trimethoprim without a prescription. (Henderson et al. 2014)

Quantitative methods are also widely used in evaluating the impact of interventions to improve medicines use or pharmacy practice. The WHO has developed a range of tools that are designed for use in developing countries (Action Programme on Essential Drugs 1993; Hardon et al. 2004; Department of Essential Drugs and Medicines Policy 2007), but can also be useful in high-income countries. These include indicators that can be used to assess access to medicines and quality use of medicines. Holloway and Henry (2014) present the results of many studies using these indicators.

3.3 Quantitative Data Gathering Methods in Pharmacy Practice

3.3.1 Existing Data

In spite of the enormous amount of money and time invested in providing medicines, surprisingly little is known about who uses medicines, what medicines they use and how. The impact of simply describing medicines use should not be underestimated. This information is useful to policymakers and funders, health professionals and patients. As outlined in the chapter on qualitative research, this research can give important insights into these questions. Complementing this, quantitative methods can test hypotheses derived from qualitative methods, estimate quantitative indicators of medicines use and explore relationships amongst variables.

Much data is routinely collected by governmental organisations, healthcare providers and insurers, which can be used for large-scale quantitative research. Comparing medicines use amongst groups raises important questions of access and equity in the provision of health services as well as medicines. Documenting prescribing practices allows researchers to raise important questions about the quality and safety of prescribing and the medicalisation of society.

When a new medicine is licensed, comparatively little is known about its long-term effects and any rare side effects. Post-marketing surveillance is crucial for gathering more information about these. Spontaneous reports of adverse effects provide signals that often need to be followed up with more systematic research. Linking data on medicines use with routinely collected data on other health outcomes provides a powerful tool to detect even quite rare adverse effects and determine the level of risk.

Exploring the impact of policies and policy changes on medicines use is extremely important and provides policymakers with feedback about the impact of their decisions. Documenting changes in medicines use is also an important part of many evaluations of health sector interventions, not just those directed at improving medicines use.

3.3.2 Sources of Existing Data

3.3.2.1 Administrative Data

Very large datasets about prescription medicines are rarely collected purely for research purposes. Most often they are collected for administrative purposes: usually related to funding of medicines themselves or of the tasks involved in prescribing or dispensing them. It is important to bear this in mind when dealing with administrative data, because it means that the data are unlikely to be ideal for research: they may have some important variables missing, they may be incomplete or they may be inaccurate in some systematic way. For example, if people are eligible for some benefit (such as cheaper prescriptions or another kind of assistance) if they have Condition A, this is likely to lead to a gradual inflation in the number of diagnoses of Condition A, as patients and their doctors who are uncertain about the diagnosis tend to record it as Condition A, and others simply defraud the system by erroneously recording Condition A.

The type and quality of data available in each country depends on the health system, and in particular in most countries it depends on how many prescription medicines are paid for, and who receives publicly funded medicines. Data from insurance companies are sometimes available to researchers (such as Ververs et al. 2006), but it is more common to get data from public funders, i.e. governments or social insurance agencies (Acquaviva et al. 2009; Hsieh et al. 2008; Hynd et al. 2008). In some countries, particularly the USA and Canada, a relatively small proportion of the population are covered by public funding of medicines. In the USA, Medicare pays for some prescriptions for the elderly (http://www.medicare.gov/part-d/) and Medicaid pays for some prescriptions for those on low incomes and with few assets (http://www.medicaid.gov/Medicaid-CHIP-Program-Information/By-Topics/Benefits/Prescription-Drugs/Prescription-Drugs.html). Therefore, there are a lot of studies in the Medicare (Yin et al. 2008; Fick et al. 2001) and Medicaid populations (Dailey et al. 2001; Morrato et al. 2007; Gibson et al. 2004; Grijalva et al. 2008). The lack of comprehensive data from a public funder in the USA is somewhat compensated for by the existence of many large-scale panel studies, such as the Medical Expenditure Panel Survey (MEPS), the National Health and Nutrition Examination Survey (NHANES) and the National Ambulatory Medical Care Survey (NAMCS), which include questions on prescription medicines use. In Canada, public funding of medicines largely depends on the province, and in Ontario only elderly people are fully covered by state; therefore, much of the drug utilisation research in Ontario focuses on this part of the population (Piszczek et al. 2014; Foster et al. 2013). In British Columbia, data on all prescriptions are captured in the PharmaNet system whether they are funded or not, allowing research on the whole medicines-using population (Daw et al. 2012).

The availability of data on whole populations is an unintended advantage of funding medicines for large parts of population and allows governments and researchers to find out a great deal more about medicines use than would otherwise be the case. In the UK, New Zealand, Australia and many other countries, the whole population is covered by public drug funding. Therefore, in these countries it is possible to describe the medicines use of the whole population. However, even in these countries it is crucial to find out exactly how the funding system works, because it may lead to gaps in the data available. For example, in New Zealand only subsidised prescriptions are entered in the national dataset. In the 1990s, patients had to pay either $5 or $15 per prescription item, depending on their income level. When a person with a higher income received a prescription for a cheap medicine or a short course (such as 3 days of an antibiotic), they paid for this privately because it was less than the $15 prescription charge. No record of these private prescriptions entered the national dataset. In 2002, we found that 35.6 % of prescriptions for antibiotics were missing from this dataset (Norris et al. 2006). Attempts to use the national dataset to compare antibiotic use amongst people by socio-economic status at that time would be futile because data capture varied by socio-economic status.

Researchers in Scandinavian countries are very fortunate to have register data which includes an enormous amount of information about people's lives and their consumption of prescription medicines. This allows them to carry out the whole national population in research on topics like drug safety (Malm et al. 2005), the costs of medicines (and other health care) used by people with a certain condition (Ringborg et al. 2008) and inappropriate medicines use (Johnell et al. 2007).

Other sources of data on medicines use include records of primary care consultations. These are likely to also include diagnosis data, although this may be uncoded and difficult to standardise (or even read if the notes are handwritten). Computers in individual pharmacies also hold a considerable amount of data, but this is likely to be partial information about people who visit a variety of pharmacies. If computers are not linked, then it may be difficult and expensive (though not impossible; Horsburgh et al. 2010) to get data from individual pharmacy owners. The use of electronic prescribing should make obtaining data on medicines use in hospitals more practical and less labour intensive.

3.3.2.2 Gaps in Administrative Data

Diagnosis data is less frequently available than data on medicines. Where diagnosis data are available, it should be viewed with some scepticism because establishing and maintaining consistent methods of recording diagnoses is difficult. Diagnoses can also change during an episode of health care (such as between hospital admission and discharge). Medicines data which include patient identifiers can be linked to other datasets including, for example, deaths or hospital admissions, which provide some insight into patients' health conditions, but precise diagnosis data are unlikely to be available. Researchers have developed strategies to approximate diagnoses or conditions. For example, Daw et al. examined a period of 9 months before admission for an in-hospital birth (except for hospital stays over 7 days) to investigate medicines use in pregnancy (Daw et al. 2012).

Data on non-prescription medicines use is rarely recorded, and this is a significant gap, especially because many medicines which used to be prescription only are now available without prescription [e.g. statins in the UK (Stewart et al. 2007)]. This means that analysis of medicines use based on prescription data is partial and may be biased. For example, comparing use of a medicine by socio-economic status may be difficult when poorer people might choose to buy it over the counter while others pay to visit a general practitioner to get it prescribed (or vice versa if GP visits are free). It also makes comparisons by country difficult. For example, comparing statin use in Country A where all statins require a prescription with

Country B where they are available OTC would be impossible if adequate records of OTC sales are not kept in Country B.

3.3.2.3 Secondary Analysis of Data from Other Studies

Existing studies can include a wealth of information on medicines use. Often this has been under-analysed, and researchers would welcome further analysis of their data. For example, longitudinal studies, which follow up cohorts of people over time, can offer insight into changing medicines use over time and as populations age. For example, the Framingham study (https://www.framinghamheartstudy.org/), on which many calculations of cardiovascular risk are based, included data on medicines use (including herbal medicines and supplements) for both their original cohort and for their offspring.

Existing published or unpublished studies can also be used to look at trends over time in medicines use. It is important in this case to take into account different definitions of medicines (e.g. whether OTCs, vitamins and homoeopathic products are included), definitions of medicines groups (consistency is improved when researchers use a well-established system like the ATC classification), of data collection and of different populations.

3.3.2.4 Analysis of Other Documents Related to Medicines

Other datasets or documents that can be useful in pharmacy practice research include national or regional formularies, lists of subsidised medicines and advertisements for medicines. For example, Ragupathy et al. (2012) compared lists of licensed and subsidised medicines to compare aspects of access to medicines in different countries. Many studies have examined the quantity and quality of information presented in medicines advertisements (Rohra et al. 2006).

3.3.3 Direct Observation

Pharmacy practice research has tended to rely heavily on self-report data from the people involved when studying behaviours and attitudes. There are many limitations to this as outlined later in this chapter. Another approach to studying behaviour, such as communication about medicines or adherence, is to directly observe it.

Actors or researchers who present themselves as normal patients to healthcare providers and record details of their care are known by a variety of names, such as mystery shoppers, surrogate patients, undercover careseekers or simulated clients (Madden et al. 1997). This is an important and useful way to assess quality and/or consistency of care. In community pharmacy and drug stores, it has been used to explore the questions pharmacy staff ask, advice given and products recommended (Chalker et al. 2000; Driesen and Vandenplas 2009; Neoh et al. 2011).

A useful review of issues and practical advice in using this method is provided by (Madden et al. 1997). Although this is aimed at research in developing countries, it is equally useful to researchers in developed countries. Watson et al. (2006) have reviewed how this method has been used in pharmacy practice research.

There are also a range of other things that can be directly observed in pharmacy practice including interactions with real patients in pharmacies and other healthcare settings (Green et al. 2013), medicine prices and availability (Cameron et al. 2009) and medicines stored in households (Abushanab et al. 2013).

3.3.4 Self-Reported Data

Another common method of collecting data is through asking participants to report about their behaviour, beliefs, understandings and attitudes. In pharmacy practice research, this can range from reporting about medicines adherence, attitudes about pharmacists, knowledge about (specific) medicines and a wide range of other topics.

Self-reported data have a number of advantages. It is generally quite cheap to collect compared to interviewing, collecting observational data or using biological markers (e.g. of adherence). It is also often quicker to collect, as a single researcher can recruit a large number of participants in a short period of time. It also has a number of disadvantages. It is inherently more subjective, there are limits on what people may be able to report and the data may be biased. The latter issues are discussed in more detail later in this chapter.

Data may be acquired in person, over the telephone, through the mail or over the Internet. Questions can range from open-ended, free-response questions through to psychometrically validated instruments. Norris et al. (2001) asked members of the public in person, verbally, for their understanding of pharmacy terms such as analgesic using open-ended, free-response questions, with the answers coded in terms of accuracy by the research team later. To assess the perceptions of Jordanians to generic medicines, El-Dahiyat and Kayyali (2013) approached patients in a variety of clinical settings to fill out a paper questionnaire that had been assessed for face and content validity. Krass et al. (2014) report the development of a new scale for measuring attitudes to pharmacist services for diabetes, which was administered on the web and on paper, with principal components analysis and Rasch scaling used to determine validity.

A specific limitation to self-reported data is the extent to which people are accurately able to report on their behaviour or thought processes. There are a series of somewhat interrelated reasons for this. It is possible to ask participants questions to which they don't know the answer, but rather than picking an explicit "don't know" option (if available) they may speculate or simply pick a relatively neutral value. For example, a patient asked about their perception of the safety of an unfamiliar drug will not necessarily produce informative data, except to the extent that their rating might be influenced by background factors, such as general scepticism towards medicines.

Forgetting is also an issue in the accuracy of self-report. This can be especially pronounced where people are asked to self-report on their behaviour over longer time periods. These problems can be minimised by the use of "concrete-specific questions close in time" to the to-be-recalled event (Reis and Gable 2000, p. 196). Shorter recall periods can increase accuracy. Importantly, forgetting does not necessarily occur equally, with some things being more memorable than others. For example, in symptom reporting research, while the prevalence of symptoms in general is underestimated (Kooiker 1995), in particular musculoskeletal, digestive and nervous system symptoms are less likely to be remembered and therefore reported, in contrast to respiratory complaints such as colds (Marcus 1982). This can occur even in relatively short recall periods.

A final and more fundamental challenge to the accuracy of self-report is the extent to which we have accurate access to our internal mental processes (Nisbett and Wilson 1977). At first glance, this appears to be a philosophical objection, but evidence has accrued over the last 30 years that human decision and behaviour is often influenced by automatic and unconscious processes, as well as the type of conscious and deliberative thoughts that we can access. This is unfamiliar territory for many pharmacy practice researchers, but automatic processes can be thought of as a gut hunch. That is, before understanding "why", a person may become aware that they prefer a choice, with the verbal explanation coming after this automatic process. Automatic processes influence many decisions and judgements (e.g. Wilson and Schooler 1991; Halberstadt and Green 2008), and it seems likely that automatic processes underlie some self-reported pharmacy behaviours. For example, people may be likely to have automatic associations about both pharmacists and medicines, which will influence their reported attitudes, preferences and decisions, as well as those reasons they are able to verbally explain.

3.4 Challenges for Quantitative Research in Pharmacy Practice

3.4.1 Social Desirability and Sources of Response Bias

With both direct observation and self-report data, there is the possibility that the very existence of a research study can modify what is being measured. This is referred to by different names, including response bias, experimental reactivity, demand characteristics or the Hawthorne effect. To better guard against these types of effects, considering the type of effect and what direction it might take can lead to a better designed study.

A recent meta-analysis of health behaviours showed that asking people questions or measuring their behaviour can have a small change in their behaviour (Rodrigues et al. 2014). This can be because the people change their behaviour or answers to be more socially desirable or acceptable. For example, a pharmacist might spend longer counselling patients or counsel them in what they consider to be a more proper fashion. One way to counter this is to observe participants over a more extended period of time, as people tend to revert to their normal behaviour over time. Covert observation (discussed later in this chapter) may also reduce this type of change.

Question order can also change responses, with preceding questions influencing later questions, or even whether a participant completes a survey. Many survey methods textbooks outline both numerous specific problems, along with ways to address these (e.g. Krosnick and Presser 2010).

3.4.2 Covert Observation

Covert observation is an alternative method to reduce response biases. For example, in order to assess the usual standard of care in pharmacy, a mystery shopper may be more likely to elicit a typical response than where the pharmacist is aware they are being observed. For example, consultations about medicines only available after consultation with a pharmacist may not be of ideal quality when covertly observed (Norris 2002).

When using covert observation, ethical issues need to be thoroughly explored. Local ethics committees may be able to advise researchers on this. Questions include: Should informed consent be obtained from participants? What is the public good being achieved? Should individual pharmacies or staff be identified in results? How can the potential good from the study be weighed against any risk to participants?

3.4.3 Non-response

Non-response may be one of the bigger challenges facing pharmacy practice researchers today. It has been acknowledged as a problem in many disciplines (e.g. Anseel et al. 2010; Galea and Tracy 2007). Kohut et al. (2012) reported that in the USA, Pew Research Center's aggregated response rates across surveys had dropped from 36 % in 1997 to 9 % in 2012, despite increasingly intensive efforts over time to increase response. The risk with lower response rates is that the people who do respond are systematically different from those who do not respond, creating a **non-response bias** and threatening the validity of the research. Although most typically considered in the context of self-reported data, non-response can also be an issue for observational or intervention studies, for example, where a smaller proportion of pharmacies, pharmacists or patients agree to participate.

Reasons given for increasing non-response include the increasing ubiquity of surveys, such as of consumers by retailers, and the rise and rise of market research (Dillman 2002). Within practice research, specific populations are also at risk for research fatigue. Practising pharmacists, along with other healthcare professionals, are frequently targeted to participate in research and can often produce low levels of response. Though not explored in a pharmacy context, typically as workplace seniority increases, participation decreases (Anseel et al. 2010). Similarly, populations with specific characteristics (e.g. taking specific classes of medicines, having certain illnesses) can also be frequently invited to participate, and this can lead to fatigue and cynicism in these groups.

A researcher's ability to reduce external causes of participation fatigue is limited, but there are strategies within a research community that can help. Providing prompt and tailored feedback of research results can give the participants a sense that their participation has been valued, and the resulting information can be seen as a reward in its own right. Ensuring that participation in the research is not unduly onerous (or is well rewarded where it is impossible to avoid), including minimising the time and boredom potential of being involved. Performing power analysis and ensuring that a study is not overpowered also means that you are minimising the participation burden on a population. Sometimes, where a convenient contact list exists, it can be tempting to take a census approach and attempt to include the whole list, rather than taking a sample, but this temptation should be avoided. A larger sample will superficially appear to be more precise (e.g. smaller confidence intervals), but will have less validity due to being less representative. Counter-intuitively, a *smaller, more-representative* sample produces more accurate results than a *larger, less-representative* sample. The former can be achieved by attempting to recruit fewer people initially, but focusing on those who are selected to keep the response rate as high as possible. As an example, Westrick and Mount (2007) compared a mailed census of over 1,100 pharmacies, with telephone follow-up pharmacies that did not respond to the mail survey. The mail survey returned a 27 % response rate, but by telephone 84 % responded. Systematic differences were observed on some questions, illustrating non-response bias, where those who do respond were not representative of those that don't respond.

For a specific survey, there are also strategies that can be used to enhance response. In a recent meta-analysis, it was shown that the effectiveness of following up with non-responders, giving participants advance notice of the survey and mailing surveys was declining with time, but personalisation was showing increased effectiveness (Anseel et al. 2010). This may reflect the overuse of the former techniques by researchers trying to combat non-response. Surprisingly, Anseel and colleagues also found that both following up with participants and giving incentives are now associated with lower response rates, controlling for other factors. However, it may be that these strategies are more likely to be deployed in situations where a low response rate is anticipated in advance by the researcher, rather than these being causes of low response rates. Personal delivery, the survey being sponsored by an organisation, the use of identification numbers and the salience of the topic to the participants were associated with higher response rates. Personally delivered surveys have higher responses than web surveys, which produce better responses than physically mailed surveys.

The effectiveness of these strategies varies by the population being targeted. In a systematic review of physicians, financial incentives still improved response rates, as did brief, personalised questionnaires, especially where sponsored by a professional organisation (VanGeest et al. 2007). These findings may also generalise to pharmacists. Incentives are also more effective for people not in full-time work, but topic salience is less effective; and consumers are less likely to be motivated by a sponsored survey (Anseel et al. 2010). Mail may sometimes be better than the web (Shih and Xitao 2008) and doctors may prefer mailed surveys.

Even studies with high response rates can be vulnerable to bias, especially where the motivation for participating in the survey is related to survey variables (Groves and Peytcheva 2008). For example, pharmacists could be motivated to respond to a survey on service model funding, and those who choose to respond may be most interested in that service model.

With declining response rates, one response has been to consider what the minimum acceptable response rate is. However, this seems to lead to lower quality reporting of response rates, and in a review of social sciences and health research journals, the reporting of response rates was relatively poor (Johnson and Owens 2003).

3.4.4 Challenges in Using Existing Data

The more widespread availability of big data and computer systems for analysing it makes it easier for a wide range of people to access and analyse such data. This obviously has some advantages but can also cause problems. It is still important to understand the data, what it is collected for and what its limits are. If not, misinterpretations are likely.

It is important for pharmacy practice researchers to provide input into the design of information systems for gathering and analysing data about medicines use. Researchers need to provide advice to policymakers on the impact of policy or system changes on data availability.

Rigorous ethics procedures are needed, but these need to be responsive to the level of risk involved in a project. Low-risk projects should have a simpler process for ethics review than higher risk projects.

3.5 Future Trends

3.5.1 *Implicit Measures*

We discussed earlier in this chapter the limitations of self-report, with both social desirability and the extent to which people are influenced by automatic associations that they are not able to self-report, both potentially compromising the validity of such measures. One proposed class of solutions to this problem has been the development of "implicit measures". These are designed to measure automatic associations between different mental representations that influence decision-making alongside explicit "deliberative" processes (see e.g. Conner et al. 2007; Olson and Fazio 2009). There is also evidence that implicit measures can be more resistant to social desirability (Brunel et al. 2004).

Implicit measures typically use timed choice tasks and look at the reaction times for different types of choice as a way to measure automatic associations. For example, Green et al. (2014) used the Implicit Association Test (IAT) to measure unconscious, implicit, automatic associations about conventional medicines and herbal medicines. In this task, people who were able to complete the task faster when words representing conventional medicines were paired with positive words would be considered to have a positive implicit attitude towards conventional medicines. This measure explained additional variance in medicines use beyond conventional self-reported measures. It seems likely that people may also have automatic implicit attitudes towards pharmacists and that these could also be measured.

3.5.2 *The "New Statistics"*

Null hypothesis significance testing (NHST) is still the most commonly used approach in pharmacy practice research. This is where a "null hypothesis" and an "alternate hypothesis" are created. For example, an alternate hypothesis might be that "polypharmacy is associated with an increased risk of falls in an older population". The null hypothesis is then that there is no relationship or difference, in this case that "polypharmacy is not associated with an increased risk of falls in an older population". Following data collection, some *inferential* statistical test is used that produces a p value. If the p value is less than 0.05, then it is considered to be a real relationship or difference. Though NHST has been at least somewhat controversial since the p value was first proposed, there has been an increasing movement away from reliance on p values in recent years. Instead, confidence intervals and measures of effect size are used to indicate precision around an estimate of numeric values.

3.6 Steps in Starting Your Quantitative Research Project

1. Define your question
   It is important that it be specific and answerable. Questions can be too big (Does polypharmacy have negative effects?) or too small and specific to be of much interest to anyone. Being clear on what your question is at the start will help you through the rest of the research process.
2. What concepts will you need to measure to answer your question?
   As part of the process of refining your question, you need to think about what are the things you will need to know about (e.g. polypharmacy, adherence, falls).
3. Consider collecting qualitative data to inform how and what you will measure.
   If you want to know what types of reasons lead to greater variation in timing evening doses of metformin, collecting qualitative data ensures that you know the potential range of answers.
4. Is there existing data that measures your concept?
   The data you wish to collect may already exist. Or similar data might refine your question or guide your choice of measures.
5. If no, think about how best to measure each concept.
   Consider whether it is feasible, how much it will cost and if you have the time available. Behavioural measures are preferred to self-report, but they are not always possible. Consider validity, and to a lesser extent reliability.

3.7 Conclusion

Quantitative methods are extensively used in pharmacy practice, from collecting observational, behavioural or self-reported data to making use of existing datasets. Despite some challenges, especially the increasing level of potential participants not wanting to be involved in research, they provide a strong compliment to qualitative methods.

References

Abushanab AS, Sweileh WM, Wazaify M (2013) Storage and wastage of drug products in Jordanian households: a cross-sectional survey. Int J Pharm Pract 21(3):185–191. doi:10.1111/j.2042-7174.2012.00250.x

Acquaviva E, Legleye S, Auleley G, Deligne J, Carel D, Falissard B (2009) Psychotropic medication in the French child and adolescent population: prevalence estimation from health insurance data and national self-report survey data. BMC Psychiatry 9(72). doi:10.1186/1471-244X-9-72

Action Programme on Essential Drugs (1993) WHO/DAP/93.1 How to investigate drug use in health facilities: selected drug use indicators

Anderson C, Thornley T (2014) "It's easier in pharmacy": why some patients prefer to pay for flu jabs rather than use the National Health Service. BMC Health Serv Res 14:35. doi:10.1186/1472-6963-14-35

Anseel F, Lievens F, Schollaert E, Choragwicka B (2010) Response rates in organizational science, 1995-2008: a meta-analytic review and guidelines for survey researchers. J Bus Psychol 25(3):335–349. doi:10.1007/s10869-010-9157-6

Brunel FF, Tietje BC, Greenwald AG (2004) Is the implicit association test a valid and valuable measure of implicit consumer social cognition? J Consum Psychol 14(4):385–404

Cameron A, Ewen M, Ross-Degnan D, Ball D, Laing R (2009) Medicine prices, availability, and affordability in 36 developing and middle-income countries: a secondary analysis. Lancet 373 (9659):240–249. doi:10.1016/S0140-6736(08)61762-6

Chalker J, Chuc NTK, Falkenberg T, Do NT, Tomson G (2000) STD management by private pharmacies in Hanoi: practice and knowledge of drug sellers. Sex Transm Infect 76(4):299–302. doi:10.1136/sti.76.4.299

Conner MT, Perugini M, O'Gorman R, Ayres K, Prestwich A (2007) Relations between implicit and explicit measures of attitudes and measures of behavior: evidence of moderation by individual difference variables. Pers Soc Psychol Bull 33(12):1727–1740. doi:10.1177/0146167207309194

Dailey G, Kim MS, Lian JF (2001) Patient compliance and persistence with antihyperglycemic drug regimens: evaluation of a medicaid patient population with type 2 diabetes mellitus. Clin Ther 23(8):1311–1320. doi:10.1016/S0149-2918(01)80110-7

Daw JR, Mintzes B, Law MR, Hanley GE, Morgan SG (2012) Prescription drug use in pregnancy: a retrospective, population-based study in British Columbia, Canada (2001–2006). Clin Ther 34(1):239–249. doi:10.1016/j.clinthera.2011.11.025, e232

Department of Essential Drugs and Medicines Policy (2007) WHO Operational package for assessing, monitoring and evaluating country pharmaceutical situations: guide for coordinators and data collectors. World Health Organisation. http://www.who.int/iris/handle/10665/69927

Dhalla IA, Mamdani MM, Gomes T, Juurlink DN (2011) Clustering of opioid prescribing and opioid-related mortality among family physicians in Ontario. Can Fam Phys 57(3):e92–e96

Dillman DA (2002) Presidential address: Navigating the rapids of change: some observations on survey methodology in the early twenty-first century. Public Opin Q 66(3):473–494

Driesen A, Vandenplas Y (2009) How do pharmacists manage acute diarrhoea in an 8-month-old baby? A simulated client study. Int J Pharm Pract 17(4):215–220. doi:10.1211/ijpp.17.04.0004

El-Dahiyat F, Kayyali R (2013) Evaluating patients' perceptions regarding generic medicines in Jordan. J Pharm Policy Pract 6(1):3. doi:10.1186/2052-3211-6-3

Fick DM, Waller JL, Maclean JR, Heuvel RV, Tadlock J, Gottlieb M, Cangialose CB (2001) Potentially inappropriate medication use in a Medicare managed care population: association with higher costs and utilization. J Manage Care Pharm 7(5):407–413

Foster PD, Mamdani MM, Juurlink DN, Shah BR, Paterson JM, Gomes T (2013) Trends in selection and timing of first-line pharmacotherapy in older patients with Type 2 diabetes diagnosed between 1994 and 2006. Diabet Med 30(10):1209–1213. doi:10.1111/dme.12214

Galea S, Tracy M (2007) Participation rates in epidemiologic studies. Ann Epidemiol 17(9):643–653. doi:10.1016/j.annepidem.2007.03.013

Gibson PJ, Damler R, Jackson EA, Wilder T, Ramsey JL (2004) The impact of olanzapine, risperidone, or haloperidol on the cost of schizophrenia care in a medicaid population. Value Health 7(1):22–35. doi:10.1111/j.1524-4733.2004.71272.x

Green JA, Brown K, Burgess J, Chong D, Pewhairangi K (2013) Indigenous and immigrant populations' use and experience of community pharmacies in New Zealand. J Immigr Minor Health 15(1):78–84. doi:10.1007/s10903-012-9572-z

Green JA, Hohmann C, Lister K, Albertyn R, Bradshaw R, Johnson C (2014) Implicit and explicit attitudes towards conventional and complementary and alternative medicine treatments: introduction of an implicit association test. J Health Psychol doi:10.1177/1359105314542818

Grijalva CG, Chung CP, Stein CM, Mitchel EF, Griffin MR (2008) Changing patterns of medication use in patients with rheumatoid arthritis in a Medicaid population. Rheumatology 47 (7):1061–1064. doi:10.1093/rheumatology/ken193

Groves RM, Peytcheva E (2008) The impact of nonresponse rates on nonresponse bias: a meta-analysis. Public Opin Q 72(2):167–189. doi:10.1093/poq/nfn011

Halberstadt J, Green J (2008) Carryover effects of analytic thought on preference quality. J Exp Soc Psychol 44(4):1199–1203. doi:10.1016/j.jesp.2008.03.008

Hardon A, Hodgkin C, Fresle D (2004) How to investigate the use of medicines by consumers. World Health Organisation, Geneva

Henderson E, McNab E, Sarten R, Wallace E (2014) Pharmacist satisfaction with trimethoprim training and the impact on clinical practice. University of Otago, Dunedin

Holloway KA, Henry D (2014) WHO essential medicines policies and use in developing and transitional countries: an analysis of reported policy implementation and medicines use surveys. PLoS Med 11(9). doi:10.1371/journal.pmed.1001724

Horsburgh S, Norris P, Becket G, Crampton P, Arroll B, Cumming J, Herbison P, Sides G (2010) The equity in prescriptions medicines use study: using community pharmacy databases to study medicines utilisation. J Biomed Inform 43(6):982–987. doi:10.1016/j.jbi.2010.08.004

Hsieh S-C, Lin I-H, Tseng W-L, Lee C-H, Wang J-D (2008) Prescription profile of potentially aristolochic acid containing Chinese herbal products: an analysis of National Health Insurance data in Taiwan between 1997 and 2003. Chin Med 3:13. doi:10.1186/1749-8546-3-13

Hynd A, Roughead EE, Preen DB, Glover J, Bulsara M, Semmens J (2008) The impact of co-payment increases on dispensings of government-subsidised medicines in Australia. Pharmacoepidemiol Drug Saf 17(11):1091–1099. doi:10.1002/pds.1670

Johnell K, Fastbom J, Rosén M, Leimanis A (2007) Inappropriate drug use in the elderly: a nationwide register-based study. Ann Pharmacother 41(7-8):1243–1248. doi:10.1345/aph. 1K154

Johnson T, Owens L (2003) Survey response rate reporting in the professional literature. In: 58th Annual meeting of the American Association for Public Opinion Research, Nashville, TN

Kohut A, Keeter S, Doherty C, Dimock M, Christian L (2012) Assessing the representativeness of public opinion surveys. Pew Research Center, Washington, DC

Kooiker SE (1995) Exploring the iceberg of morbidity - a comparison of different survey methods for assessing the occurrence of everyday illness. Soc Sci Med 41(3):317–332

Krass I, Costa D, Dhippayom T (2014) Development and validation of the Attitudes to Pharmacist Services for Diabetes Scale (APSDS). Research in Social and Administrative Pharmacy. doi:10.1016/j.sapharm.2014.04.005

Krosnick JA, Presser S (2010) Question and questionnaire design. In Handbook of Survey Research (2nd Ed.). West Yorkshire, England: Emerald, (pp 263–314)

Madden J, Quick J, Ross-Degnan D, Kafle K (1997) Undercover careseekers: simulated clients in the study of health provider behavin developing countries. Soc Sci Med 45(10):1465–1482

Malm H, Klaukka T, Neuvonen PJ (2005) Risks associated with selective serotonin reuptake inhibitors in pregnancy. Obstet Gynecol 106(6):1289–1296. doi:10.1097/01.AOG. 0000187302.61812.53

Marcus AC (1982) Memory aids in longitudinal health surveys - results from a field experiment. Am J Public Health 72(6):567–573

Morrato EH, Dodd S, Oderda G, Haxby DG, Allen R, Valuck RJ (2007) Prevalence, utilization patterns, and predictors of antipsychotic polypharmacy: experience in a multistate Medicaid Population, 1998–2003. Clin Ther 29(1):183–195. doi:10.1016/j.clinthera.2007.01.002

Neoh CF, Hassali MA, Shafie AA, Awaisu A (2011) Nature and adequacy of information on dispensed medications delivered to patients in community pharmacies: a pilot study from Penang, Malaysia. J Pharm Health Serv Res 2(1):41–46. doi:10.1111/j.1759-8893.2010. 00026.x

Nisbett RE, Wilson TD (1977) Telling more than we can know - verbal reports on mental processes. Psychol Rev 84(3):231–259

Norris PT (2002) Purchasing restricted medicines in New Zealand pharmacies: results from a "mystery shopper" study. Pharm World Sci 24(4):149–153

Norris P, Simpson T, Bird K, Kirifi J (2001) Understanding of pharmacy-related terms among three ethnic groups in New Zealand. Int J Pharm Pract 9(4):269–274. doi:10.1111/j.2042-7174. 2001.tb01058.x

Norris P, Funke S, Becket G, Ecke D, Reiter L, Herbison P (2006) How many antibiotic prescriptions are unsubsidized? NZ Med J 119(1233):5

Olson MA, Fazio RH (2009) Implicit and explicit measures of attitudes: The perspective of the MODE model. In: Petty RE, Fazio RH, Brinol P (eds) Attitudes: insights from the new implicit measures. Pyschology Press, New York, pp 19–63

Piszczek J, Mamdani M, Antoniou T, Juurlink D, Gomes T (2014) The impact of drug reimbursement policy on rates of testosterone replacement therapy among older men. PLoS One 9(7):1–6. doi:10.1371/journal.pone.0098003

Ragupathy R, Aaltonen K, Tordoff J, Norris P, Reith D (2012) A 3-dimensional view of access to licensed and subsidized medicines under single-payer systems in the US, the UK, Australia and New Zealand. PharmacoEconomics 30(11):1051–1065. doi:10.2165/11595270-000000000-00000

Reis HT, Gable SL (2000) Event-sampling and other methods for studying everyday experience. In: Reis HT, Judd MC (eds) Handbook of research methods in social and personality psychology. Cambridge University Press, New York, pp 190–222

Ringborg A, Martinell M, Stålhammar J, Yin DD, Lindgren P (2008) Resource use and costs of type 2 diabetes in Sweden – estimates from population-based register data. Int J Clin Pract 62(5):708–716. doi:10.1111/j.1742-1241.2008.01716.x

Rodrigues AM, O'Brien N, French DP, Glidewell L, Sniehotta FF (2014) The question-behavior effect: genuine effect or spurious phenomenon? A systematic review of randomized controlled trials with meta-analyses. Health Psychol. doi:10.1037/hea0000104

Rohra DK, Gilani AH, Memon IK, Perven G, Khan MT, Zafar H, Kumar R (2006) Critical evaluation of the claims made by pharmaceutical companies in drug promotional material in Pakistan. J Pharm Pharm Sci 9(1):50–59

Shih TH, Xitao F (2008) Comparing response rates from web and mail surveys: a meta-analysis. Field Methods 20(3):249–271. doi:10.1177/1525822X08317085

Stewart D, John D, Cunningham S, McCaig D, Hansford D (2007) A comparison of community pharmacists' views of over-the-counter omeprazole and simvastatin. Pharmacoepidemiol Drug Saf 16(12):1290–1297. doi:10.1002/pds.1481

VanGeest JB, Johnson TP, Welch VL (2007) Methodologies for improving response rates in surveys of physicians: a systematic review. Eval Health Prof 30(4):303–321. doi:10.1177/0163278707307899

Ververs T, Kaasenbrood H, Visser G, Schobben F, de Jong-van den Berg L, Egberts T (2006) Prevalence and patterns of antidepressant drug use during pregnancy. Eur J Clin Pharmacol 62(10):863–870. doi:10.1007/s00228-006-0177-0

Watson M, Norris P, Granas A (2006) A systematic review of the use of simulated patients and pharmacy practice research. Int J Pharm Pract 14(2):83–93. doi:10.1211/ijpp.14.2.0002

Westrick SC, Mount JK (2007) Evaluating telephone follow-up of a mail survey of community pharmacies. Res Soc Admin Pharm 3(2):160–182. doi:10.1016/j.sapharm.2006.06.003

Wilson TD, Schooler JW (1991) Thinking too much: introspection can reduce the quality of preferences and decisions. J Pers Soc Psychol 60(2):181

Yin W, Basu A, Zhang JX, Rabbani A, Meltzer DO, Alexander GC (2008) The effect of the medicare. Part D: Prescription benefit on drug utilization and expenditures. Ann Intern Med 148(3):169–177. doi:10.7326/0003-4819-148-3-200802050-00200

Chapter 4
Qualitative Methods in Pharmacy Practice Research

Susanne Kaae and Janine Marie Traulsen

Abstract Qualitative research within pharmacy practice is concerned with understanding the behavior of actors such as pharmacy staff, pharmacy owners, patients, other healthcare professionals, and politicians to explore various types of existing practices and beliefs in order to improve them. As qualitative research attempts to answer the "why" questions, it is useful for describing, in rich detail, complex phenomena that are situated and embedded in local contexts. Typical methods include interviews, observation, document analysis, and netnography. Qualitative research has to live up to a set of rigid quality criteria of research conduct to provide trustworthy results that contribute to the further development of the area.

4.1 Why Qualitative Methods in Pharmacy Practice?

4.1.1 Introduction

Qualitative research within the health sciences has developed as a means to gather an in-depth understanding of human behavior, as well as to find the underlying reasons, attitudes, and motivations that govern such behavior. Qualitative research has grown out of a variety of disciplines such as sociology, anthropology, history, education, and linguistics. The qualitative approach is concerned with the why and how of people's decision making; this means that the studies usually consist of small and focused samples. There are a variety of qualitative research methods, such as interviews, observation, document analysis, and netnography, which are often divided into different types.

In pharmacy practice research, qualitative methods are most often used in research whose goal is to identify, improve, and develop current practices, for example, to explore various types of existing practices and beliefs. This is done

---

S. Kaae (✉) · J.M. Traulsen
Faculty of Health and Medical Sciences, Department of Pharmacy, University of Copenhagen, København, Denmark
e-mail: susanne.kaae@sund.ku.dk; janine.traulsen@sund.ku.dk

to understand attitudes, values, and perspectives underlying these practices (either by an individual or a group of people) by asking questions such as:

- Which practices work?
- Which don't work and why?
- What are the perceptions of the role of pharmacy?
- What are the perceptions of the role of the pharmacist?

Typical research questions include:

- What are the facilitators and barriers to service implementations?
- What are the perceptions of pharmacy staff, of patients, and of other healthcare professionals with regard to existing practices?
- Do they have suggestions for improvement?

For years there has been a focus in research on patient-centered care. For pharmacy practice research, this means being aware of and trying to understand where patients are "coming from." What and who informs and influences the patient's views about medicine and treatment? Qualitative methods can contribute to answering questions such as:

- How is communication with patients characterized?
- What are effective means of communicating with patients?

The basic assumption among researchers who use qualitative methods is that people make sense out of their experiences, thus creating their own reality, and are capable of sharing those experiences with others. Further, it is assumed that what people say is valid, reliable, and meaningful. Qualitative studies are not seeking to verify some "truth"; they assume that there are multiple truths, realities, and meanings, and the goal is to try to understand how people understand themselves.

Qualitative research is usually conducted in the subject's natural setting whenever possible, for example, the information is collected from the patient in the hospital or home or at the community pharmacy. The "data" produced by qualitative methods is a record of how people express their feelings, what they say they believe, and what they do.

In general, qualitative methods produce specific information on the particular cases studied. More general conclusions are presented only as propositions (informed assertions). When it comes to studying pharmacy practice, there is no right or wrong approach, no right or wrong method; the rule of thumb is to find the appropriate method for answering the research questions. Often, a combination of quantitative and qualitative approaches is the most appropriate: this is known as triangulation. For example, a survey to explore and identify new trends in pharmacy practice, followed by the thoughts and experiences of pharmacy personnel expressed through interviews with practitioners.

4.1.2 Steps in Qualitative Research

All scientific research consists of systematically gathering data on a specific topic in order to answer a specific question(s). Thus, research, including qualitative research, consists of various phases which can roughly be divided up into the conceptual phase, the design and planning phase, the empirical data-generation phase (preparation and data gathering), the analytic phase, and the dissemination phase. Qualitative studies differ from all other research (quantitative as well as experimental) in the way the different phases are carried out with the exception usually of the dissemination phase.

There are four essential aspects of qualitative analysis which ensure both high research quality of the individual phases and the links between. First, the participant selection must be well reasoned and the inclusion must be relevant to the research question. Second, the methods must be appropriate for the research objectives and setting. Third, the methods—which can include field observation, interviews, and document analysis—must be comprehensive enough to provide rich and robust descriptions of the events studied. Fourth, the data must be appropriately analyzed and the findings adequately corroborated by using multiple sources of information, more than one researcher to collect and analyze the raw data, another researcher checking to establish whether the participants' viewpoints were adequately interpreted, or by comparing with existing social science theories.

4.2 Interviews

Interviews are a common and useful method when investigating the subjective understandings, feelings, values, attitudes, experiences, and/or ideas of persons affected by—or trying to change—pharmacy practice (e.g., patients, healthcare professionals including pharmacy staff, and policy makers). Through interviews, critical issues in current practices can be identified and thereafter addressed and resolved. Interviews can likewise detect well-functioning practices to support these further. Examples of topics in pharmacy practice covered by interviews include the experiences of pharmacy staff with newly introduced cognitive services or tools such as asthma services or programs for electronic transmission of prescriptions (Emmerton et al. 2012), the perception of pharmacy customers of the role of pharmacies and pharmacists (Cavaco et al. 2005), or patients' reasons for accepting cognitive services (Latif et al. 2011).

Interviews are a type of conversation between the researcher and one or several interviewees for the purpose of exploring the lifeworld perspective of the interviewee(s).

4.2.1 Types of Interviews

Interviews vary according to the degree of structure, i.e., the extent to which the interviewee will influence the direction and content of the conversation. Interviews also vary according to the number of interviewees. Interviews with several participants are called group or focus group interviews.

4.2.1.1 Individual Interviews

Individual interviews are usually divided into three types: fully structured, unstructured, and semi-structured. There is no strict line between these and, depending on the research question, they can be mixed.

Structured interviews bear a strong resemblance to questionnaires with predefined questions and categories of answers in which there can be no deviation. When conducting a structured interview, the researcher will read aloud the questions and tick the answer boxes. A structured interview usually pertains to the methodological principles of quantitative research.

In contrast, unstructured interviews are characterized by the researcher asking as few questions as possible and avoiding steering the answers of the interviewee in a certain direction. Ideally, the flow of the interview is formed by the interviewee talking freely and in depth, i.e., creating a narrative—about their experiences with the theme in question.

The most commonly used interview form is the semi-structured interview, where the researcher focuses on relatively few, specific questions. However, the order and weight of the questions depends on the answers of the interviewee, as the purpose is to explore the deeper perspective of the interviewee. Often the researcher probes (asks the interviewee to elaborate further on an answer they have given) in order to get a better understanding of the issue at hand.

4.2.1.2 Focus Group Interviews

Originally conceived as a tool for market research, focus group discussions are a qualitative method which has increasingly gained importance in health services research. Focus group interviews are often preferred when the interaction between the different participants (ping-pong exchanges of opinions or provoking each other) are believed to produce data and insights that would be less accessible without the interaction found in a group. They provide nuanced data by asking open-ended questions about complex issues, for example, group norms such as pharmacy organization culture (Morgan 1988; Smith 1998). They can also stimulate nuanced reflections, which are otherwise difficult to catch, for example, patients' experiences of pharmacy visits. They are well suited for exploratory work.

To be able to stimulate group interaction, it is recommended that between six and ten persons participate (Hassell and Hibbert 1996). The form the group interview takes will often be a mixture of the unstructured and semi-structured interview. Although the researchers will probably have several research questions to be answered, they will allow the discussions between participants to move freely (Hassell and Hibbert 1996).

4.2.2 Preparing Interviews

Several methodological decisions have to be made before conducting the interview, for example, the structure of the interview guide, i.e., the themes, the number and types of questions, and how many and which participants to recruit. In addition, consideration must also be taken as to how to record data for later analysis and where to conduct the interview. Finally, ensuring the consent of the interviewee is very important.

The interview guide is the tool used by researchers to organize and keep track of the development of the interview and to ensure that all relevant questions have been answered. The themes of the interview guide can come from a variety and mixture of different sources. Sources include literature reviews, theory, or expert knowledge. It is important that all themes in the interview guide can be justified.

For semi-structured and unstructured interviews, it is usually recommended to ask open-ended questions to stimulate rich and nuanced answers, which can then be followed by more closed questions to illustrate the specific perspective of the participant. Kvale (1996) describes nine types of questions that can be used during an interview, including the technique of "silence" to give the interviewee time to reflect and express her-/himself. Asking "interpretation questions," i.e., clarifying whether the understanding of the researcher is aligned with the perceptions expressed by the interviewee, is also recommended (Kvale 1996).

4.2.2.1 Sampling

Participant sampling is another vital step to create valuable results. As interviews are characterized by creating substantial amounts of data, researchers often have to include a restricted number of participants. One purpose of qualitative research is to identify patterns with regard to similarities of feelings, attitudes, or experiences of people pertaining to a certain group. This requires a minimum of number of participants in order to ensure that all relevant patterns are found and appear consistently. Hence, recruitment continues until no new patterns are identified; this is known as data saturation, which requires that the analysis is carried out parallel to the data-collection phase. For semi-structured interviews, between 15 and 25 interviews are often necessary in order to achieve saturation.

The researcher must also reflect on who the interviewee represents. Does the participant illustrate a rare case, a critical case, or a typical case in relation to what is being investigated? Does the researcher aim for maximum or minimum variation between the cases/interviewees? Often sampling is affected by practical issues including limited access; one option is "snowballing," whereby you ask participants and experts in the field if they could recommend potential participants who fulfill the inclusion criteria.

4.2.2.2 Conducting the Interview

As patients' accounts in unstructured and semi-structured interviews are detailed and rich and often beyond the immediate comprehension of the researcher, noting down the interviewee's answers during the interview is not sufficient for capturing all the relevant information. This is why interviews should be audio-recorded. It is also important to create a trusting environment during the interview in order to allow the interviewee to feel safe to express their true opinions. Therefore, reflecting about where to conduct the interview to create this atmosphere is crucial.

Conducting pilot studies is often not necessary if a sound interview guide has been developed. As lifeworld accounts are complex and not fully predictable, conducting interviews of an inductive nature, i.e., applying learning from one interview to the next to probe, for example, more accurately, is highly recommended.

The ethics in doing interviews concern, in particular, adequately informing the interviewee about the purpose of the research project. In addition, it is important to protect the anonymity of the interviewee throughout the research process and be aware of the asymmetry of power in the interview situation where the researcher often defines the process, e.g., to be sensible not to ask and probe about matters which the interviewee may feel uncomfortable talking about.

4.2.3 Analyzing Interviews

The first step in the analysis process is to transcribe the audio recordings into written data. Keeping the exact wording is essential, as well as including supplementary notes in the transcribed text if the interviewee showed a special physical reaction at some point during the interview (body language). Smaller pauses and sounds like "oh..." could be left out.

There is no strictly defined way to analyze transcribed interviews. Common approaches include meaning condensation, theoretical analysis, and grounded analysis.

Meaning condensation, which according to Kvale (1996, p. 192) "entails an abridgement of the meanings expressed by the interviewees into shorter formulations" is often linked directly to the developed and well-argued themes of the interview guide. Within each theme of the interview guide for each of the interviewees, quotes pertaining to this particular theme are highlighted and moved to a special table in order to obtain an overview of the process (e.g., by using software). The researcher should at this point be open to new, interesting, and at times unexpected statements made by the interviewee that cannot be directly linked to the existing themes. When the entire interview has been coded in this way, the different quotes for one interviewee within one theme are condensed by the researcher, interpreting in her/his own words, as briefly as possible, the meaning expressed by the interviewee. When this process has been conducted for each individual participant, patterns of similarities or differences between participants can be identified (Kvale 1996).

Based on the initial coding, the researcher might also try to go beyond the self-understanding of the interviewee to understand, for example, which factors characterize or drive and influence the perspective of the interviewee. This type of analysis is known as "critical common sense" (Kvale 1996).

Other analytical approaches involve theoretical analysis, i.e., interpretation of transcripts through the application of a specific and relevant theory, or the technique of grounded theory which generates new theory by looking upon the transcripts without pre-assumptions. These hypotheses or ideas of patterns and the meaning of patterns can then be tested by applying them to all included cases in order to refine it or, if not fully consistent with the data material, to discard the idea and test others.

4.2.4 Strengths and Weaknesses

The strength of the interview is to illustrate patterns of perceptions, attitudes, ideas, etc. of a group of "actors," for example, within the field of pharmacy practice pinpointing similarities and differences between participants. Interviews reflect participants' own accounts of actions in real life, which should not necessarily be understood as what actions actually take place (Kaae et al. 2010). If the goal is to describe actions taking place, methods such as observations are more suitable.

4.3 Observation

Observation is increasingly gaining recognition within pharmacy practice research. As a research method, it entails the observation and description of a subject's behavior in their natural environment. In pharmacy practice, observations have been used to study, for example, pharmacy organization in relation to the impact of technology on the workflow of staff members (Walsh et al. 2003), communication between pharmacy staff and patients (van Hulten et al. 2011), and the behavior of patients when they are in the pharmacy (Mobach 2007).

Observation pertains to both quantitative and qualitative methodology. When using observations for qualitative research purposes, studies are often engaged with describing behavioral patterns of actors within the pharmacy practice field. This could be characterizing the leadership style of a pharmacy owner (Kaae et al. 2011) or communication behavior, i.e., "the roles" of the pharmacist and patient during the interaction or "how the two parties interact" (Murad et al. 2014).

4.3.1 Types of Observation

Different types of qualitative observation exist, depending on whether or not the researcher takes part in the activities being observed. Hence, the researcher can choose to be fully covert from the action taking place; the researcher can choose to be overt/visible but not participating in the activities, or they can engage in and take an active part of the actions to be investigated.

4.3.1.1 Non-participatory Observation

The idea of non-participatory observation is to capture the way certain behaviors take place in the real world without the researcher exerting any influence. This type of observation can be covert or overt according to whether the participants are aware of being observed. Non-interfering covert observation raises many practical and ethical challenges which must be addressed and resolved.

If choosing overt observation, practicalities such as where to stand in order to hear and see all relevant aspects must be considered. The risk of the so-called Hawthorne effect must be addressed, i.e., the influence the presence of the researcher has on the actors' behavior. According to the Hawthorne effect, people try to live up to the existing norms or the assumed expectations of the researcher. It has however been shown that participants display different reactions when being observed, hence it is difficult to foresee exactly if and how the observer influences the behavior of participants (McCambridge et al. 2014). It has been suggested that, when possible, the researcher should spend time with participants prior to the observation, in order to get them accustomed to the presence of the observer (Smith 1998). Using audio recordings as observation tools is an option in order to reduce the Hawthorne effect.

4.3.1.2 Participant Observation

To get a more in-depth understanding of the behaviors taking place, participant observation is relevant. An ideal opportunity for participant observation in pharmacy practice exists for the pharmacist researcher. However, observing while at the same time acting in the environment is challenging and thus according to Robson (2002) requires extensive training.

A special type of covert participant observation has been used in pharmacy practice in the case of mystery shoppers. This method is often used to assess the communication behavior of the staff at the pharmacy counter. It is mainly used for quantitative purposes.

4.3.2 Preparing the Observation

Preparing an observation study includes decisions regarding the sampling setting, i.e., where the behaviors under observation will take place, and how to collect data, as well as the period of time necessary to collect sufficient amounts of data.

Typical, representative, or unique cases could be included depending on the research questions (see also "Preparation of the interview"). The number of different settings as well as settings within a setting should be considered before starting the observation. If, for example, exploring communication at the counter, it should be decided what the number and characteristics of included pharmacies should be. Additionally, how many and what members of staff should be observed. It is also important to decide the time of day when the observations will take place. Finally, the number of different encounters at the counter or when to stop observation has to be determined. This often necessitates parallel data collection and analysis.

The collection instrument for observation can take several forms. Based on the works of Spradley, Robson (2002) suggests nine dimensions to observe, all of which have to be described thoroughly initially in order to obtain rich and nuanced data. The levels are space, actors, activities, objects, acts, events, time, goals, and feelings. Hence, the description includes both physical elements and the immediate interpretation of goals and feelings of the people under investigation. The advantage is that the context of the behaviors is then registered along with the behaviors themselves. As behaviors are indisputably dependent on the context in which they take place, this factor can then be described and analyzed.

The scheme designed by Robson (2002) will in most cases have to be supplemented with new categories/dimensions pertaining to specific elements of interest. For example, when observing communication at the pharmacy counter, nonverbal behavior, spatial behaviors (if actors move closer or further away from each other), extra-linguistic behavior (e.g., speed of speaking or loudness), and linguistic behaviors (actual content and structure of talk) could all be integrated. Use of audio or video recordings might also provide useful supplementary data. These tools will inevitably register a variety of details during the action which could never be obtained to the same degree when taking notes by hand (Murad et al. 2014).

4.3.3 Analyzing the Observation

When using audio or video recordings, the first step in the analysis could be to transcribe actions into written accounts. Coding directly on recordings is also feasible. Then the nine categories developed by Robson (2002) could be used as the first step in the analysis.

Units of behavior are then defined. The unit can be defined in many ways—one patient–staff encounter at the counter or the actions of the pharmacy owner during 1 day, or one patient's activities in the waiting area of the pharmacy before they are called to the counter. The next step is either to select verbal statements and/or contemporary behavior within the unit or start coding these to be able to characterize the typical nature of the observed behavior within the unit.

After coding the data according to the first set of categories, the researcher can then start looking more into the meaning of the content of the different codes. Which codes are linked and in which ways—what really defines the actions within one code? Contextual factors can be considered here as well. Do behaviors differ according to differences in the context? New meanings and codes are then developed and renamed and finally turned into a total understanding of the characteristics of the first unit. The unit can then be compared with other units to explore similarities and differences between them.

4.3.4 Strengths and Weaknesses of Observations

Observations are useful to explore what people actually do instead of relying on what people say they do. In some cases, peoples' perceptions of their actual actions coincide with what others register (Fedder et al. 1998). In case of discrepancies, observations are often believed to be "truthful" compared to self-reported practices reported in questionnaires or interviews. However, expressed perceptions should never be discarded as false, but rather understood to represent another angle to the case, i.e., how people perceive or want to be perceived in a certain situation. As people are often unaware of their actions or can never explain in detail how they actually act, observations are useful in registering this.

Observations are only a limited resource for initiating practice improvements because they don't allow the practitioners to reflect on their own behavior, for example, the opportunity to provide reasons and arguments for acting in a particular way. Hence, the reasoning and perceptions of the involved actors of their behavior hold very useful information as to how they can be motivated into changing practices in the future. A very fruitful method of triangulation is first to carry out observations and then ask interviewees to comment directly on the observations made (Watson, Kaae et al. 2010).

4.4 Documentary Methods

A document is a piece of written, printed, or electronic matter that provides information or evidence which relates to some aspect of the social world and often serves as an official record. Documents reveal what people do or did and what they value. Often the behavior revealed in the document occurred in a natural setting which gives this type of data a strong validity.

Document analysis is the method of using documents as the object of study. The goal of the analysis is to find and interpret patterns in data, to classify patterns, to interpret the text, and (when possible) to generalize the results. Within pharmacy practice, documentary methods are, for example, useful to explore the development of policies influencing practice. One example includes the analysis of how and why publicly reimbursed cognitive services are agreed upon. Such insight can be used to advocate for more services.

A documentary study can either be quantitative or qualitative; it all depends on the research questions. Qualitative methods of document analysis involve interpreting the information provided in the material through descriptive and analytic means, in particular studying the context and the multiple meanings that can be found in the documents. Document analysis as a research method often avoids ethical issues, in that most often the documents being analyzed are in the public domain.

4.4.1 Types and Sources of Documents

The document sources are many and varied and can be found in a variety of places, for example, literature reviews—the process of reading, analyzing, evaluating, and summarizing scholarly literature. Medical documents (including patient journals) are frequently the object of study in pharmacy practice studies. In research that focuses on the patient perspective, personal documents can be used such as patient diaries and copies of their correspondence with health professionals.

Official documents such as government publications, legal documents, documents of public hearings, guidelines, or reports are often the source of policy analysis. For example, document analysis of a particular pharmaceutical policy—such as the problem of counterfeit drugs—might include white papers or reports produced by the ministry of health, as well as position papers produced by the World Health Organization or other international organizations. The intention of most official documents is for them to be read as objective statements of fact; however, in research, documents are regarded as socially produced and serve as evidence or proof and therefore can reveal underlying meanings and motives.

A documentation review or analysis can include—in addition to written documents—visual documents such as photographs, posters, TV, and film, as well as sound recordings. These sources of visual and audio material could, for example, be the source of a study which explores or evaluates the message of health or prevention campaigns.

4.4.2 Preparing for the Documentary Analysis

Most important when preparing document studies is to identify and then decide on exactly what documents you need/want to analyze. In other words, based on your research question(s) what documents can provide answers, or at least partial answers, to these questions.

Further, it is important to keep order in your documents and your notes. Sometimes it is useful to scan the documents onto a computer and use a qualitative analysis package.

4.4.3 Analyzing Documentary Material

The first step in analyzing the documentary material is to roughly sort out the documents, weeding out those that are non-relevant. Then it is a good idea to summarize the contents of the relevant documents.

Next, go back to your main and supplementary questions to see if you have found answers. You move from raw data (the documents themselves) to an understanding and/or interpretation of the material by looking for repetition and trying to find patterns.

A useful tool in document analysis is a worksheet. Basic categories include the title of the document, author, potential for author bias, the source, and date published. There should be space in the worksheet for notes whereby you address the following questions:

- What are the important facts?
- What inferences can be made from this document?
- What is the main point/idea?
- How can this be used in my research question? (Does it in any way answer my research questions or contribute to this?)
- Was there any unexpected, yet relevant, information?

The goal is to find an explanation and understanding of the questions addressed in your project. The answer can take many forms. For example, an analysis of package inserts for a particular medicine could reveal that "The majority of the problems with package inserts are most likely due to communication problems—in other words, customers do not understand the advice provided in the inserts because the language is too technical."

4.4.4 Strengths and Weaknesses

In general, documentary studies are useful when a document exists that is relevant to your research question; when you reach the realization that if you did not analyze this (these) document(s), you would have a hole in your research; and when it is not possible to observe or do interviews with your population. Though useful to use computers to help organize and sort data, no computer can manage your data—it is up to you to devise a system of filing and recall for all your documents and notes (Traulsen and Klinke 2005).

4.5 Netnography

Netnography is a relatively new concept in the field of qualitative research and has gained popularity and impetus in the field of marketing research. Robert V. Kozinets (an anthropologist by training) is a professor in marketing and a social media expert who has championed netnography as a method and written extensively on the subject since 1995. He defines it as the use of online communities, such as newsgroups, blogs, forums, social networking sites, podcasting, video casting, photo-sharing communities, and virtual worlds, for research purposes (Kozinets 2010). Some call netnography a method and others a discipline; basically, it is using the computer as a tool to support research and the Internet as a source of generating/providing data.

Initially devised to investigate consumer behavior, netnography is a useful tool/method in pharmacy practice research for studying online cultures and communities such as patient groups and organizations or to do marketing and consumer research. Another field of pharmacy practice research that can benefit from this method is studies of organization and management in community and hospital pharmacies.

Netnography is more naturalistic and unobtrusive than other qualitative methods such as focus groups or interviews. Netnography explores cultural phenomena (such as blogs, Facebook groups, and other Internet-based social media, tweets, etc.) where the goal of the research is to observe communities and social groups from the point of view of the subject of the study—what some call "writing the culture of the group." Netnography is capable in providing information on the symbolism, meanings, and consumption patterns of online consumer groups. In particular, netnography is a suitable method for sensitive research areas, since the Internet offers good possibilities for anonymity.

Social media opens great opportunities for pharmacy practice research, making it easy to get in contact with and establish dialogs with patients, patient associations, as well as pharmacists and healthcare professionals. For example, if one is interested in understanding the increase in use of antidepressants among young women, one could set up a blog and/or a "chat room" and invite young women to join. One recent initiative includes a study which set up a pharmacy-based nationwide online tele-pharmacy chat service offering free pharmacy counseling to all, followed by an analysis of the types of enquires in order to identify the needs of customers and therein improve pharmacy services to citizens (Ho et al. 2014).

4.5.1 Using Computers and the Internet in Qualitative Research

Whereas previously research was an extremely time-consuming and work-intensive process, over the years computers and the Internet have positively contributed to the research process. For example, the overall advantages include the expedient and speedy handling of data, the increase in data storage capabilities, a consistent increase in accuracy (computer errors are inevitably human errors), the possibility to automate many functions, and last but not least diligence—computers don't get tired or lose their concentration.

Computers and the Internet have become invaluable in all types and phases of research; these include using the Internet to search for literature and the computer to store relevant articles, data, and text. Software packages and apps are available to assist in designing, planning, and analyzing research projects. Data collection (empirical work) is made easy in that computers can store data in Word files or lay them out in Excel spreadsheets. Software has been developed to assist in the audio uptake, storage, and transcription of interviews.

In general, information obtained through the Internet can be analyzed the same way as other documentary material (see Documentary Methods). Whereas data consist of discrete entities that are described objectively without interpretation (e.g., transcriptions of interviews or text found in a document), data must be organized, structured, and interpreted. They must then be synthesized so that interrelationships can be identified and formalized. Whereas a majority of studies can benefit from simple word-processing programs to record and analyze qualitative data, software programs are available for more sophisticated and complex text analysis, such as "NVivo" for qualitative data research software.

And last but not least, the contributions of computers and the Internet to the dissemination phase include the availability of word-processing programs including standard (and customized) layouts for both articles and posters, the possibility of instantly producing portable data formats (PDF) files, the possibility to store published material on the world wide web, and access to the social media and online research groups which are invaluable tools for disseminating research results.

4.5.2 Strengths and Weaknesses

Computers and the Internet have positively contributed to the research process, in particular at handling data—which is very different from the goal of research, which is the creation of new knowledge. Computers cannot do this; they can only help in the various stages of the process. A potential problem with conducting research over the Internet is that you cannot always be sure who you are communicating with and whether they are who they claim to be.

4.6 Validity, Reliability, and Transferability in Qualitative Studies

Qualitative research, as all scientific research, has to live up to a set of rigid quality criteria of research conduct in order to provide trustworthy results that contribute to the further development of pharmacy practice. This includes validity, reliability, and transferability of the research process and results. As pharmacy practice research is situated within different research traditions including natural sciences, social sciences, and humanities, several conflicting or supplementary perceptions of exactly which quality criteria to apply and how to apply them exist. This challenge is reflected in the pharmacy practice literature.

Aside from specific quality criteria, research in pharmacy practice should also be assessed by its contribution to the development of the field. This depends on the research questions, which often rely on an in-depth knowledge of the field. The pharmacy profession has been criticized for reproducing an unexamined and noncritical professional ideology by pharmacists who turn a blind eye toward their own shortcomings (Almarsdottir et al. 2014).

4.6.1 Validity

Validity is measured by whether or not the researcher has managed to present adequately the real-life phenomenon she or he intended to investigate. Ensuring validity includes validation of every step of the research process, from formulating relevant research questions to the dissemination of results. How this is managed is again a question of which research tradition the researcher identifies with.

Transparency is a crucial element in building up validity, as no process undertaken in a study is justified by itself. To obtain transparency, a thorough description of all relevant actions undertaken during the project is needed, including solid arguments for the choices made. Solid argumentation may include a description of the pre-assumptions of the researcher. Eliciting understandings and decisions made during the research project also helps to bridge the different phases to each other in order to ensure, for example, that the data-collection tool is in line with the research questions as well as with a relevant theory and review of the literature in the field.

Another important quality element in qualitative research is obtaining richness of data which allow for interpretation that goes beyond purely descriptive accounts. This calls for research methods which are sensitive to details.

Finally, being open to finding unexpected patterns in the collected data is also important for the validity of a qualitative study.

4.6.2 Reliability

Reliability is whether two independent researchers using the same methods, including data-collection tools and analysis, would arrive at the same results. Considering the endless complexity and richness of data within qualitative research, producing results which make relevant contributions to the objective of the research project appears more important than obtaining reliability. According to Kvale, placing too much emphasis on reliability can reduce the creativeness of the researcher (Kvale 1996).

The reliability of data analysis is often described as a quality asset of qualitative projects when the researchers involved reach consensus on the results. However, having a group of researchers who don't manage to obtain consensus on the results could likewise be argued to be an important contribution to research (Malterud 2001). In this case, different possible understandings of the studied practices can be presented which yield an even deeper insight into the phenomenon. Kvale advocates that all too often, too few interpretations are given (Kvale 1996).

4.6.3 Transferability

The transferability of results is relevant because one of the main purposes of research is pooling knowledge in order to get a better insight into relevant areas in order to develop these further. Results pertaining to pharmacy practice research often show strong resemblances between different countries, which makes the issue of transferability highly relevant. One example is the implementation of pharmaceutical care, where barriers such as the attitude of the pharmacist (Mak et al. 2012; Gastelurrutia et al. 2008) or lack of recognition by other healthcare professionals (McDonough and Doucette 2001; Bradley et al. 2012) have been independently identified in several countries across different continents.

Transferability is of course directly linked to the cases included in the study—the pharmacists, patients, pharmacies, etc. Who has been involved in the study? Whom do they represent? Can it be argued that other actors with similar profiles exert the same behavior, ideas, and perceptions? It has been argued that the reader of the study and not the writer is often better at assessing whether results in one setting are transferable to another, as the reader often knows best what the relevant comparable setting is. This requires applying the principle of transparency in order for the reader to make an adequate assessment.

As the goal of sampling in qualitative observation is not to generalize results but to identify patterns of behavior, one well-chosen case could in theory demonstrate features and categories that are relevant for a number of other cases (Mays and Pope 1995). Hence, spending time and effort to include the most relevant cases in a study could prove very valuable as well as applying partial sampling. Selection bias, i.e., including cases and people who are more engaged in the topic than those abstaining from participating, is often unavoidable. Rather than trying to change what can't be circumvented, it is important to describe the biases when writing up the results, and then try to assess the influence they exert over the results.

4.7 Strengths and Limitations of Qualitative Studies

4.7.1 Strengths

Qualitative research attempts to answer the "why" questions and is therefore useful for describing, in rich detail, complex phenomena that are situated and embedded in local contexts; for example, what are the reasons underlying the inappropriate use of antibiotics? When used combined with and parallel to quantitative data collection, it helps explain why a particular response was given, and it provides depth and detail by recording attitudes, feelings, and behaviors—thus creating a detailed picture about why people act in certain ways and their feelings about these actions.

The openness and flexibility of qualitative research has one major advantage. It creates openness since it is carried out in an informal, relaxed atmosphere that invites participants to be open and honest, encouraging them to expand on their responses. This in turn can open up new areas of interest not initially considered, with the added advantage of allowing respondents to answer questions in as much detail as they want.

Qualitative research collects data in naturalistic settings, making it possible to get more valid information about respondents' attitudes, values, and opinions since it opens the possibility for people to explain. Qualitative approaches are especially responsive to local situations, conditions, and stakeholders' needs.

4.7.2 Limitations

The major limitation of qualitative research is that fewer people are usually studied. This has several consequences; for example, the results are unlikely to be representative of a particular population, making it impossible to generalize. This means that the results can be difficult to directly compare or generalize to other people/patient types; other settings or other findings. Because the results are often unique to the relatively few people included in the study, the results are often reported in exact numbers rather than percentages.

Qualitative research is extremely dependent on the skills of the researcher, particularly when conducting individual interviews, focus groups, and observation. There is always the danger that the results can be easily influenced by the researcher's personal biases and idiosyncrasies.

With regard to resources, qualitative studies are time-consuming and labor-intensive—in terms of both data collection and data analysis.

Critics say that qualitative research has lower credibility with many administrators and policy makers, who often prefer percentages, statistics, and tables.

4.8 Summing Up

Qualitative research answers the "why" questions by establishing close personal contact to the person(s) being studied; it emphasizes understanding through the in-depth study of people's words, actions, and records by being responsive to local situations, conditions, and stakeholders' needs. Although qualitative research only studies a limited number of persons and is time-consuming and labor-intensive, it provides a more complete, detailed description about respondents' attitudes, values, and opinions, therein providing valuable information that can lead to valuable improvements in pharmacy practice.

References

Almarsdottir AB, Kaae S, Traulsen JM (2014) Opportunities and challenges in social pharmacy and pharmacy practice research. Res Soc Adm Pharm 10(1):252–255

Bradley F, Ashcroft DM, Noyce PR (2012) Integration and differentiation: a conceptual model of general practitioner and community pharmacist collaboration. Res Soc Adm Pharm 8:36–46

Cavaco AM, Dias JP, Bates IP (2005) Consumers' perceptions of community pharmacy in Portugal: a qualitative exploratory study. Pharm World Sci 27(1):54–60

Emmerton LM, Smith L, LemAy KS, Krass I, Saini B, Bosnic-Anticevich SZ, Reddel HK, Burton DL, Stewart K, Armour CL (2012) Experiences of community pharmacists involved in the delivery of a specialist asthma service in Australia. BMC Health Serv Res 12:164. doi:10.1186/1472-6963-12-164

Fedder DO, Levine DL, Patterson Russell R et al (1998) Strategies to implement a patient counseling and medication tickler system — a study of Maryland pharmacists and their hypertensive patients. Patient Educ Couns 11:53–64

Gastelurrutia MA, Benrimoj SI, Castrillon CC et al (2008) Facilitators for practice change in Spanish community pharmacy. Pharm World Sci 31(1):32–39

Hassell K, Hibbert D (1996) The use of focus groups in pharmacy research: processes and practicalities. J Soc Adm Pharm 14(4):169–177

Ho I, Nielsen L, Jacobsgaard H, Salmasi H, Pottegård A (2014) Chat-based telepharmacy in Denmark: design and early results. Int J Pharm Pract. doi:10.1111/ijpp.12109

Kaae S, Søndergaard B, Haugbølle LS, Traulsen JM (2010) Development of a qualitative exploratory case study research method to explore sustained delivery of cognitive services. Pharm World Sci 32:36–42

Kaae S, Søndergaard B, Haugbølle LS, Traulsen JM (2011) The relationship between leadership style and provision of the first Danish publicly reimbursed CPS—a qualitative multi-case study. Res Soc Adm Pharm 7:113–121

Kozinets R (2010) Netnography: doing ethnographic research online. Sage, London

Kvale S (1996) Interviews: an introduction to qualitative research interviewing. Sage, London. ISBN 0-8039-5819-6

Latif A, Boardman H, Pollock K (2011) Reasons involved in selecting patients for a Medicines Use Review (MUR): exploring pharmacist and staff choices. Int J Pharm Pract 19 (Suppl1):31–33

Mak VS, Clark A, Poulsen JH, Udengaard KU, Gilbert AL (2012) Pharmacists' awareness of Australia's health care reforms and their beliefs and attitudes about their current and future roles. Int J Pharm Pract 20(1):33–40

Malterud K (2001) Qualitative research: standards, challenges, and guidelines. Lancet 358 (11):483–488

Mays N, Pope C (1995) Observational methods in health care settings. BMJ 311:182–184

McCambridge J, Witton J, Elbourne D (2014) Systematic review of the Hawthorne effect: new concepts are needed to study research participation effects. J Clin Epidemiol 67(3):267–277

McDonough RP, Doucette WR (2001) Developing collaborative working relationships between pharmacists and physicians. J Am Pharm Assoc 41(5):682–692

Mobach MP (2007) Consumer behavior in the waiting area. Pharm World Sci 29(1):3–6

Morgan DL (1988) Focus groups as qualitative research. Sage, London

Murad MS, Chatterley T, Guirguis LM (2014) A meta-narrative review of recorded patient-pharmacist interactions: exploring biomedical or patient-centered communication? Res Soc Adm Pharm 10:1–20

Robson C (2002) Real world research. A resource for social scientists and practitioner-researchers. Chap 11: Observational methods, 2nd edn. Blackwell, Oxford

Smith F (1998) Focus groups and observation studies. Int J Pharm Pract 6:229–242

Traulsen JM, Klinke BO (2005) Project handbook—from idea to project—a handbook for pharmacy projects. The Danish University of Pharmaceutical Sciences, Copenhagen, 27 pp (English). ISBN 87-990703-1-6

van Hulten R, Blom L, Mattheusens J, Wolters M, Bouvy M (2011) Communication with patients who are dispensed a first prescription of chronic medication in the community pharmacy. Patient Educ Couns 83(3):417–422

Walsh KE, Chui MA, Kleser MA, Williams SM, Sutter SL, Sutter JG (2003) Exploring the impact of an automated prescription-filling device on community pharmacy technician workflow. J Am Pharm Assoc 51(5):613–618

Further Reading

Denzin NK, Lincoln YS (2010) The SAGE handbook of qualitative research, 4 edn. Sage, London. ISBN 978-1-41297-417-2

Flick U (2009) An introduction to qualitative research, 4 edn. Sage, London. ISBN 978-1-84787-323-1

Garfield S, Hibberd R, Barber N (2013) English community pharmacists' experiences of using electronic transmission of prescriptions: a qualitative study. BMC Health Serv Res 13:435. doi:10.1186/1472-6963-13-435

Giacomini MK, Cook DJ (2000) Are the results of the study valid? For the Evidence-Based Medicine Working Group. JAMA 284(3):357–362. doi:10.1001/jama.284.3.357

Kozinets RV (1998) Netnography: initial reflections on consumer research investigations of cyberculture in NA. In: Alba JW, Wesley Hutchinson J (eds) Advances in consumer research, Vol 25. Association for Consumer Research, Provo, UT, pp 366–371

Kozinets RV (2002) The field behind the screen: using netnography for marketing research in online communities. J Market Res 39(1):61–72

Lincoln YS, Guba EG (1985) Naturalistic inquiry, Chap. 11: Establishing trustworthiness. Sage, London, pp 289–331. ISBN 0-8039-2431-3

Thurmond V (2001) The point of triangulation. J Nurs Scholarsh 33(3):254–256. http://www.ruralhealth.utas.edu.au/gr/resources/docs/the-point-of-triangulation.pdf

Chapter 5
Action Research in Pharmacy Practice

Lotte Stig Nørgaard and Ellen Westh Sørensen

Abstract Action research (AR) is based on a collaborative problem-solving relationship between researcher and client, and the aims of this research are to solve the problem and to generate new knowledge. The chapter describes and shows how several different methods might be used for data collection in an AR-based study. Concepts related to AR are described; in addition, the multifaceted role of the action researcher is described, along with a set of data quality criteria for evaluating the quality of an AR-based study. Then follows a thorough description of a Danish AR-based pharmacy practice study. The chapter concludes with a list of experience-based recommendations for others who are interested in running an AR-based study. This is followed by an Appendix describing four different AR-based studies.

Keywords Action research • Denmark • Pharmacy practice • Researcher role • Data quality • Strengths • Weaknesses • Recommendations

5.1 Action Research as a Research Approach

We both started our professional careers in community pharmacy as pharmaceconomists/community pharmacists and worked there for several years before moving to academia. The focus both in pharmacy practice and in social pharmacy for the past 30–35 years has been on *changing* the role of pharmacy into service-oriented tasks and putting emphasis on the patients or users. One of the ways this can be done is by engaging practitioners (pharmaconomist, students, community pharmacists, etc.) in the change process in pharmacy practice, not only by studying change from the "outside," but by taking part in the change process and establishing partnerships. And this is what action research (AR) is all about: involvement and changing practice in a direction wanted by the involved actors.

L.S. Nørgaard (✉) • E.W. Sørensen
Department of Pharmacy, Section for Social and Clinical Pharmacy, Copenhagen University, Universitetsparken 2, Copenhagen, Denmark
e-mail: lotte.norgaard@sund.ku.dk; ellen.westhsorensen@sund.ku.dk

> We have been fortunate to work together with pharmacy practitioners in a variety of projects, starting in the 1980s, with the purpose of implementing changes with them (Sørensen 1986, 1988, 1993; Børsting et al. 1989; Sørensen and Winther 1996). We continued in the 1990s and 2000s to work together with 100 Danish internship pharmacies and the internship students in the Pharmacy University study from 1998 to 2001 and in the Medisam study from 2007 to 2011. In addition, practitioners in pharmacy practice have welcomed the AR strategy in their master thesis writing (Agerholm and Sørensen 2006).

In recent years, a good number of cases concerning processes and outcomes of AR studies involving pharmacists and pharmacy practice have been described in international journals. Books about the theory and practical guidelines have also been appearing in the last decade, both about AR in general and especially in healthcare.

5.2 What is Action Research ?

There are several definitions of AR. It is, traditionally, defined as an approach to research that is based on a collaborative problem-solving relationship between researcher and client and that aims at both solving a problem and generating new knowledge. The key idea is that AR uses a scientific approach to study the resolution of important social and organizational issues together with those who experience these issues directly (Coghland and Brannick 2005).

Other terms used for AR are "participatory action research," "participatory research," and "community-based participatory research." AR is thus a strategy, a research design, and a methodology—along with other research designs such as case studies, surveys, and field experiments. No methods are "wrong" or "right" in an AR study. Several methods might be used and typically are used (for an example see the PU study [below] and the Appendix).

Hart and Bond (1995) have given excellent descriptions of the characteristics of AR. AR is educative and aims at improvements and involvement; it is problem focused, context specific, and future oriented, and it involves a change intervention. It involves a cyclic process in which research, action, and evaluation are closely interlinked. It is also founded on a research relationship in which those involved are participants in the change process.

AR draws on existing methodological approaches to practice change, such as continuous quality improvement (CQI) and total quality management (TQM). TQM is a structured organizational process for involving personnel in planning and executing continuous stream improvements in systems to provide quality health care that meets or exceeds customer expectations. Improvement plans are used as a tool for running a process change in CQI, TQM, and AR. AR can be distinguished from TQM and CQI by its explicit focus on research and participation, its democratic basis, and its proximity to practice (Mclaughlin and Kaluzny 1994). Therefore, AR is a type of change strategy and is well suited for research, especially in an organizational setting. AR is designed specifically to bridge the gap between theory, research, and practice (Holter and Schwartz-Barcott1993).

To give an idea of AR studies carried out in pharmacy practice, we commend reading the Appendix, in which we describe different AR case studies. The four studies described below have the following characteristics in common: an organizational approach, a focus on the process, a focus on learning, and cooperation with practitioners on several levels.

5.3 AR: Its Origin and Related Concepts

Action Research has developed from a form of rational social management to a more democratic and empowering approach to change. Related developments have been going on in organizational research, in community development, in education, and in nursing.

Action Research in its traditional sense has its origin in applied behavioral sciences and has developed in organizational context. This approach comes from the work of the social psychologist Kurt Lewin (1890–1947), who is recognized as the founder of AR. Other concepts are used for AR, for instance:

Participatory AR (PAR) is an approach that has developed from sociology. It is explained by Fals-Borda (2001), who focuses on how communities as sociopolitical systems enact social change. It involves egalitarian participation by a community to transform some aspects of its situation or structures. It focuses on concerns of power and powerlessness and how the powerless are excluded from decision-making, and it moves to empowering people to construct and use their own knowledge. Examples of AR projects using the term PAR are, for instance, those by Van Buul et al. (2014) and Bradley (2013).

Participatory research (PR) is explained as the co-construction of research through partnerships between researchers and people affected by and/or responsible for action on the issues under study (see Jagosh et al. [2012] and Lalonde et al. [2014]).

Community-based PR (CBPR) takes place in community settings and involves community members in the design and implementation of research projects. Examples of CBPR are works by Tapp et al. (2014), Rudolph et al. (2010), and Jagosh et al. (2012).

Other approaches to AR include "action learning," "action science," and "reflective practice" (Coughlan and Brannick 2005). The use of these concepts is closely connected to different research communities.

5.4 The Role of the Action Researcher

The action researcher's role is to implement the AR method in such a manner as to produce a mutually agreeable outcome for all participants in a domain/an organization, with the process being maintained by them afterward (O'Brien 1998). To accomplish this, it may necessitate the adoption of many different roles at various stages of the process, including those of a planner, a leader, a catalyzer, a consultant, a facilitator, a teacher, a critic, a designer, a listener, an observer, a synthesizer, a legitimizer, and/or a reporter. Thus, the roles of an action researcher are manifold, but indeed challenging.

The main role, however, is to nurture local leaders to the point where they can take responsibility for the process. When this point is reached, they understand the methods and are able to carry on when the initiating researcher leaves. In many AR situations though, the researcher's role is primarily to take the time to facilitate dialogue and foster reflective analysis among the participants, provide them with periodic reports, and write a final report when the researcher's involvement has ended (O'Brien 1998).

5.5 Data Quality in Action Research

An AR study is a case-study and is not easily (and not even necessarily) generalizable according to criteria from the natural scientific paradigm. Quality criteria for AR are validity and whether learning and change have taken place and only to a minor extent generalizability (Launsø and Rieper 2005; Roberts et al. 2006).

Reason and Bradbury (2001) argue that the quality of an AR study can be judged from the following questions:

- Is the study explicitly both aimed at and grounded in the world of practice?
- Is the study being explicitly and actively participative in nature: research with, for, and by people, rather than "on" people?
- Is the study drawing on a wide range of knowledge—including intuitive, experiential, and presentational as well as conceptual—and linked to form theory?
- Is the study worthy of the term "significant"?
- Is the study emerging toward a new and enduring infrastructure?

In the AR study you can benefit from selecting the points you want to be judged against, based on these criteria.

Change is difficult to achieve, though, especially sustainable changes. Therefore, an AR study is not only to be judged solely on the changes achieved, but on what has been *learned* from the experience of undertaking a work. It is therefore important to describe the work in textual details (Meijer et al 2004).

As an AR researcher, you must also consider how best the findings can be validated and tested for reliability (Tanna et al. 2005). By answering the following questions you can be aided in creating a detailed data quality description of your study (Waterman et al. 2001):

- Were the phases of the project clearly outlined?
- Were the participants and the stakeholders clearly described and justified?
- Was consideration given to the local context while implementing change?
- Was the relationship between researchers and participants adequately considered?

All this clearly shows that the data quality criteria developed for AR are very different from traditional quality criteria we know from traditional quantitative and qualitative studies.

5.6 Strengths and Weaknesses of AR

The strengths of AR are its participatory and democratic basis and its starting point in practice. Because it is educative and it enables participants to handle complex problems, you have "many" researchers to do the job. Also, the diversity in knowledge and skills in a project group can be an important ingredient for the success of an AR study. In an AR study, there is room for learning in the project group and especially "learning from our mistakes."

But there are of course also weaknesses in an AR study. None of the individual participants in a steering group get to decide. The collective process makes therefore decision-making procedures relatively complex, and the collective decision-making by the various parties is therefore much more time-consuming for all parts compared to traditional project management. That also means that the leaders must be aware of *when* it is necessary to use the collective form of decision-making and *when* to make decisions in a smaller forum.

5.7 Experiences from the Danish Pharmacy–University Study

In the following, we will focus in more detail on the working process in one of our AR projects which ran between 1998 and 2001: The Pharmacy–University Study. The Pharmacy–University (PU) Study was selected for description because the reader can easily access further information about the study in the scientific literature (see Sørensen and Haugbølle 2008).

5.8 Context and Background

The project background is Danish pharmacies and Danish pharmaceutical education in 2000 (Table 5.1). During their pharmacy internship, pharmacy interns from Copenhagen University back in 1998 performed a small research project in a community pharmacy. Pharmacy staff was challenged by questions from the students; these questions were related to pharmacy practice and the development of pharmacy practice influencing the two others (see Fig. 5.1).

Table 5.1 The Danish pharmacy context in 2000, when the PU study was conducted

Number of community pharmacies in Denmark	288
Population served per pharmacy	18,450 inhabitants
Average pharmacy staff per pharmacy	1 proprietor pharmacist, 2.2 community pharmacists, and 8.6 pharmacy technicians (converted into full-time employees)
Prescription control	Typically the pharmacist, although about 70 % of pharmacy technicians are authorized to control prescriptions
Staff counseling	Proprietor pharmacist, community pharmacists, pharmacy technicians, pharmacy technician students, and pharmacy students from university
Pharmacists' training	Content of the 5-year Master of Science in Pharmacy curriculum of 1988: • *Mathematics, physics, chemistry, toxicology*: 89 ECTS points (approx.1.5 full-time study years taken primarily during semesters 1–4) • *Anatomy, biochemistry, pharmacology, clinical pathology, microbiology etc.*: 58 ETCT points (approx. 1 full-time study year taken primarily during semesters 4–6) • *Drug formulation and production, etc*: 34 ECTS points (approx. 0.5 full-time study year taken during semesters 5–7) • *Social pharmacy, management and organization, occupational health, economics*: 24 ECTS points (approx. 0.4 full-time study year taken primarily during semesters 6–7) • *Interdisciplinary theme period*: 6.5 ECTS points (semesters 2 and 4) • *Pharmacy internship (hospital pharmacy or community pharmacy)*: 30 ECTS points (0.5 full-time study year in semester 8) • *Elective subjects*: 30 ECTS points (0.5 full-time study year taken in semester 9) • *Master's thesis*: 30 ECTS points (0.5 full-time study year taken in semester 10) The Faculty of Pharmacy is the only academic institution in Denmark that offers an MSc program in community pharmacy. The Faculty admits 230 undergraduate students a year
Pharmacy technicians' training	Takes 3 years (20 weeks at the Danish College of Pharmacy Practice, the rest in a pharmacy)

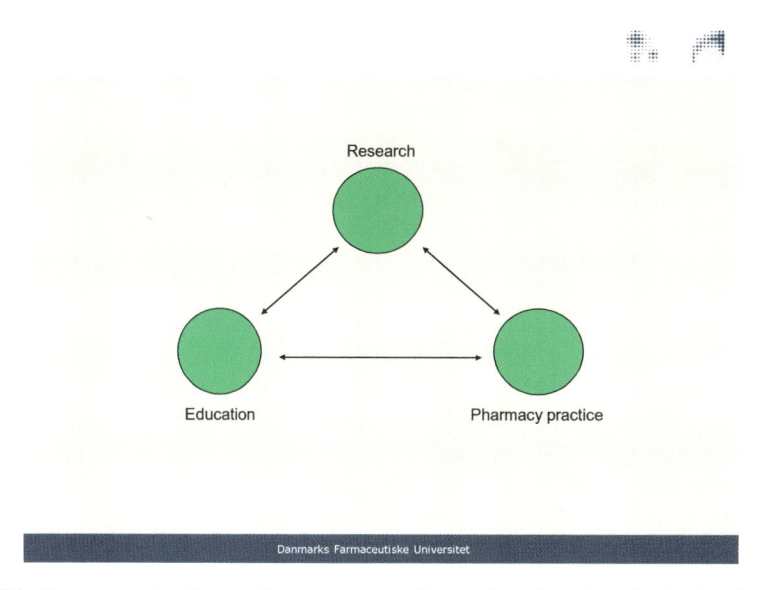

Fig. 5.1 Research, education, and pharmacy practice are interdependent in the development process

The ideas for the study were discussed with the pharmacy supervisors at a yearly supervisor meeting, since we knew the importance of taking a research starting point from *practice* ideas and challenges.

The objectives of the PU-study were:

For community pharmacies: to form a basis for improving the pharmacy's advice to patient groups.
For the pharmacy students: to get involved in the development of pharmacy advice to patients, to gain insight into patients' perspectives on illness and medicines, and to gain experience in carrying out research.
For the researchers: to implement and evaluate AR as a way of carrying out development studies in pharmacy practice.

5.9 Roles of the Involved Persons

The participants in the study were a steering group consisting of researchers, pharmacy students, and pharmacy staff.

The steering group (between 12 and 18 people, researchers, students, pharmacists) worked out project plans and data-collection tools, analyzed data, and disseminated them as indicated below.

The researchers were the initiators, fundraisers, and resource persons for research methodology; they had a secretariat, and they were decision-makers in relation to teaching and disseminators in relation to research.

During the initial phases of the study, the researchers' role was mostly of a planning, facilitating, and designing kind. Explicitly during the yearly supervisor meetings and during steering group meetings, our researcher roles were to be leaders, observers and to catalyze processes.

The pharmacy students were the local leaders of the project in their internship pharmacy.

They introduced the project, presented the results, and collected data for the project.

Research interviews were carried out with *patients* about their perceptions and actions in relation to their illness and medicines.

The internship pharmacies who accepted the invitation hosted the activities, and they also gained benefit from this research process. *Pharmacy staff* completed a questionnaire about their own knowledge and activities in relation to a specific patient group and were invited to take action in the pharmacy on the basis of the new knowledge presented to them by the pharmacy students concerning patients' perception and staff's perception on medicine use.

5.10 Methods

Several methods were used for producing data in the PU study. First of all, questionnaires were used for evaluating pharmacies' activities and for evaluating internship students' knowledge and perceptions. Then, qualitative interviews were used for evaluating students' knowledge and perception and for evaluating participating pharmacists' and steering group members' perspective on the study. Finally, agendas and referees from steering group meetings and supervisor meetings were used for evaluating the process in the steering group and at supervisor meetings.

5.11 Results

The results section is divided into two:

Principles Used in Carrying Out the Study

- The AR cycle
- AR project management
- Focus on stakeholders in the study
- Focus on study start-up
- Action, reflection, and learning processes
- Wide use of existing structures

Outcome for Participants and Long-Term Implications

- For participating pharmacies
- For students and education
- For researchers and the steering group
- Long-term implications

5.11.1 Principles Used in Carrying Out the Study

In connection with carrying out the PU study, the steering group gained experience in using the following principles:

5.11.1.1 The AR Cycle

The PU study was conducted in six different cycles consisting of four phases each: diagnosis, planning, taking action, and evaluation. The first cycle is shown in Fig. 5.2.

The initial idea from the angina pectoris study in 1999 was repeated in 2000 and 2001 with two other groups of chronic patients (people with type 2 diabetes and asthma patients). These two groups were selected because they were the focus of campaigns conducted by the Danish Pharmaceutical Association (DPA) in the years in question. All proprietor pharmacists in Denmark are members of the DPA.

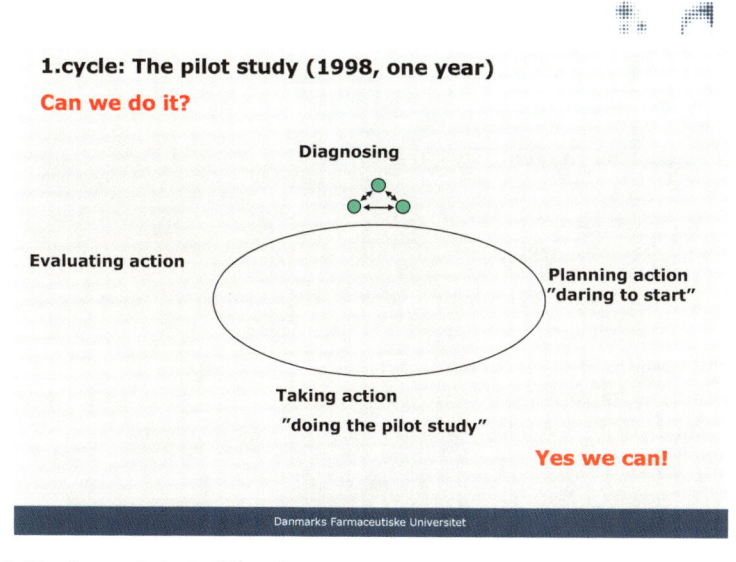

Fig. 5.2 The first cycle in the PU study

The selection of the two latter patient groups was not the original idea of the steering group, however. The steering group would have preferred to follow up on the angina pectoris sub-study from 1999 by conducting an observation study of the advice given to angina pectoris patients at the pharmacy counter, on the basis of problems identified in the initial study. However, the supervisors at the internship pharmacies were more interested in studies coordinated with the Danish Pharmaceutical Association's campaigns.

In the cycles that followed, the angina pectoris study was repeated with minor adjustments for people with type 2 diabetes and asthma patients. Several new issues were identified from the steering group's evaluation of actions, such as better interview training of interns, that the management needs a secretariat and a coordinator, and that the manuals used in the study should be disseminated to all pharmacies.

5.11.1.2 AR Project Management

The steering group was composed of people from the university, Pharmakon (the Danish College of Pharmacy Practice), the Danish Pharmaceutical Association, the 100 internship pharmacies, and the more than 450 pharmacy interns (who boosted coordination of the activities in the participating pharmacies). As one of the steering group members put it: *"When we do things together, they really hang together. It is easier for us to deal with them [in the pharmacies], because it doesn't seem like many different projects."*

Members of the steering group were positive about the AR working form and would like to use it in future studies, because, for instance, "you set your own agenda," there is no fixed "recipe," and there is room for informal meetings—discussion and spontaneity.

5.11.1.3 Focus on Stakeholders in the Study

Stakeholders were identified at the start of the study and followed during the study. Key stakeholders were evaluated in the introductory analysis in terms of:

– Their support for the study and in what form (driving force, resources, formal approval, social acceptance)
– Problems and barriers (obstacles, resistance, limitations)
– Expectations (negative and positive)
– Goal (the perfect situation)

5.11.1.4 Focus on Study Start-Up

Start-up was slow, since the authors of this book chapter were aware that the study needed the acceptance and interest of the participating parties, of which the most important were the internship pharmacies represented by the supervisors. The idea of a cooperative project between the university and the internship pharmacies, and the potential benefit to both parties, was presented at the annual preceptor days held in 1998, where the supervisors approved the initiative and suggested possible topics. Another important prerequisite was acceptance by the university department where the two authors of the chapter were occupied. For instance, the department provided secretarial help for the project.

5.11.1.5 Action, Reflection, and Learning Processes

All activities were subject to evaluation and subsequent reflection in the steering group and among participants at the annual supervisor days. Reflection gave rise to adjustments, changes, and concluding some parts of the project. For example: the steering group became more aware of providing better coordination of the project with the other activities initiated in the entire pharmacy sector.

The basic tenet of the project was the *learning aspect* for all parties involved. The steering group considered the supervisors practical knowledge and researchers' theoretical knowledge as equal prerequisites for being able to carry out the project. The steering group accepted that there might be mistakes in the process, and this was seen as a potential learning experience for the entire steering group. Therefore, it was accepted that the steering group members selected tasks based on areas of interest rather than individual strengths exclusively.

Not all parties learned equally much from the project. Whereas the researchers and practitioners in the steering group in particular entered into a lengthy learning process, the individual pharmacies tended to see the PU study as one of many options offered to them, and they did not want to take on further obligations. Similarly, the students found it attractive to be able to participate in the project during their internship, as long as it didn't demand too much of their time.

5.11.1.6 Wide Use of Existing Structures

The existing structure used as the basis for the study was the university's pharmacy internship program. The project was presented to the advisory board, which gave their approval and support. There was an additional need for a steering group as well as various ad hoc working groups (interview group, questionnaire group, process group, hospital group, and dissemination group). Members of the working groups were also members of the steering group. Once the working groups were organized, the steering group's meetings could be limited to twice a year. Using the existing structure enabled us to carry out the study at a minimal amount of extra cost.

5.11.2 Outcome for Participants and Long-Term Implications of the Study

5.11.2.1 For Participating Pharmacies

Following the study, 85 % of the participating pharmacies made decisions for change in 1999, with a major emphasis on staff-oriented activities such as teaching of staff, meetings with staff about coronary heart disease and medication, and development and revision of material and protocols for counseling angina pectoris patients and patients with other coronary heart diseases. Patient-oriented activities included increased focus on handing out brochures, improvement of distribution, and arranging local citizen meetings about cardiovascular disease. Fewer pharmacies made changes the following 2 years, namely, 48 % in 2000 and 47 % in 2001, primarily because the pharmacies had already started making changes in response to the results from 1999.

Interviews with supervisors revealed that the PU study had influenced the choice of the pharmacies' activities, in terms of a stronger focus on the medicine use of the different patient groups. The following comment from one of the interviewed preceptors backs this up:

> Well in any case, I think it has been really exciting to have the extra resources in the form of students in house to tackle this kind of project in depth. We are curious; we want to know how the patients feel and what they experience, of course we do…[even] if we don't have the time to get involved with projects like this in depth. So it's something of a gift, if I may put it that way, to have the students do it…the staff get something out of it that way…we thought we were better than we were, and we were certainly not as good as people could expect of any of us. [Patients] didn't use us as much as we thought. That came as a shock.

It was evident from study results that the self-confidence of pharmacy staff in providing patient information was low initially, and that they lacked knowledge about medicine and the patients' medicine use process. Identifying drug-related problems and carrying out medication reviews was slowly becoming staff practice, and they became more focused on providing advice to patients and being qualified to do so through presentations of the study results at pharmacy staff meetings.

5.11.2.2 For Students and Education

During the study period, the students gained practice as project leaders and consultants in the pharmacies. They also carried out patient interviews, filled out medication profiles, and identified drug-related problems. These clinically oriented tasks were accordingly integrated into the internship for all pharmacy students. The participating students' knowledge about the patient group's pharmacotherapy, medication, illness, and patient behavior was significantly better than that of students who did not contribute to the study. Only a few (9.3 %) of the students were negative about similar studies in the future (Sørensen et al. 2005).

5.11.2.3 For Researchers and the Steering Group

The PU study provided teachers and leaders of the pharmacy internship program with in-depth knowledge about the pharmacies' status in giving advice to three different patient groups. They also gained insight into medication and illness-related knowledge, perception, and behavior for the same patient groups (Haugbølle et al. 2002a,b; Haugbølle and Sørensen 2006). Another change in knowledge came from the insight the study provided into effective learning methods for students during pharmacy internships (Sørensen et al. 2005), and new knowledge and experience acquired by the leaders from steering an action-oriented study (Sørensen and Haugbølle 2008). The total amount of publications were: five international scientific peer-reviewed papers, 31 international and national conference presentations, nine Danish articles in professional journals, four Danish research reports, and one home page. In addition, the study helped bring about genuine collaboration between the institutions in pharmacy practice research and development.

5.11.2.4 Long-Term Implications

Concerning changes in dissemination products, the PU study gave rise to numerous reports, oral presentations, poster presentations, a home page, etc. In addition, and also due to the focus of the study, since 2004 all Danish pharmacy students have practiced clinical pharmacy during their 6-month internship period, including themes on drug-use profile, drug-related problems, and patient counseling.

5.12 Recommendations for How to Plan Your Own Action Research Study

On the background of our AR-based experiences, we have made the following list of recommendations and comments regarding conducting an AR study.

When planning a pharmacy practice research study, there is a need to write a standard project description (introduction, background, aim, research questions, design, methods, and plan for the project). This is also usual in other forms of research; however, in an AR-based study we recommend the involvement of practitioners from the very beginning when the aim and research questions are being formulated.

1. *Swear the stakeholders in.*

    You start up by describing a preliminary purpose and background of the study, e.g., "... a desire to do an implementation of medicine service in a hospital ward, because the hospital have given high priority to patient-oriented information, and in this particular ward they want to focus on medication information" (Sørensen and Mak 2011). Your next step as a researcher is to find out about the context, meaning the setting, the ones who are involved in the study, what areas of interest are involved, who will be actors in the study, and who will support the study. You must also try to figure out who will be against or even will try to stop the study. Then, you decide whom to invite into a project group, and you consider if you should invite a group of persons for external cooperation. "In a community pharmacy, one of the pharmacists made a masters thesis in the area of developing the skills and practice for identification and registration of drug-related problems for the pharmacy staff. Here the project group consisted of: the project leader, the proprietor, a pharmacist and a pharmacoeconomist, all employed in the pharmacy" (Agerholm and Sørensen 2006).

    You arrange a meeting where you invite the stakeholders for a discussion. The purpose is for the stakeholders to come to an agreement about the purpose of the study.

2. *Start at the right time.*

    When should you initiate the study? You as a researcher might have your timeline and know exactly when you would like to start up, but in the hospital ward or in the pharmacy they have quite another agenda. They might be unable to start producing data exactly at the time convenient for you. Perhaps the organization is to move to a new building soon, which will postpone the initiation of the study, or a new leader who is eager to make changes might be starting that month, which fortunately goes hand in hand with the start of the study.

3. *Map the organizational structure.*

    It is important to map the organization in which you do AR. Who is the leader(s) (formal and informal)? What are the organization's (the ward, the community pharmacists) purpose and tasks? What are the staff's competencies? Is there any cooperation with other parts of the organization? You must also find out what other activities you are "competing" with, because time is needed for this new study and it has to suit the other activities at the place.

4. *Involve, share, let go of control, divide tasks, and compromise.*

    You are working together with the project group with regard to setting the diagnosis and formulating the research questions and issues. In contrast to other types of studies, you are not the only one to define these. And you need to realize that you might have to "kill your darlings" because some issues which

may be important for you may, however, not be considered useful from the practitioners' point of view.
5. *Use existing structure.*
It is always time-consuming, especially for the practitioners, to put new meetings into the busy daily work schedule. Therefore, it is wise to find out how to integrate information and discussions about this project into the current existing communication channels. This could be in monthly or weekly meetings, in newsletters or in minutes, etc.
6. *Set up milestones.*
It is overwhelming to plan changes in an organization which will run over a long period of time—maybe even years. In our own AR studies we planned for at least 3 years, and the masters thesis projects we supervised ran for more than a year.
7. *Plan–do–observe–reflect (make room for reflection).*
The AR-cycle elements are diagnosing, planning, action, and evaluation. The AR cycle is an important part of the action research concept. Problems, and methods for solving them, are formulated as the study moves along. You might have to go through several cycles, in order to make progress. In the first cycle, the pilot, you try out what is really possible in daily life for the practitioners. What you have learned from this will equip all of you to make the next cycle better, and it will suit all the participants.
8. *Answer the question: What are the engines for change?*
Find out how motivated the participants are, either the individual, being engaged in their own professional career and the development of the pharmacist professional role, or motivation coming from the environment, e.g., third-party payment of pharmaceutical services. Such influences can be a very strong motivation for the change process if they go hand in hand.
9. *Focus on disseminating products.*
An important task for the AR researcher is to plan dissemination of various kinds of information based on the study, not only papers in international journals or a masters thesis for the researcher.
10. *Be aware: It is time-consuming.*
Though we are very enthusiastic about the AR-based way of doing research, even we have to admit an AR-based study takes a lot of time, and normally lasts years.

The pilot circle can be very disappointing sometimes, because neither the researcher nor the practitioners have at all reached the expectations set up in the beginning, but once you have evaluated your plan and actions you get accustomed to this way of working—and then get a better understanding of the situation.

The above recommendations were written in 2005, where we ran a workshop entitled "Developing participatory action research in pharmaceutical care" (Haugbølle and Sørensen 2006). The workshop was run as part of the "4th International Working Conference on Pharmaceutical Care Research" and was organized by the Pharmaceutical Care Network Europe (PCNE). The overall aim of the workshop was to develop ways to implement pharmaceutical care using AR. During the workshop, the 13 workshop participants from nine different European countries made a significant contribution to the further development of a recommendation list from our action-oriented university-based studies, which resulted in the ten recommendations regarding conducting AR in pharmacy practice. Since 2005, the recommendation list has been used for several other AR studies in pharmacy practice.

We are convinced that researchers who consider conducting AR-oriented studies in pharmacy (or in another field for that matter) will improve both the process and the outcome of the study by following the above recommendations.

Appendix: Four Examples of AR-Based Pharmacy Practice Research Studies

Study 1: Pharmacists' Role in Improving Awareness About Folic Acid: A Pilot Study on the Process of Introducing an Intervention in Pharmacy Practice (Meijer et al. 2004)

Objective To determine whether a multiple intervention program aimed at improving women's awareness of folic acid was feasible in community pharmacy practice, to identify adjustments in organization and materials that could improve feasibility, and to assess how the target group experience the intervention. *Setting:* a core team in each of four community pharmacies in the eastern region of the Netherlands.

Methods An AR study was undertaken in which four community pharmacies participated. In each pharmacy, a core team (one pharmacist and one to two technicians) was responsible for the organization and implementation of the intervention. The intervention had several possible levels. As a minimum, pharmacy staff added a label about folic acid to the box of dispensed oral contraceptives (OCs) and handed out a leaflet about folic acid. The intervention was discussed during core team meetings every 6 weeks. Modifications were made based on the experience of the pharmacy team, on responses from pharmacy customers, and on the results of a questionnaire sent to women 1 week after they visited the pharmacy with an OC prescription. This cycle of planning, action, observation, and reflection was repeated twice.

Results The minimum intervention was carried out by all four pharmacies. Other activities differed: two pharmacies introduced a maximum client age limit for handing out the leaflet, two installed an electronic information display, three worked with posters and window displays, and in two pharmacies the pharmacy technicians wore project badges, and an information portfolio was placed in the pharmacy public area. From the target group, 44 % were positive about the label, 49 % were neutral, and 4 % were negative. Over half (56 %) of the target group stated that they appreciated the public health information given through the pharmacy.

Conclusion Working with core teams seemed to be a successful strategy to implement practice change. By discussing and modifying the intervention during each research cycle in the core team meetings, an optimal intervention was reached that fitted in with the existing organization within the pharmacy and possible barriers were overcome. Feedback from the target group was mainly positive, and motivated the core teams to continue.

Study 2: Collaborative Medication Management Services: Improving Patient Care (Gilbert et al. 2002)

Objective To implement and evaluate a collaborative medication management service model. *Setting:* the study was conducted from March 1999 to March 2000, with the participation of 1,000 patients, 63 pharmacists, and 129 general practitioners from six Divisions of General Practice in South Australia.

Methods The design of the study was PAR, in which researchers worked with participants to design, implement, and evaluate the service, allowing researchers and participants to solve problems that arose as the research progressed. The PAR process involved GPs, pharmacists, and consumers in a series of workshops, focus groups, and feedback sessions. A collaborative service delivery model, involving a preliminary case conference, a home visit, and a second case conference, was agreed through discussions with medical and pharmacy organizations, and then implemented. Outcome measures were medication-related problems, actions recommended, actions implemented, and outcomes after actions taken.

Results Overall, 2,764 problems were identified. The most common medication-related problem (17.5 % of all problems) was the need for additional tests. Thirty-seven percent of problems related to medicine selection, 20 % to patient knowledge, and 17 % to the medication regimen. Of 2,764 actions recommended to resolve medication-related problems, 42 % were implemented. Of the 978 problems for which action was taken and follow-up data were available, 81 % were reported to be "resolved," "well managed," or "improving."

Conclusion A collaborative service delivery model was agreed upon through discussions between pharmacists and doctors and accordingly implemented. The implementation model was successful in engaging GPs and pharmacists and in assisting in the resolution of medication-related problems.

Study 3: Roles and Competencies of District Pharmacists: A Case Study From Cape Town (Bradley 2013)

Objective The aim of this study (a PhD thesis) was to explore the contribution of substructure and sub-district pharmacists to health system development and how to support them in their roles, by considering their roles and related competencies in the South African health system and by piloting an intervention to enhance their competencies. *Setting:* The managers in Cape Town City Health and Metro District Health Services, together with the district and sub-district pharmacists in the period from 2008 to 2011.

Methods Participatory action research (PAR) was used as the approach to partner with pharmacists and managers in both organizations between 2008 and 2011. The partnership benefitted from the contextual and practice experiences of the health services stakeholders and the researcher's evolving research expertise. Including a broad stakeholder group was considered important for developing the shared learning and understanding that would translate into action and change in the organizations. The flexible and emergent approach of PAR was considered to be suited to a complex health system in the midst of change. After an initiation stage, the research evolved into a series of five iterative cycles of action and reflection, each providing increasing understanding of the roles and related competencies of substructure and sub-district pharmacists and their experiences as they transitioned into these new management positions in the two organizations. The research centered around two series of three interactive workshops facilitated by researchers and attended by both pharmacists and managers. Semi-structured interviews and focus groups were conducted at various stages during the research, to inform conceptualization and supplement workshops and, later on, to reflect on the experiences of substructure and sub-district pharmacists.

Results and Conclusion The research identified five main roles each for substructure and sub-district pharmacists. Four of these roles are the same for each: (1) substructure (sub-district) management; (2) planning, coordination, and monitoring of pharmaceuticals, HR, budget, and infrastructure; (3) information and advice; and (4) quality assurance and clinical governance. Their fifth role is different though: research for substructure pharmacists and dispensing at clinics for sub-district pharmacists. But although they look similar, there were substantial differences between substructure and sub-district pharmacist roles in the two organizations. Five competency clusters were identified for both cadres, each with several competencies: professional pharmacy practice, health system/public health, management, leadership, personal, interpersonal, and cognitive. Although the competencies appear similar, there were differences between the roles, so that the different cadres required different competencies within these competency clusters. Transitioning into these new management positions was an emergent process, which entailed pharmacists changing from performing technical and clinical functions associated with professional pharmacy practice to coordinating pharmaceutical services across the substructure or sub-district. They moved from working in a pharmacy to being a member of a multi-professional team in a substructure or sub-district. Adjusting to these new management positions took time and was facilitated by several personal and organizational factors which varied in the two organizations. Managers and pharmacists mentioned the positive contribution of the PAR in assisting with this transition through the development of shared understanding of the DHS and the roles and functions of pharmacists working in these management positions.

Study 4: "Medisam—A Model of Cooperation Between Patients, General Practitioners and Pharmacists for Medicines Review and Reconciliation" (see www.farma.ku.dk/index.php?id=7913, Kaae et al. (2011, 2014) and Sørensen et al. (2009, 2011)

Objective The aim of the study was to develop, implement, and evaluate a model of cooperation for medicines review and reconciliation involving patients, pharmacists, and general practitioners in a multi-professional dialogue aimed at solving drug-related problems by involving the patients in decision-making around their medication.

Setting The education pharmacies at the University of Copenhagen (app. 90), the pharmacy students (app. 170), and their pharmacist tutors, the physicians, and patients being involved in the home medication review. The project was run in the period 2008–2011, starting with a pilot study in 2007.

Methods The project was carried out in cooperation between internship pharmacies, their pharmacy students, and the Faculty of Pharmaceutical Sciences. The working method of the project was based on AR principles, where research is focused on solving problems together with those who experience the problems, i.e., in this case the patients, pharmacists, and general practitioners. The project was carried out in a 3-year period, using the main steps of the AR cycle, starting in 2007 where the detailed project plans were elaborated, tested, and evaluated and continued the following 3 years. All internship pharmacies and their pharmacy students were each year invited to join the project. The pharmacist and general practitioner agreed on those patients who should be offered a medicines review and reconciliation. Methods used for data collection were: registration forms for drug-related problems, medication reconciliation forms, patient interviews, case summaries, minutes of various meetings, etc. Data about the AR process were collected each year using written material from meetings in the project group, yearly meetings with tutors, and questionnaires to the pharmacy students, supplemented with qualitative interviews with representatives for the students.

Data about the pharmacist–GP collaboration were collected in 2011 by conducting semi-structured interviews with pharmacy students along with their supervisors and with the connected physicians, in two separate interviews.

Results A collaboration model for home medication review was developed. The model has been practiced as a compulsory part of pharmacy education at the education pharmacies at the University of Copenhagen since 2010. A database (www.medisam.dk) was developed during the project. The database was used by the students for registering the prescribed and used medicines, the drug-related findings, and recommended interventions at the patient level and used by the researchers for quantitative analysis of the data. New knowledge was gained in the following areas: cooperation between GPs, pharmacists, pharmacy education, and patients, implementation of medication review by using AR, the collaborative working relation between pharmacist and physician (theoretical perspectives), and communications around medication review in community pharmacy.

Conclusion The study has taken a direction in accordance with the expressed needs of all participants. Conclusively, medication review has become a sustainable daily practice at the education pharmacies since 2010.

References

Agerholm H, Sørensen EW (2006) Developing community pharmacy by detecting drug related problems—an action research project. Poster, FIP: Salvador, Bahia, Brazil

Børsting I, Nielsen JCR, Sørensen EW (1989) Apotek på en anden måde: Nyt fra Samfundsvidenskaberne. København

Bradley HA (2013) Roles and competencies of district pharmacists: a case study from Cape Town. PhD thesis. http://hdl.handle.net/11394/3255

Coghlan D, Brannick T (2005) Doing action research in your own organization, 2nd edn. Sage Publications, London

Fals-Borda O (2001) Participatory (action) research in social theory: origins and challenges. In: Bradbury H, Reason P (eds) Handbook of action research. Sage Publications, London, pp 27–37

Gilbert AL, Roughead EE, Beilby J, Mott K, Barrarr JD (2002) Collaborative medication management services: improving patient care. Med J Aust 177:189–192

Hart E, Bond B (1995) Action research for health and social care. Open University Press, Buckingham

Haugbølle LS, Sørensen EW (2006a) Drug-related problems in patients with angina pectoris, type 2 diabetes and asthma – interviewing patients at home. Pharm World Sci 28:239–47

Haugbølle LS, Sørensen EW (2006) Workshop IV: developing participatory action research in pharmaceutical care. In: 4th international working conference on pharmaceutical care research—beyond the pharmacy perspective. Workshop leadership and lectures, Hillerød, February 2005

Haugbølle LS, Sørensen EW, Gundersen B, Lorentzen L, Petersen KH (2002a) Basing pharmacy counselling on the perspective of the angina pectoris patient. Pharm World Sci 24(2):71–78

Haugbølle LS, Sørensen EW, Henriksen HH (2002b) Medication- and illness-related factual knowledge, perceptions and behaviour in angina pectoris patients. Patient Educ Couns 47:281–289

Holter IM, Schwartz-Barcott D (1993) Action research: what is it? How has it been used and how can it be used in nursing? J Adv Nurs 18:298–304
Jagosh J et al (2012) Uncovering the benefits of participatory research: implications of a realist review for health research and practice. Milbank Q 90(2):311–46
Kaae S, Sørensen EW, Nørgaard LS (2011) Exploring communications around medication review in community pharmacy. Int J Clin Pharm 33:529–536
Kaae S, Sørensen EW, Nørgaard LS (2014) Evaluation of a Danish pharmacist student—physician medication review collaboration model. Int J Clin Pharm 36(3):615–622
Lalonde L et al (2014) Development of an interprofessional program for cardiovascular prevention in primary care: a participatory research approach. Sage Open Medicine. DOI: 10.1177/2050312114522788
Launsø L, Rieper O (2005) Forskning om og med mennesker [Research on and with people. In Danish only]. NNF Arnold Busck, Copenhagen
Mclaughlin CP, Kaluzny AD (1994) Continuous quality improvement in health care. Aspen, Gaithersburg, MD
Meijer WM, de Smit DJ, Jurgens RA, de Jong-van den Berg LTW (2004) Pharmacists' role in improving awareness about folic acid: a pilot study on the process of introducing an intervention in pharmacy practice. Int J Pharm Pract 12:29–35
O'Brien R (1998) An overview of the methodological approach of research. http://web.net/~robrien/papers/xx%20ar%20final.htm. Viewed 21 August 2014
Reason P, Bradbury H (2001) Introduction: inquiry and participation in search of a world worthy of human aspiration. In: Reason P, Bradbury H (eds) Handbook of action research. Sage Publications, London, pp 1–14
Roberts AS, Benrimoj SI, Chen TF, Williams KA, Aslani P (2006) Implementing cognitive services in community pharmacy: a review of facilitators used in practice change. Int J Pharm Pract 14:163–170
Rudolph AE et al (2010) A community based approach to linking injection drug users with needed services through pharmacies: an evaluation of a pilot intervention in New York City. Aids Educ Prev 22(3):238–251
Sørensen EW (1986) The pharmacy organisation under change. Paper. 4th Social Pharmacy Workshop, Uppsala
Sørensen EW (1988) Experiments in changing the pharmacy. Paper. 5th Social Pharmacy Workshop, Prague
Sørensen EW (1993) Conducting social action research. Presentation, 10th November. Department of Social and Behavioural Pharmacy, University of Wisconsin-Madison
Sørensen EW, Haugbølle LS (2008) Using an action research process in pharmacy practice research—a cooperative project between university and internship pharmacies. Res Social Adm Pharm 4:384–401
Sørensen EW, Mak V (2011) Action research as an implementation strategy in pharmacy practice. Workshop presentation, Nordic Social Pharmacy Workshop, Reykjavik, June
Sørensen EW, Winther L (1996) Conducting pharmacy practice research, part 1: research consultancy and action research. Paper. 9th Social Pharmacy Workshop, Madison
Sørensen EW, Haugbølle LS, Herborg H, Tomsen DV (2005) Improving situated learning in pharmacy internship. Pharm Educ 5:223–33
Sørensen EW et al (2009) Implementation of medication review using an action research method. Abstract and presentation. Nordic Social Pharmacy Conference, Oslo
Sørensen EW et al (2011) Implementation of a home medication review (HMR) collaboration model for pharmacies and pharmacy students—using action research. Abstract, poster and workshop. Nordic Social Pharmacy Conference, Reykjavik
Tanna KN, Pitkin J, Anderson C (2005) Development of the specialist menopause pharmacist (SMP) role within a research frame work. Pharm World Sci 27:61–7

Tapp H et al (2014) Adapting community based participatory research (CBPR) methods to the implementation of an asthma shared decision making intervention in ambulatory practices. J Asthma 51(4):380–90

Van Buul LW et al (2014) Participatory action research in anti-microbial stewardship: a novel approach to improving antimicrobial proscribing in hospitals and long-term care facilities. J Antimicrob Chemother. doi:10.1093/jac/dku068

Waterman H, Tillen D, Dickson R, De Koning K (2001) Action research: a systematic review and guidance for assessment. Health Tech Assess 5

Chapter 6
Participatory Action Research in Pharmacy Practice

Hazel Bradley

Abstract Participatory action research is part of a broad family of approaches and includes as its distinctive features action, reflection and partnership. In participatory action research, knowledge is created in the interplay between research and practice, thus requiring researchers to work with practitioners as active researchers and agents of change through iterative cycles of action and reflection. The purpose of participatory action research is to understand and effect change through generating new learning and knowledge whilst empowering participants. The approach facilitates in-depth understanding of issues in complex settings, which is perhaps not possible with narrower, traditional research approaches. Participatory action research's emergent nature is particularly suited to research in changing circumstances, such as professional development of pharmacists or developing pharmacy services in new settings.

This chapter describes the key features of the participatory action research approach, describes innovative participatory processes and methods and discusses critical issues of the approach including ethical concerns, quality and generalisability. The benefits and challenges and application of participatory action research are highlighted. Finally, I illustrate the application of the participatory action research approach through my own experience of conducting a case study to identify roles and competencies of district and sub-district pharmacists in Cape Town.

Keywords Participatory action research • Action • Reflection • Participation • Emergence • Quality • Pharmacy practice

---

H. Bradley (✉)
School of Public Health, University of the Western Cape, Private Bag X17, Bellville, 7535
South Africa
e-mail: hbradley@uwc.ac.za, http://www.uwc.ac.za/Faculties/CHS/soph

6.1 Introduction to Participatory Action Research as a Research Approach

Participatory action research is part of a broad family of approaches and includes as its distinctive features action, reflection and partnership (Huang 2010; Reason and Bradbury 2008). In participatory action research, knowledge is created in the interplay between research and practice, thus requiring researchers to work with practitioners as active researchers and agents of change through iterative cycles of action and reflection (Huang 2010). This contrasts with the more traditional research approaches in which research is conducted on research subjects rather than collaborating with them as partners. Participatory action research's purpose is, therefore, not only to understand but also to effect change through generating new learning and knowledge and empowering participants (Loewenson et al. 2011).

6.1.1 Historical Roots of Participatory Action Research

There are varying opinions as to the origin of participatory action research, with one strand emerging from the utilitarian approach of action research in Europe and the USA in the middle of twentieth century. This arises primarily out of the work of the German social psychologist, Kurt Lewin. Other strands have emerged from community-based participatory research which developed in the public health field in recognition of the importance of social determinants on disease and from rapid and participatory rural appraisal which evolved in 1970s (Loewenson et al. 2014).

Participatory action research, however, is generally acknowledged to have its roots in emancipatory-empowerment research of Paulo Freire and others who used participatory action research in 1970s to encourage poor and oppressed communities to examine and analyse structural reasons for their oppression (Baum et al. 2006; De Koning and Martin 1996). After gaining some ground in Latin America, Freire assisted others in southern Africa to design educational and health programmes using similar emancipatory-participatory action research principles.

6.1.2 Current Fields of Participatory Action Research

Given its origins, it is not surprising that participatory action research has been extensively used in low- and middle-income countries (LMICs) in the fields of community health and development. The use in developed countries is increasing especially in the fields of health promotion and evaluation (Baum et al. 2006; Minkler and Wallerstein 2003). More recent approaches have been used in health services research, both in LMICs and developed countries, particularly in health improvement initiatives and professional development (Iles and Sutherland 2001; Waterman et al. 2001). Some recent examples from LMICs include the development and implementation of clinical record keeping systems in three hospitals in Jordan and health policy and systems work in Southern and Eastern Africa (Khresheh and Barclay 2007; Loewenson et al. 2011).

In pharmacy practice research, the participatory action research approach was successfully used in Uganda to develop a user-friendly adverse event report form to capture information on events associated with anti-malarials (Davis et al. 2012). In professional development, the approach was useful in developing knowledge and understanding practitioners' new roles and practices, including new pharmacist roles (Tanna et al. 2005).

Several researchers have advocated support for participatory action research as a complementary methodology to other research approaches used in the health services, with some saying that participatory action research may fill the theory–practice gap in health care (Meyer et al. 2000). At a global level WHO Options for Action/Changing Mindsets launched in 2012 promoted stronger collaboration between decision makers and researchers and the importance of co-production of knowledge, thereby lending further credibility to the participatory action research approach.

6.2 Key Features of Participatory Action Research

Whilst there is no one accepted definition of participatory action research, a number of key characteristics have been identified which include:

- Participation
- Cyclical spiral process—spiral of continuous and overlapping cycles
- Emergence
- Reflection and reflexivity

6.2.1 Participation

Participation is a fundamental characteristic of participatory action research, with some linking the participative nature to the democratic process (Greenwood and Levin 1999). Several different aspects of participation should be considered.

Level of Participation Participation can occur at any or every stage of the research from setting the agenda, clarifying the research focus, undertaking fieldwork and analysing findings, through to managing the research, advocacy and using the results (Laws et al. 2003; Reason 2006). Several typologies have emerged on the degree of participation, developed mainly from work on engagements with communities; these include a *ladder of participation* schematised by Arnstein describing a continuum of increasing stakeholder involvement (Reed 2008). Some researchers maintain that authentic participatory action research means participation by researcher and participants at all stages of research, and especially in the initiation phase, whilst others have a more pragmatic stance and say that in their opinion participation should be in areas most relevant to the research project (Bless and Higson-Smith 2004; Reason 2006).

Positionality of Researcher Another consideration related to participation is the positionality of the researcher in the research. Herr and Anderson (2005) described a continuum of six positions from insider to outsider in the setting. One of the middle positions, reciprocal collaboration (insider–outsider teams) is mostly closely aligned to the ideal in participatory action research. Other issues of positionality relate to hierarchical positions within the organisation and the dominance of groups, such as race, religion, gender or age, and it is also important to note that positions sometimes change during the research process itself.

Establishing and Maintaining Participation Co-operative and trusting relationships are key qualities required for participatory action research, and previous experiences of working together contribute significantly to initiation of studies adopting this approach (Calnan and Rowe 2006). The practicalities of maintaining participation over protracted periods pose a serious challenge for participatory action research, and strategies including regular communication, realistic expectations of time and levels of engagement, as well as flexibility and tenacity of the researcher are essential. Coglan and Casey, 2001 as cited in Waterman et al. (2001) coined the terms *performing* and *backstaging* as important for securing and maintaining participation. *Performing* is where the action researcher plays the formal role in organising meetings, and *backstaging* is the work done behind the scenes to encourage attendance and commitment.

6.2.2 Cyclical, Spiral Process

Another typical feature of participatory action research is the cyclical process where cycles of activities form a spiral of continuous and overlapping cycles of action and reflection. Each cycle consists of a small scale intervention or changes in understanding. Gummesson calls them hermeneutic spirals where each turn of the spiral builds on understanding of the previous turn (Dick et al. 2009).

6.2.3 Emergence

Emergence is another central feature of participatory action research. Emergence signifies that during the research, there may be changes in the questions, relationships and purposes of the research (Reason 2006). This evolutionary research process emerging out of a period of collaborative engagement is suited to complex situations and environments in transition or where there is a desire for change (Gilson 2012). This aspect of participatory action research makes it particularly useful in pharmacy practice research, which occurs in the context of complex health systems and where new pharmacists' roles are emerging in many settings around the globe.

6.2.4 Reflection and Reflexivity

Reflection and reflexivity (self-reflection) are integral parts of participatory action research. Reflection has been defined as "*(making) meaning of the situation in ways that enhance understanding*" (Boud et al. 1985). The approach is already established in professional pharmacy practice where reflection and reflective practice are increasingly included as attributes of competent practitioners and are seen as assisting professionals in complex and changing health systems where they continually need to update skills and solve complex problems (Mann et al. 2009; Schon 1983). Several countries, including the UK and South Africa, include reflection as part of their Continuing Professional Development (CPD) cycle for pharmacists. Two dimensions of reflection have been identified: iterative and vertical. In the iterative dimension, the process of reflection is triggered by experience which produces new understanding and the potential to act differently in response to experience (Boud et al. 1985). The vertical dimension includes different levels of reflection on experience, with surface level reflection being more descriptive and deeper levels of reflection being more analytical and critical (Mann et al. 2009).

Reflexivity or self-reflection is the recognition of the researcher's presence in the research study and the interplay between the researcher, the research context and the data. McNiff and Whitehead (2010) write of the importance of the researcher demonstrating critical engagement at every stage of the research including awareness of historical, political and cultural forces that have led to the researchers' current situation and the way they think.

6.3 Participatory Action Research Processes and Methods

Quantitative and qualitative research methods, described in detail in other chapters, may be used in participatory action research, although qualitative methods are more usual. However, participatory action research also uses a range of participatory processes and methods. Many of these new methods are not familiar to research academics or practitioners and are highlighted in Table 6.1.

Table 6.1 Selected participatory methods and tools and application to pharmacy practice research

Methods	Use in PAR process	Application to pharmacy practice research
Participatory mapping—those involved draw maps of study setting noting physical conditions	Draw and validate information on conditions and experience Identify problem sites, analyse service access and proposals for change Can be used at different stages to present new information or monitor and evaluate action and transformation	Access to pharmacies or pharmacy services
Social mapping—similar to participatory mapping but focusses on social characteristics	Identify key social groups and processes, different needs, disease distribution, negotiation of priorities	Identification and prioritisation of key medicines and services required in an area
Pictures or photovoice	Trigger discussion on conditions, system performance, causes and actions to be taken Useful for raising sensitive issues	Highlight infrastructure challenges in managing medicines supply Discussions on sexual, reproductive and mental health
Venn diagrams—series of interrelated circles that indicate relationships, status in the community and interactions. The size of the circle and position indicates relationships between actors	Mapping, reviewing and discussing features of diagram to examine relationships between actors and services	Examine relationship between different actors and pharmaceutical services
Spider-grams—visual tools for identifying and analysing relationships. 'Body' may be focus of issue and legs different factors that are impacted by situation. Can use two spiders, one for positive and one for negative impacts	Draw evidence on determinants or outcomes of a situation, problematise issues and analyse links across determinants or outcomes as an input to problem solving	User fees on use of pharmaceutical services, positive and negative impacts
Ranking and scoring—individual features can be written onto cards and sorted	Used for scoring preference parameters and satisfaction with services. Comparisons can be made through scores or by grouping	Preference for different contraceptive methods or satisfaction with pharmaceutical services
Seasonal calendar—drawn up by participants to show seasons experienced and changes associated, including health burden	Information on seasonal patterns used to analyse relationship including movement of people and disease burden	Quantification of medicines and vaccines requirements at different sites and times of year
Life histories, narratives and storytelling—used to represent experiences	Methods of exploring practice, settings and situations	Understand valuable cultural contexts and interpretations regarding medicines use

(continued)

Table 6.1 (continued)

Methods	Use in PAR process	Application to pharmacy practice research
Problem trees—structured ways of collectively unpacking levels of problems	Used to analyse causes, with pods as problems, branches as immediate causes and trunk or roots as underlying structural causes. Ground is political systems and values	Unpack issues relating to access to medicines or lack of qualified pharmacists
Human sculpture—used to portray people taking roles of actors involved in a health problem with the sculpture showing how they relate to each other. The location, positioning and height of actors reveal dimensions of power and interaction	Used to analyse relationships within health system and identifying changes to be made to address needs of specific groups	Analyse needs of youth in accessing sexual and reproductive health services

Source: Loewenson et al. (2014) and author

6.4 Issues and Challenges in Participatory Action Research

6.4.1 Logistical Aspects

Several aspects of participatory action research, already highlighted, bring practical challenges to the execution of this research approach. The collaborative learning environment provides great opportunities for sharing complementary expertise, but it also requires considerable trust on the part of researcher and health services partners. Likewise whilst the contextual nature of the approach facilitates deep insights, evolving settings undergoing structural re-organisation add to the complexity of the research (Loewenson et al. 2011).

6.4.2 Ethics in Participatory Action Research

Addressing ethical issues in participatory action research is critical to minimise any risks to the research participants and researchers. As with other research approaches, ethical considerations are important at all stages of participatory action research from planning, throughout execution and to reporting and dissemination. However, in addition to meeting legal and ethical standards required for all researches, the participatory and emergent nature of the participatory action research approach bring its own particular challenges. Research protocols should be as clear and explanatory as possible and cover all relevant ethical aspects.

Some of the critical ethical issues that require consideration while conducting a partcipatory action research project include:

- At the beginning of the research, it is critical to establish **shared goals and agreed processes and methods**, although it is quite usual that as the research progresses, the goals and research process may need to be re-negotiated.
- **Nature of participant involvement** including the roles and responsibilities of researcher and participants should be clarified at the outset, again recognising that they may change during the research.
- **Informed voluntary consent** needs to be obtained for the research. In most situations, individual written consent is required, although under some circumstances, group or verbal consent may be agreed. However, as participatory action research is often conducted within organisations or communities, it is particularly important that no one feels coerced into participating for any reason.
- Whilst consent is required at the beginning of the research, as participatory action research is often a lengthy and emergent engagement, it often needs to be **re-negotiated** at stages throughout the research if the research goals or processes changes over time.
- **Respect and privacy** are key ethical principles, but it is important to point out to participatory action research participants that **protection of identity and individual confidentiality** cannot be guaranteed.
- Sensitivity to commitments and availability of participants may necessitate halting the research processes at some stages and **rescheduling** for later date.
- Agreement on regular reporting of progress to key stakeholders and **reporting and dissemination** of findings should be agreed at the outset. Particular consideration should be given to appropriate presentation formats to meet both participants' and researchers' requirements. This should include sensitivity to language, culture and presentation style, which could be in the form of oral presentations, written reports or academic publications.

6.4.3 Quality in Participatory Action Research

A critical issue in all research is quality, and this is particularly the case in participatory action research which has been labelled as "unscientific" by some academics and practitioners. Several terms are used to evaluate quality in research —validity, trustworthiness, authenticity and credibility (Herr and Anderson 2005; Marti and Villasante 2009). Whilst validity is the term preferred by positivists (using in quantitative methods) and trustworthiness by naturalistic researchers (using in qualitative methods), researchers have suggested that neither is suitable for participatory action research as they do not account for the action or the participative engagement (Herr and Anderson 2005).

Several researchers favour the use of the term **quality** and emphasise the importance of measuring quality in action research against criteria relevant to the approach (Marti and Villasante 2009; Reason 2006). Herr and Anderson (2005) suggested five validity criteria. Each criterion is linked to what may be generally agreed as goals of action research, and these criteria provide useful starting points for examining quality in participatory action research.

- Outcome validity (achievement of action-oriented outcomes)
- Process validity (sound and appropriate research methodology)
- Democratic validity (results relevant to local setting)
- Catalytic validity (education of both researcher and participants)
- Dialogic validity (generation of new knowledge)

Reason (2006) in his publication *Choice and Quality in Action Research* introduced four dimensions of AR, which represented fairly similar criteria but added an evolutionary process. The dimensions include pursuing worthwhile purposes, democracy and participation, many ways of knowing and emergent development. Viswanathan et al. (2004) also developed guidelines for quality for their systematic review of community-based participatory research assessing three broad areas: quality of research methods, quality of community involvement and whether projects achieved their intended outcomes. Perhaps illustrative of the complexity of achieving high-quality research in this field, when measured using conventional research quality criteria, few studies were rated highly for both participation and research quality, thereby highlighting the challenge for those engaging in this type of research.

6.4.4 Generalisabilty or Transferability in Participatory Action Research

Generalisability, known as external validity in fixed designs, may be considered in a number of ways in participatory action research. As participatory action research generates new knowledge on particular issues or situations within a defined context, its purposive sampling and the inclusion of groups with common social feature limit generalisation to other settings. However, researchers have proposed that in participatory action research insights, concepts, learnings or motivations for action and reflection may be **transferred** to other settings, even if specific findings are not transferred (Gilson 2012). Another way to address generalisability in participatory action research would be through multi-country or site research that identifies common knowledge across different countries or sites.

6.5 Benefits and Challenges of Using the Participatory Action Research Approach

Whilst participatory action research provides considerable benefits for both researchers and practitioners, there are significant challenges which tend to make the approach more suited to experienced researchers who have established links with practitioners with whom they wish to engage with in research. It is less suited to undergraduate pharmacy students whose research projects are typically of a short duration. Those who want to use participatory action research for their masters or doctoral studies are advised to seek out others with experience to support them during their engagement with this rather complex but nevertheless rewarding approach. Several useful books have been written to guide students and the ones I found particularly useful are *Doing and writing action research* by McNiff and Whitehead (2010) and *The action research dissertation: a guide for students and faculty* by Herr and Anderson (2005).

Here I am summing up the approach by highlighting the benefits and challenges of participative action research:

6.5.1 Benefits

Participatory action research provides several critical benefits for pharmacy practice and health services research. The participative approach facilitates shared or collaborative learning between the researcher and practitioner and between the practitioners themselves as the research progresses. As the participants are embedded in the contextual setting, they bring rich learnings to the research which contributes to deeper understandings being generated by the research. The cyclical nature of the research means that these understandings can be translated into improvements or changes during the actual research process itself. Another benefit of participatory action research is that its flexibility makes it suitable for investigating complex and evolving situations.

6.5.2 Challenges

On the other hand, participatory action research poses significant challenges. It is a complex approach, which is largely unfamiliar to academics and practitioners in pharmacy practice and health services research. It is helpful to have support from someone who has prior experience of using this approach, but this is sometimes difficult given the limited experience in the field. Several challenges relate to the partnership relationship, a critical feature of the approach. These include prior relationship between the researcher(s) and participants and knowledge of the research context, as trust between partners is critical to the initiation and long-term sustainability of the research.

Even though shared goals, processes and some timelines may have been agreed at the outset, the emergent process means that they have to be re-negotiated from time to time which can raise difficult issues. The length of time required for this type of research has implications for both the researcher and participants in terms of use of resources and for the different expectations of the research. The researchers have publications as one of their goals whilst health services participants often are most interested in quick answers. Ethical permission and funding are additional challenges for participatory action research studies.

This research approach demands particular characteristics of the researcher (and the participants) including flexibility, tenacity and patience. Writing up participatory action research for publication in peer-reviewed journals is also challenging as is presenting this type of research in a suitable format for a Master or PhD thesis report.

6.6 Roles and Competencies of District and Sub-district Pharmacists: A Case Study from Cape Town, South Africa

In Table 6.2 below, I summarise my own participatory action research study about district and sub-district pharmacists' roles in Cape Town, which I conducted as my doctoral study, and illustrate key features of the approach in the second column. The research was initiated in response to concerns of the health services manager of the two PHC organisations in Cape Town about the roles and competencies of newly appointed district and sub-district pharmacists in their organisations. My prior relationship with pharmacists and managers of both organisations contributed to the initiation of the research and facilitated maintaining the partnership over 4 years. Although it was a challenging experience, working collaboratively with the health service partners turned out to be rewarding, and significant changes in understanding and practice emerged throughout the engagement (Bradley 2013).

Table 6.2 Research illustrating key participatory action research features

Research: roles and competencies of district and sub-district pharmacists: a case study from Cape Town, South Africa	Participatory action research features
Introduction This research focused on the emergence of district and sub-district pharmacists in Cape Town by considering their roles and related competencies and the support required to establish them in these new positions. The research was carried out in partnership with Metro District Health Services (MDHS) and City Health. Both organisations provide services across the whole of the Cape Metro. The research took place as MDHS was dividing the Cape Town Metro District into four districts, and the research is embedded in these unfolding developments. The four districts were created to be closer in size to WHO health districts than the large Metro District, which was considered unmanageable. Consequently, districts and district pharmacists in this study should be considered equivalent to districts and district pharmacists in other settings	Suitable for research into evolving professional pharmacy roles Partnership between researcher and health services organisations Health organisations undergoing re-structuring and change
Methods I used a participatory action research approach to partner with pharmacists and managers in both organisations between 2008 and 2011. The partnership benefitted from the contextual and practice experiences of the health services stakeholders and from my evolving research expertise. Including a broad stakeholder group was considered important for developing the shared learning and understanding that would translate into action and change in the organisations. The flexible and emergent approach of participatory action research was considered suited to a complex health system in the midst of change	4-year engagement Benefits of collaborative learning Shared experiences bringing new understanding leading to change Complex context
Overview of cycles of action and reflection After an initiation stage, the research evolved into a series of five iterative cycles of action and reflection, each providing increasing understanding of the roles and related competencies of district and sub-district pharmacists and their experiences as they transitioned into these new management positions in the two organisations. The research centred around two series of three interactive workshops I facilitated. These were attended by both pharmacists and managers, in which I contributed information from published literature and documentary reviews. Semi-structured interviews and focus groups were conducted at various stages during the research. This was to inform conceptualization and supplement workshops. The interviews and focus groups in years three and four were useful opportunities to reflect on the experiences of district and sub-district pharmacists	Initiation stage strengthened by prior relationship between researcher and health services personnel Participatory methods and processes triangulated with other data collection methods Ongoing iterative data collection and analysis processes

(continued)

Table 6.2 (continued)

Research: roles and competencies of district and sub-district pharmacists: a case study from Cape Town, South Africa	Participatory action research features
Results and discussion The research identified five main roles each for district and sub-district pharmacists. Four of these roles are the same for each: • District [Sub-district] management, as part of the management team • Planning, co-ordination and monitoring of pharmaceuticals, human resources, budget and infrastructure • Information and advice • Quality assurance and clinical governance • But their fifth role is different: • Research, for district pharmacists. Dispensing at clinics for sub-district pharmacists	Key outcomes identified
Although the roles look similar, there were substantial differences between district and sub-district pharmacist roles in the two organisations. Their roles were shaped by the differences in leadership and governance, as well as by the services provided by the two organisations. District pharmacists were generally involved in strategic level management functions, whilst sub-district pharmacists combined sub-district management activities with dispensing in clinics. Essentially the two cadres were working at different management and leadership levels, with district pharmacists working at middle management level and sub-district pharmacists straddling first level and middle management levels.	Nuances uncovered through depth of understanding of context
Five competency clusters were also identified for both cadres, each with several competencies. • Professional pharmacy practice • Health system/public health • Management • Leadership • Personal, interpersonal and cognitive competencies	Key outcomes identified
Whilst professional pharmacy practice competencies were particularly valued by district and sub-district managers, overall, district and sub-district pharmacists required management and leadership competencies. Along with the more technical management and leadership competencies, both organisations recognised the importance of 'softer' competencies for pharmacists moving into these management positions. These softer competencies included personal and interpersonal competencies such as professionalism, relationship building and teamwork and cognitive competencies such as problem solving, decision making and communication	Full range of competencies identified and nuances between organisations

(continued)

Table 6.2 (continued)

Research: roles and competencies of district and sub-district pharmacists: a case study from Cape Town, South Africa	Participatory action research features
Transitioning into these new management positions was an emergent process, which entailed pharmacists changing from performing technical and clinical functions associated with professional pharmacy practice to co-ordinating pharmaceutical services across the district or sub-district. They moved from working in a pharmacy to being a member of a multi-professional team in a district or sub-district. Adjusting to these new management positions took time and was facilitated by several personal and organisational factors which varied in the two organisations. Mangers and pharmacists mentioned the positive contribution of the participatory action research in assisting with this transition through the development of shared understanding of the DHS and the roles and functions of pharmacists working in these management positions. This research also assisted with practical aspects including the development of new job descriptions	Length of engagement facilitated deeper understanding of pharmacists roles and competencies in emerging organisational structures Benefits of collaborative learning Integration of understanding into change
Implications and conclusions Several implications for developing competencies in district and sub-district pharmacists emerged during the research. First, although competency frameworks for district and sub-district pharmacists are useful for selecting new staff, conducting performance appraisals and identifying learning needs, the competency framework needs to be tailored for each setting. Second, a mixture of traditional training options, including academic qualifications and short courses, as well as innovative on-the-job support such as mentoring and coaching are required to support district and sub-district pharmacists and other similar cadres in these positions	Practical implications of research findings highlighted and realistic suggestions offered

References

Baum F, MacDougall C, Smith D (2006) Participatory action research. J Epidemiol Community Health 60(10):854–857. doi:10.1136/jech.2004.028662

Bless C, Higson-Smith C (2004) Fundamentals of social research methods: an African perspective, vol 3. Juta, Cape Town

Boud D, Keogh R, Walker D (1985) Reflection: turning experience into learning. Kogan Page, London

Bradley HA (2013) Roles and competencies of district pharmacists: a case study from Cape Town. University of the Western Cape. Retrieved from http://hdl.handle.net/11394/3255

Calnan M, Rowe R (2006) Researching trust relations in health care: conceptual and methodological challenges–an introduction. J Health Organ Manag 20(5):349–358

Davis E, Chandler C, Innocent S, Kalumuna C, Terlouw D et al (2012) Designing adverse event forms for real-world reporting: participatory research in Uganda. PLoS One 7(3):e32704

De Koning K, Martin M (1996) Participatory research in health: issues and experiences. Zen Books, London

Dick B, Stringer E, Huxham C (2009) Final reflections, unanswered questions. Action Res 7 (1):117–120. doi:10.1177/1476750308099601

Gilson L (2012) Health policy and systems research: a methodology reader. WHO, Geneva

Greenwood D, Levin M (1999) Introduction to action research: social research for change. Sage, London

Herr K, Anderson G (2005) The action research dissertation: a guide for students and faculty. Sage, Thousand Oaks, CA

Huang HB (2010) What is good action research. Action Res 8(1):93–109

Iles V, Sutherland K (2001) Organisational change: a review for health care managers, professionals and researchers. Service Delivery and Organisation Research and Development Programme, London

Khresheh R, Barclay L (2007) Practice-research engagement. Action Res 5(2):123–138

Laws S, Harper C, Marcus R (2003) Research for development: a practical guide. SAGE, London

Loewenson R, Flores W, Shukla A, Kagis M, Baba A, Ryklief A, Mbwili-Muleya C, Kakde D (2011) Raising the profile of participatory action research at the 2010 global symposium on health systems research. MEDICC Rev 13(3):35–38, Retrieved from http://search.ebscohost.com/login.aspx?direct=true&db=rzh&AN=2011218020&site=ehost-live

Loewenson R, Laurell AC, Hogstedt C, D'Ambruoso L, Shroff Z (2014) Participatory action research in health systems: a methods reader. EQUINET, Harare, p 336

Mann K, Gordon J, MacLeod A (2009) Reflection and reflective practice in health professions education: a systematic review. Adv Health Sci Educ 14(4):595–621

Marti J, Villasante T (2009) Quality in action research: reflections for second-order inquiry. Syst Pract Action Res 22(5):383–396

McNiff J, Whitehead J (2010) Doing and writing action research. Sage, London

Meyer J, Pope C, Mays N (2000) Using qualitative methods in health related action research. Br Med J 320(7228):178–181, Retrieved from http://search.ebscohost.com/login.aspx?direct=true&db=a9h&AN=2895217&site=ehost-live

Minkler M, Wallerstein N (eds) (2003) Community based participatory research for health. Jossey-Bass, San Francisco, CA

Reason P (2006) Choice and quality in action research practice. J Manag Inq 15(2):187–203, Retrieved from http://search.ebscohost.com/login.aspx?direct=true&db=sih&AN=21000778&site=ehost-live

Reason P, Bradbury H (2008) Concluding reflections: whither action research? In: Reason P, Bradbury H (eds) The SAGE handbook of action research, 2nd edn. SAGE, London

Reed MS (2008) Stakeholder participation for environmental management: a literature review. Biol Conserv 141(10):2417–2431

Schon D (1983) The reflective practitioner. Basic Books, New York, NY

Tanna N, Pitkin J, Anderson C (2005) Development of the specialist menopause pharmacist (SMP) role within a research framework. Pharm World Sci 27(1):61–67

Viswanathan M, Ammerman A, Eng E (2004) Community-based participatory research: assessing the evidence report/technology assessment no 99. Agency for Healthcare Research and Quality, Rockville, MD

Waterman H, Tillen D, Dickson R, de Koning K (2001) Action research: a systematic review and guidance for assessment. Health Technol Assess 5(23)

Chapter 7
Mixed Methods Research in Pharmacy Practice

Cristín Ryan, Cathal Cadogan, and Carmel Hughes

Abstract Irrespective of the field of research, the underpinning methodologies used are critical in generating high quality data and evidence. Most importantly, the method selected should answer the research question that has been posed. It is important to accept that no single method will answer all research questions, and in the field of health services and pharmacy practice research, there may be a number of questions that will form part of an overarching programme or project. In such circumstances, more than one method will be required to answer all the research questions within a single project or programme, an approach known as mixed methods.

This chapter provides an overview of the current definition of mixed methods research and the advantages and limitations of this approach. The importance of mixed methods research in pharmacy practice and the required consideration when designing and analysing a mixed methods research study or programme are outlined. The various typologies of mixed methods research using illustrative examples from the pharmacy practice research literature are described, and guidance is provided on choosing the most applicable typology for a given research question.

Keywords Mixed methods • Mixed methodology • Multi-methods • Multi-strategy • Mixed methodology • Sequential explanatory • Sequential exploratory • Concurrent design • Convergent parallel • Embedded design • Pharmacy practice

7.1 Introduction

Irrespective of the field of research, the underpinning methodologies used are critical in generating high quality data and evidence. Most importantly, the method selected should answer the research question posed (Sackett 1997). Traditionally, research studies have been designed using single method research designs. However, single method research studies often report various limitations and

C. Ryan (✉) • C. Cadogan • C. Hughes
School of Pharmacy, Queen's University Belfast, Belfast, Northern Ireland
e-mail: c.ryan@qub.ac.uk; c.cadogan@qub.ac.uk; c.hughes@qub.ac.uk

weaknesses in their study design, for example, single study designs do not consider multiple viewpoints and perspectives (Johnson et al. 2007; Driscoll et al. 2007).

Consequently, the practice of using more than one research method, or a mixed methods approach as it is more commonly termed, to answer the research question posed has become increasingly popular. This enables the expansion of the scope or breadth of research to offset the weaknesses of using any approach alone (Driscoll et al. 2007). Mixed methods research is now a recognised research paradigm in the health services and pharmacy practice research fields. This is evidenced by the publication of a dedicated journal of mixed methods research, the *Journal of Mixed Methods Research* http://mmr.sagepub.com/. This journal aims to act as an impetus for creating bridges between mixed methods researchers and to provide a platform for the discussion of mixed methods research issues and the sharing of ideas across academic disciplines (Tashakkori and Creswell 2007).

Despite the relative novelty of this approach in the health services research arena, the process of using more than one research method within a single study or a research programme has been conducted for decades in other research fields. As noted above, mixed methods research adds further insights to research questions which would otherwise not be answered if a single research approach was used. Whilst this chapter focuses on mixed methods research in pharmacy practice, a mixed methods approach may not always be appropriate. It is important to refer back to the research question posed, and to let the research question guide the study design. The selection of study design should be considered in tandem with the way in which the research question is asked, and in some instances, single study designs may be preferable. Sackett emphasises the importance of letting the research question guide the study design, stating that *'the question being asked determines the appropriate research architecture, strategy, and tactics to be used-not tradition, authority, experts, paradigms or schools of thought'* (Sackett 1997).

A variety of terms have been used to describe the mixed methods research approach including 'integrated', 'hybrid', 'combined', 'mixed research', 'mixed methodology', 'multi-methods', 'multi-strategy' and 'mixed methodology' (Bryman 2006; Johnson et al. 2007; Driscoll et al. 2007). Throughout this chapter, we will use the term 'mixed methods' to describe research approaches which use more than one research method to answer the research question posed.

This chapter provides an overview of the current definition of mixed methods research, the advantages, the limitations and the importance of this research approach in pharmacy practice. We also outline the required considerations when designing and analysing a mixed methods research study or programme, and describe the various typologies of mixed methods research. We refer to illustrative examples from the pharmacy practice research literature and provide guidance on how to choose the most applicable typology for a given research question.

We conducted a literature search to inform the content of this chapter using the following electronic databases; International Pharmaceutical Abstracts, MEDLINE and Web of Science, using the following search terms: 'mixed methods', 'pharmacy, 'triangulation', parallel design, 'embedded design' and 'sequential design'.

Searches were restricted to include only full-text papers published in English language within the last 10 years (2004–2014).

7.2 Current Definition of Mixed Methods Research

As the field of mixed methods research is still evolving, several researchers believe that the definition of mixed methods research should remain open to allow for its development and refinement, as the practice of mixed methods research grows across academic disciplines (Johnson et al. 2007). However, there is a general consensus that mixed methods research typically involves both a qualitative and a quantitative component embedded within a single study or research programme (Tashakkori and Creswell 2007; Creswell et al. 2004).

Johnson et al. (2007) approached 19 experts in the field and invited them to propose a definition of mixed methods research to ensure a common and uniform understanding of the term. They subsequently summarised their findings and proposed the following definition:

> Mixed methods research is the type of research in which a researcher or team of researchers combines elements of qualitative and quantitative research approaches (e.g. use of qualitative and quantitative viewpoints, data collection, analysis, inference techniques) for the broad purpose of breadth and depth of understanding and corroboration (Johnson 2007).

In addition, they also specified that mixed methods research is a specific programme of research: '*A mixed methods study would involve mixing within a single study; a mixed method program would involve mixing within a program of research and the mixing might occur across a closely related set of studies*' (Johnson 2007).

It is difficult to provide a step-by-step guide as to how to undertake a mixed methods study. It will be driven by the research question, and therefore, the most appropriate methods should be selected in order to achieve this. However, broadly, consideration should be given to the precise type of quantitative and qualitative methods to be employed, what order data collection should be undertaken, the types of data collection tools to be used and methods of analysis.

Mixed methods research is therefore a synthesis that can include findings from both qualitative and quantitative research and, importantly, the integration of the findings from each research strand. Integration refers to the interaction between the different research strands (Ó Catháin et al. 2010). We outline an approach to integrating findings from different strands of research at the end of this chapter.

7.2.1 Advantages of Mixed Methods Research

The use of a mixed methods approach to research is especially useful in understanding contradictions between quantitative results and qualitative findings. For example, within a large research programme on prescribing errors, junior doctors rated their level of confidence in a variety of prescribing-related tasks, e.g. selecting the most appropriate dose, as very high, overall, in a questionnaire study (Ryan et al. 2013), despite prior indication that they were responsible for a large proportion of prescribing errors identified in a related prevalence study (Ryan et al. 2014). To explore this contradiction and to examine the disparity between doctors' perceived level of confidence and the fact that prescribing errors were often made during the study period, analysis of the qualitative work revealed that doctors were not always made aware of their errors. Prescribing charts were often amended by other prescribers, without providing feedback to the original prescriber (Ross et al. 2012).

Mixed methods approach allows participants' point of view to be reflected, provides methodological flexibility and encourages multi-disciplinary team working. For example, a research study conducted to evaluate the extension of prescribing rights to pharmacists consisted of a number of linked phases, which were qualitative and quantitative in nature (McCann et al. 2011, 2012a, b). The research team consisted of pharmacists, a general practitioner (GP) and an economist. This mix of disciplines contributed to a more holistic overview of the research topic and ensured that the research objectives would be met. The study phases consisted of a cross-sectional questionnaire which was completed by qualified prescribing pharmacists (McCann et al. 2011). The questionnaire provided the quantitative baseline and background data that were explored in subsequent qualitative phases (McCann et al. 2012a, b). Pharmacists, physicians and other health-care professionals with a vested interest in prescribing participated in interviews which revealed the advantages and disadvantages of prescribing in greater depth than would have been gleaned from a quantitative questionnaire alone (McCann et al. 2012a). However, further qualitative work with patients, via focus groups, who had experienced prescribing by a pharmacist was even more revealing (McCann et al. 2012b). Patients not only recognised the importance of pharmacist input but also cited limitations to this new model of care, particularly pharmacists' focus on one medical condition at a time. This issue had been highlighted in much of the pharmacist prescribing literature before, but never from the perspective of patients. Using these various methodologies within one study enabled a more comprehensive and deeper understanding of how pharmacist prescribing had evolved and provided evidence for policy makers as to how this model of care could be extended into more mainstream practice.

7.2.2 Disadvantages of Mixed Methods Research

Mixed methods approaches to research are labour-intensive and require a broader range of research expertise across a multidisciplinary team than those needed to conduct a single method study. Mixed methods studies are complex to plan and conduct and can pose challenges in ensuring methodological rigour of individual study components. Furthermore, the integration of data from a number of different sources can be challenging and complex as detailed below.

7.3 Mixed Methods Research in Pharmacy Practice

The use of mixed methods research in pharmacy practice research has been fuelled by a transition in the focus of health services research from a practitioner-centred approach to more of a patient-centred approach. For example, this has been highlighted by research into the development of community pharmacy-based interventions targeting alcohol use. Early work did not report any patient involvement during intervention development (Fitzgerald et al. 2008). However, a recent study by Krska and Mackridge (2014) describes the use of a mixed methods approach using telephone interviews with key stakeholders and survey data with patients/public to develop their intervention. Additionally, in intervention and implementation research, there is an increasing drive for theoretically derived evidence to inform the development of interventions with a growing emphasis on the science underpinning intervention development. This is illustrated by the United Kingdom's (UK) Medical Research Council's (MRC) influential guidance on the development of complex interventions (Medical Research Council 2008), which is increasingly being used in the design of pharmacy practice interventions (Fig.7.1).

This has been adopted by pharmacy practice researchers as health-care interventions are, in general, complex (utilising several components, rather than a single active 'ingredient') and involve a variety of health-care professionals. Furthermore, as pharmacy practice interventions are often targeted at individual patients, effective interventions need to be tailored to these individuals accordingly.

Each phase of the MRC framework requires the application of different research methods. For example, in order to develop an intervention to improve medication adherence, researchers should firstly identify the extent of the problem of non-adherence (e.g. by quantifying the level of non-adherence) in the Development component, and then identify an appropriate theoretical basis to underpin the development of the intervention. In the Feasibility/Piloting component, the MRC recommends that retention, recruitment and sample size should be estimated (quantitative methods), and intervention procedures should be tested (quantitative and/or qualitative methods). This highlights the important role of mixed methods research in pharmacy practice intervention design as the research question could not be addressed using one method alone.

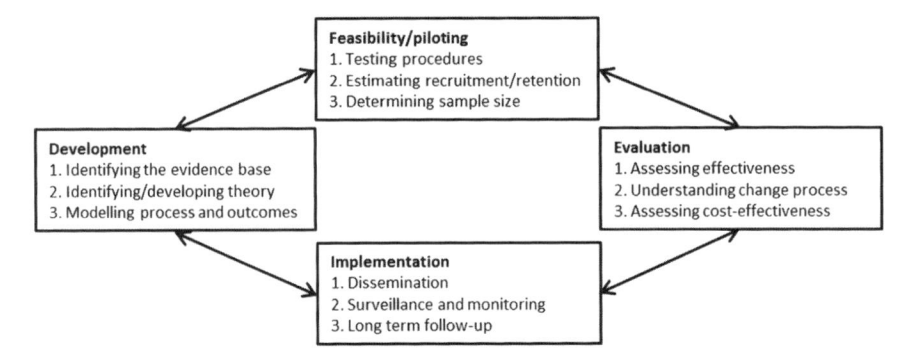

Fig. 7.1 MRC framework for the development of a complex intervention

In order to assess the effectiveness of an intervention, specific outcome measures need to be compared before and after the intervention, e.g. the level of adherence (quantitative) as part of the Evaluation component. For the change processes to be identified and understood, i.e. those mechanisms which led to changes in adherence, qualitative methods should primarily be employed to seek participants' views and experiences of the intervention. Finally, an assessment of cost-effectiveness would be quantitative in nature.

The final component of the framework (Implementation) which comprises monitoring, surveillance and long-term follow up of the intervention, qualitative and quantitative methods can be used either alone or in combination, but the chosen methods are largely dependent on the intervention being tested and the outcomes of interest. As conveyed by Fig.7.1, these various phases are not necessarily constrained by a rigid sequence, but can be iterative in nature. This type of framework is ideal for the application of mixed methods.

7.4 Typologies of Mixed Methods Research

As stated previously, the choice of research methodology to adopt for a given study depends entirely on the research question. Within mixed methods research, there are a variety of categories, otherwise known as typologies, which help to formalise the approach taken and which add rigour to research projects (Bryman 2006). There are a number of classification matrices by which mixed methods research designs are described, with no one method having superiority over the other (Driscoll et al. 2007). However, each classification suggests that the factors below should be considered when deciding on the typology to use (Bryman 2006; Driscoll et al. 2007; Ó Catháin et al. 2010; Hadi et al. 2013):

- Order of data collection: Are the qualitative and quantitative data collected independently or sequentially?
- Priority: Which type of data has priority, i.e. quantitative or qualitative data?

- Integration: What is the purpose of integration, e.g. triangulation (combining the findings from a mixed methods approach) (See Sect.7.5)?
- Number of data strands: How many constituent research components are involved?

The following section will describe four of the most common mixed methods typologies used in pharmacy practice research (*concurrent design, explanatory sequential design, exploratory sequential design and the embedded design*), with examples of studies that have used these approaches. Advantages and disadvantages of each approach will also be noted.

7.4.1 Concurrent Design

The 'concurrent mixed methods' design describes an approach whereby both qualitative and quantitative data are collected concurrently, in separate, but related studies. This typology is also referred to as the 'convergent parallel design', 'current triangulation', 'simultaneous triangulation' and 'parallel study' (Hadi et al. 2013). Each study is given equal priority, findings are integrated only at the interpretation stage, i.e. studies are seen as separate entities during both data collection and analysis. This approach is useful for validating qualitative data with quantitative data and vice versa. This design facilitates the development of an overall understanding of the research question. For example, Ryan and colleagues used this study design type in the research programme on prescribing errors previously referred to. Whilst there were several components to this research programme, an observational prevalence study (Ryan et al. 2014) and a semi-structured interview study with junior doctors (Ross et al. 2013) were conducted concurrently. Each study was analysed separately, but data were interpreted together. The interview study offered some explanations as to why various types of errors identified in the prevalence study occurred. For example, the prevalence study revealed that errors of omission (i.e. drugs not being prescribed) at admission to hospital were one of the commonest types of errors encountered (Ryan et al. 2014). Findings from the semi-structured interviews somewhat explained these errors, in that interviewees noted difficulties in accessing prescribing information from primary care at the point of patient admission.

7.4.2 Sequential Design

Sequential design studies involve the collection of data on an iterative basis, i.e. data collected in one phase contributes to the data collection in the next phase (Driscoll et al. 2007). Subsequent phases provide more detailed data on findings from earlier phases and can help to generalise findings by verifying and augmenting study results. Sequential design studies can be either **explanatory** or **exploratory** (Hadi et al. 2013). In **explanatory** sequential design studies, the first phase consists of quantitative data collection, and this is followed by a qualitative study, the aim of which is to explain the findings from the quantitative study. The collection of quantitative data first allows application of statistical methods to determine which findings to augment in the next phase (Driscoll et al. 2007). For example, in the first phase of a study investigating prescribing errors in Scottish hospitals, the researchers defined the prevalence of prescribing errors and in the second phase, the researchers conducted semi-structured interviews with prescribers to determine the causes and under what circumstances the prescribing errors identified in phase one occurred (Ryan et al. 2014). At study completion, i.e. at the end of the qualitative study, data were triangulated to provide a wider understanding of the occurrence of prescribing errors.

Ramsay and colleagues (2014) used a mixed methods approach to evaluate the effects of a ward-level medication safety scorecard to influence medication safety and the factors that influenced the use of the scorecard. A mixed methods approach was used to gain an understanding of how and why the intervention influenced staff behaviour and whether there were any unintended consequences and which factors were influential (Ramsay et al. 2014). The quantitative component (a controlled before and after study) assessed the performance of this safety scorecard, while the qualitative component involved interviews with hospital staff exploring governance of medication safety, experiences of scorecard feedback and explored implementation issues. Each component, i.e. the qualitative and quantitative aspects, was analysed separately in the first instance and the findings were then triangulated. Using this methodological approach allowed for the evaluation of the efficacy of the score card, as well as considerations of contextual factors that might influence the implementation of this patient safety initiative (Ramsay et al. 2014).

Similarly, **exploratory** sequential design studies also consist of two distinct phases. The first phase consists of a qualitative study, to explore the research question in depth. Based on analysis of the qualitative data, a quantitative study is then developed to test the findings. For example, a semi-structured interview approach is currently being used to investigate health-care professionals' views of and attitudes towards medicines management in intermediate care facilities. Based on these findings, a quantitative study will be designed, to further explore medicines management issues, e.g. prescribing quality, in these facilities. This stepwise approach facilitates a logical elucidation of the main issues and challenges which are faced by those who work in these types of facilities. An interpretation of quantitative findings without an understanding of the contextual factors may lead to invalid or biased conclusions.

Adopting a sequential design approach allows researchers to investigate emergent and unexpected themes in more detail. However, this approach can be time consuming.

7.4.3 The Embedded Design

The embedded design consists of both a qualitative and a quantitative phase. However, in contrast to the previously mentioned typologies, in the embedded design, one research method is designated as the key method, and the other component of the research adopts a supportive role. In essence, whilst the qualitative and quantitative components of the research study are based on the same broad topic, each research component in the embedded design answers a different research question. This design is often used in randomised controlled trials, where the quantitative component of the research study is the main focus (key role) in terms of intervention outcomes. However, the qualitative components (supportive role) can provide important process evaluation information in terms of issues such as implementation. The qualitative component of the research project can be incorporated into the study at any time point, e.g. at the beginning to help in the design of the intervention, during the intervention to explore participants' experiences or after the intervention to help to explain results. This is illustrated by a study which evaluated the impact of a pharmaceutical care model regarding the prescribing of psychoactive medications in older nursing home residents (Patterson et al. 2010). The original model of care (described as the Fleetwood model) had been developed in the United States (US) by the American Society of Consultant Pharmacists for application by pharmacists in the US nursing home context (Cameron et al. 2002). However, as the model of care in US nursing homes is very different to the rest of the world, this care model required adaptation before it could be used in non-US nursing homes. Thus, a qualitative study was undertaken in Northern Ireland to allow this adaptation to take place (Patterson et al. 2007). Semi-structured interviews or focus groups were held with GPs, nursing home managers, pharmacists and advocates of older people. The American Fleetwood model was explained to all participants who were then asked for their views and opinions on how such a model could be adapted for use in the UK setting. Participants recognised that for such a model of care to work outside of the US, consideration would need to be given as to how pharmacists would access medical records, prescribers and nursing home residents in order to implement this care model to its full potential. The resultant changes to the model enabled it to be successfully employed in 22 nursing homes as part of a randomised trial. Indeed, the adapted model of care proved to be effective and cost-effective (Patterson et al. 2010, 2011) and has since been rolled out in nursing homes across Northern Ireland.

7.5 Integrating Findings in Mixed Methods Research

Mixed methods research does not simply involve the collection of qualitative and quantitative data; integration of findings is a central part of mixed methods research. As previously noted, integration refers to the interaction between the different research strands, and this can be achieved through the triangulation of data (Ó Catháin et al. 2010).

Triangulation was initially conceptualised as a means of validating findings but the focus has since changed and triangulation is increasingly seen as a means of enriching and completing knowledge (Flick 2009). Triangulation has been described as a process of using different methods to study a problem in order to gain a more complete picture (Ó Catháin et al. 2010). This can involve the combination of multiple qualitative methods or the combination of qualitative and quantitative methods (Flick et al. 2012). Through the use of different research methods, triangulation seeks to exploit the strengths and neutralise the limitations that are inherent to each method (Jick 1979). In mixed methods research, integration can occur at different levels of the research process, e.g. study design, methods, interpretation and reporting (Fetters et al. 2013). In this chapter, we focus on the integration of findings at the level of interpretation using a triangulation-based approach, once each dataset has been analysed separately, as is a common practice in mixed methods health-care studies (Östlund et al. 2011).

Triangulation looks to explore convergence, complementarity and dissonance between the findings of each method (Farmer et al. 2006). Convergence and dissonance refer to the extent to which findings from each method agree or disagree, respectively. Complementarity occurs where findings from different methods provide complementary information on the same issue. The triangulation of data from different methods offers important advantages in that it can generate richer data, uncover unexpected findings that can provide opportunity for enriching explanations and ultimately increase confidence in research findings (Jick 1979).

Triangulation has been classified into four different types (Denzin 1989): methodological triangulation (use of different research methods or data collection techniques), theory triangulation (use of different theoretical perspectives), data triangulation (use of multiple data sources or groups of research participants) and investigator triangulation (use of multiple researchers in data analysis). However, various authors have noted that little guidance has been provided to date on performing triangulation (Jick 1979; Morgan 1998; Östlund et al. 2011). Given the range of typologies in mixed methods research, as detailed earlier in this chapter, there is no single approach to triangulation that can be applied to all mixed methods research. However, as outlined in Farmer's triangulation protocol, there are a number of basic steps that can be followed in order to provide methodological transparency where triangulation is used in any given research context (Farmer et al. 2006). This triangulation protocol is considered to provide the most detailed account of how to triangulate data and is applicable to mixed methods in health research (Ó Catháin et al. 2010).

The triangulation of data within mixed methods research requires decisions about the weighting given to each dataset. As noted by Jick (1979), in the absence of guidelines for systematically ordering data decisions regarding the weighting of different study components, decisions are likely to be subjective. Farmer et al. (2006) propose that decisions about weighting should be based on the contribution of the different components to the research question.

The use of a triangulation protocol can help to improve the quality and reporting of mixed methods research and to address deficiencies that have been identified in the existing mixed methods literature relating to pharmacy practice (Hadi et al. 2014), as well as the wider health-care literature (Östlund et al. 2011). The application of the triangulation protocol is exemplified below by reference to a current, ongoing research project to develop an intervention to improve appropriate polypharmacy in older patients in primary care.

7.5.1 Case Study: Application of a Triangulation Protocol in a Mixed Methods Project with a Sequential Design

The triangulation protocol outlined below was adapted from the work of Farmer et al. (2006) and developed as part of an ongoing mixed methods research project seeking to develop an intervention to improve appropriate polypharmacy in older patients in primary care. The project has several phases, consisting of a Cochrane systematic review (Patterson et al. 2014), semi-structured interviews of health-care professionals (general practitioners, community pharmacists) and patient focus groups. Triangulation will be based on the completed analysis of interview and focus group data. The topic guide for each qualitative component of the project (interviews and focus groups) will be based primarily on an established framework which consists of 12 theoretical domains relevant to changing health-care professionals' behaviour (Michie et al. 2005). The findings of the Cochrane review will also be used to inform part of the topic guides. The main aim of the analysis is to identify the principal barriers and facilitators to changing target behaviours in health-care professionals, namely, prescribing and dispensing, in order to achieve the desired outcome (i.e. appropriate polypharmacy) through integration of the findings from each dataset. This will allow for different perspectives on the same research question. An established taxonomy of behaviour change techniques (Michie et al. 2013) will then be used to target these domains and elicit desired changes in target behaviours. Intervention delivery and related outcome assessments will be informed by the findings of the updated Cochrane review.

Prior to triangulation, each qualitative dataset will be independently analysed by two researchers using the framework method (Ritchie and Spencer 1994). Qualitative analysis of each dataset will follow a deductive approach, and the theoretical framework (Michie et al. 2005) used to develop the topic guides will be served as a coding framework. The subsequent paragraphs relate to the triangulation of the findings from each dataset.

Triangulation will involve multiple investigator triangulation, methodological triangulation and data source triangulation. As a single theoretical framework is being used to analyse the individual datasets, theoretical triangulation will not be conducted and integration of the datasets will focus on the prominence of the framework domains (themes) across the datasets. Although the intervention will target health-care professionals, it will also need to be beneficial to patients. Thus, the findings from each dataset (health-care professionals and patients) will be weighted equally.

1. **Sorting**: Findings from each dataset will be reviewed in order to identify key domains within the theoretical framework that need to be targeted as part of the intervention. A convergence coding matrix will be developed to compare the presence, frequency and examples of domains across the datasets. This will allow differences and similarities between datasets to be summarised.
2. **Convergence coding**: The convergence coding matrix will be applied to determine convergence of findings across the datasets on two levels: first, in terms of the prominence of domains and, second, in terms of the convergence of coverage (i.e. level of agreement/disagreement across the datasets) and examples for each domain. Convergence will be characterised using predefined criteria according to the degree and type of convergence. For example, where there is full agreement between the findings on both of the above levels of comparison (i.e. prominence and coverage), this will be characterised as 'agreement'. The criteria will also cover cases where one dataset covers the domain or example but others do not (silence) and cases where there is disagreement across the individual datasets (dissonance).
3. **Convergence assessment**: All comparisons across the datasets will be reviewed to provide a comprehensive assessment of the level of convergence. Any cases where researchers' views on convergence or dissonance differ will be documented.
4. **Completeness assessment**: Findings from the datasets will be compared to create an overarching summary of the findings highlighting both unique and similar contributions to the research question. In the context of this research project, the patients' perspectives will help to broaden the range of findings relevant to the research question. For example, patients may highlight additional barriers to, or facilitators of, the prescribing and/or dispensing of appropriate polypharmacy which may not have been raised by health-care professionals.
5. **Researcher comparison**: Formal assessments will be used to compare the level of agreement between the researchers in terms of the degree of convergence across the datasets. Any disagreements will be resolved by consensus through discussion with another researcher.
6. **Feedback**: Triangulated results will be presented to the other members of the research team for discussion. A consensus-based approach will be used within the team to agree on the specific domains of the theoretical framework that should be targeted as part of the intervention.

This thorough and painstaking process is expected to yield rich and informative results which will highlight multiple perspectives on an important issue within primary care, i.e. polypharmacy. A single focus on a single constituency, e.g. GPs, would have provided a narrow and limited view. Any subsequent intervention development would have considered only this single view, and the resultant intervention may have little impact on important outcomes. Researchers should be aware that adopting this kind of triangulation protocol will be time consuming, but the findings in subsequent types of phases of research should be much more meaningful.

7.6 Conclusion

Using a variety of methods to answer a research question can add further context and explanations to findings and interpretations. We have outlined a variety of mixed methods typologies that are used in pharmacy practice research. It is important to note there is no preferred typology that pharmacy practice researchers should adopt. Instead, researchers should ensure that the methodological approach chosen in a study is suitable for the research question posed. The growing recognition of the contribution of mixed methods to pharmacy practice research should ensure that studies are addressing key research questions in a comprehensive and meaningful way.

References

Bryman A (2006) Integrating quantitative and qualitative research: how is it done? Qual Res 6:97–113

Cameron K, Feinberg JL, Lapane KL (2002) Fleetwood project Phase III moves forward. Consult Pharm 17:181–198

Creswell JW, Fetters MD, Ivankova NV (2004) Designing a mixed methods study in primary care. Ann Fam Med 2:7–11

Denzin NK (1989) The research act: a theoretical introduction to sociological methods. Prentice Hall, Englewood Cliffs, NJ, ISBN 10: 0137743815; ISBN 13: 9780137743810

Driscoll DL, Appiah-Yeboah A, Salib P, Rupter DJ (2007) Merging qualitative and quantitative data in mixed methods research: how to and why not. Ecol Environ Anthropol 3:19–27

Farmer T, Robinson K, Elliott SJ, Eyles J (2006) Developing and implementing a triangulation protocol for qualitative health research. Qual Health Res 16:377–394

Fetters MD, Curry LA, Creswell JW (2013) Achieving integration in mixed methods designs–principles and practices. Health Serv Res 48:2134–2156

Fitzgerald N, McCaig DJ, Watson H, Thomson D, Stewart DC (2008) Development, implementation and evaluation of a pilot project to deliver interventions on alcohol issues in community pharmacies. Int J Pharm Pract 16:17–22

Flick U (2009) Qualitative research at work II: triangulation. In: Flick U (ed) An introduction to qualitative research, 4th edn. Sage, London

Flick U, Garms-Homolova V, Herrmann WJ, Kuck J, Rohnsch G (2012) "I can't prescribe something just because someone asks for it...": using mixed methods in the framework of triangulation. J Mixed Methods Res 6:97–110

Hadi MA, Alldred DP, Closs SJ, Briggs M (2013) Mixed-methods research in pharmacy practice: basics and beyond (part 1). Int J Pharm Pract 21:341–345

Hadi MA, Alldred DP, Closs SJ, Briggs M (2014) Mixed-methods research in pharmacy practice: recommendations for quality reporting (part 2). Int J Pharm Pract 22:96–100

Jick TD (1979) Mixing qualitative and quantitative methods: triangulation in action. Adm Sci Q 24:602–611

Johnson RB, Onwuegbuzie AJ, Turner LA (2007) Towards a definition of mixed methods research. J Mix Methods Res 1(2):112–133. doi:10.1177/1558689806298224

Krska J, Mackridge AJ (2014) Involving the public and other stakeholders in development and evaluation of a community pharmacy alcohol screening and brief advice service. Public Health 128:309–316

McCann L, Haughey S, Parsons C, Lloyd F, Crealey G, Gormley G, Hughes CM (2011) Pharmacist prescribing in Northern Ireland–a quantitative assessment. Int J Clin Pharm 33:824–831

McCann L, Haughey S, Parsons C, Lloyd F, Crealey G, Gormley G, Hughes CM (2012a) "They come with multiple morbidities" – a qualitative assessment of pharmacist prescribing. J Interprof Care 26:127–133

McCann L, Haughey S, Parsons C, Lloyd F, Crealey G, Gormley G, Hughes C (2012b) A patient perspective of pharmacist prescribing: "crossing the specialisms-crossing the illnesses". Health Expect. doi:10.1111/jgs.12101

Medical Research Council (2008) Developing and evaluating complex interventions: new guidance http://www.mrc.ac.uk/documents/pdf/complex-interventions-guidance/

Michie S, Johnston M, Abraham C, Lawton R, Parker D, Walker A (2005) Making psychological theory useful for implementing evidence based practice: a consensus approach. Qual Saf Health Care 14:26–33

Michie S, Richardson M, Johnston M, Abraham C, Francis J, Hardeman W, Wood C (2013) The behavior change technique taxonomy (v1) of 93 hierarchically clustered techniques: building an international consensus for the reporting of behavior change interventions. Ann Behav Med 46:81–95

Morgan DL (1998) Practical strategies for combining qualitative and quantitative methods: applications to health research. Qual Health Res 8:362–376

Ó Catháin AO, Murphy E, Nicholl J (2010) Three techniques for integrating data in mixed methods studies. BMJ 341:1147–1150

Östlund U, Kidd L, Wengström Y, Rowa-Dewar N (2011) Combining qualitative and quantitative research within mixed method research designs: a methodological review. Int J Nurs Stud 48:369–383

Patterson SM, Hughes CM, Lapane KL (2007) Assessment of a United States pharmaceutical care model for nursing homes in the United Kingdom. Pharm World Sci 29:517–525

Patterson SM, Hughes CM, Crealey G, Cardwell C, Lapane K (2010) An evaluation of an adapted United States model of pharmaceutical care to improve psychoactive prescribing for nursing home residents in Northern Ireland (Fleetwood NI Study). J Am Geriatr Soc 58:44–53

Patterson SM, Hughes CM, Cardwell C, Lapane K, Murray AM, Crealey GE (2011) An evaluation of an adapted United States model of pharmaceutical care for nursing home residents in Northern Ireland (Fleetwood NI Study): a cost-effectiveness analysis. J Am Geriatr Soc 59:586–593

Patterson SM, Cadogan CA, Kerse N, Cardwell CR, Bradley MC, Ryan C, Hughes C (2014) Interventions to improve the appropriate use of polypharmacy for older people. Cochrane Database Syst Rev (10):CD008165

Ramsay AIG, Turner S, Cavell G, Oborne CA, Thomas RW, Cookson G, Fulop NJ (2014) Governing patient safety: lessons learned from a mixed methods evaluation of implementing a ward level medication safety scorecard in two English NHS hospitals. BMJ Qual Saf 23:136–146

Ritchie J, Spencer L (1994) Qualitative data analysis for applied policy research. In: Bryman A, Burgess TG (eds) Analyzing qualitative data. Routledge, London

Ross S, Hamilton L, Ryan C, Bond C (2012) Who makes prescribing decisions in hospital inpatients? An observational study. Postgrad Med J 88:507–510

Ross S, Ryan C, Duncan EM, Francis JJ, Johnston M, Ker JS, Lee AJ, Macleod MJ, Maxwell S, McKay G, Mclay J, Webb D (2013) Perceived causes of prescribing errors by junior doctors in hospital inpatients: a study from the PROTECT programme. BMJ Qual Saf 22:97–102

Ryan C, Ross S, Davey P, Duncan E, Fielding S, Francis JJ, Johnston M, Ker J, Lee AJ, MacLeod MJ, Maxwell S, McKay G, McLay J, Webb D, Bond C (2013) Junior doctors' perceptions of prescribing errors: rates, causes and self-efficacy. Br J Clin Pharmacol 76:980–987

Ryan C, Ross S, Davey P, Duncan EM, Francis JJ, Fielding S, Johnston M, Ker J, Lee AJ, MacLeod MY, Maxwell S, McKay G, McLay JS, Webb DJ, Bond C (2014) Prevalence and causes of prescribing errors: the Prescribing Outcomes for Trainee Doctors Engaged in Clinical Training (PROTECT) study. PLoS One 9(1):e79802. doi:10.1371/journal.pone.0079802

Sackett DL (1997) Choosing the best research design for each question. BMJ 315:1636. http://dx.doi.org/10.1136/bmj.315.7123.1636

Tashakkori A, Creswell JW (2007) Editorial: The new era of mixed methods. J Mixed Method 1:3–7

Chapter 8
Applying Organisational Theory in Pharmacy Practice Research

Shane Scahill

Abstract This chapter introduces the most common organisational theories that could be applied by pharmacy practice researchers. These theories can be useful for framing questions and guiding research in three distinct but overlapping domains: individual (micro-level), organisational (meso-level) and environmental (macro-level). In general, pharmacy practice researchers have not made full use of the potential of management theory. Pharmacists work within organisations that are undergoing significant environmental change. Taking a systematic approach means that a well-founded yet broad research agenda that is underpinned by organisational theory can be developed. The process of theory building and testing is also outlined in this chapter. Theory building is not as simple as people are led to believe, and there can be significant anguish in making sense of large volumes of complex dialogue. The bulk of the chapter addresses the nature of theory building and testing and provides methodological considerations for those brave enough to indulge themselves in this process.

Keywords Pharmacy practice research • Theory building • Theory development • Theory testing • Ontology • Epistemology

8.1 Introduction

This chapter introduces the most common organisational theories and the process of theory building and testing. The established theories that can be applied to pharmacy practice research are in three distinct but overlapping domains: individual (micro-level), organisational (meso-level) and environmental (macro-level). The original idea for this chapter came to me via three main realisations. The first is that theory building is not as simple as people are led to believe. There was significant anguish in making sense of my large data set as I went through a process myself to develop a theory for my PhD thesis (Scahill 2012). This seems to be commonplace

S. Scahill (✉)
School of Management, Massey Business School, Massey University, Albany, Auckland, New Zealand
e-mail: s.scahill@massey.ac.nz

and is part and parcel of the theory development process. The fact that the process engages three levels (micro, meso, macro) makes it all the more challenging.

The second realisation is that, in general, pharmacy practice researchers have not made full use of the potential when applying management theory. Pharmacists work within organisations, and there is significant potential in developing a research agenda underpinned by management theory that will have implications for policy and practice. The third realisation that underpins this chapter is the notion that positivism seems to pervade over all else in the world of pharmacy. Trying to break through this positivist stronghold to publish subjectivist research can seem daunting. Pharmacy practice researchers whose epistemological bent lies at the subjective end of the research spectrum require all the support they can get.

It is expected that this chapter will help to address the challenges the research sector faces by providing a way forward and some tools for our more subjectively oriented colleagues. This chapter is structured to include a brief description of the levels of theory and a succinct summary of the tenets of each of the main theories within the levels. The bulk of the chapter, though, addresses the nature of theory building and testing and provides methodological considerations for those brave enough to indulge themselves in this process.

8.2 Levels of Organisational Theory

Theory can be applied to research within pharmacy practice at multiple levels (Fig. 8.1), and the following section provides an overview of these.

8.2.1 Micro

Micro-level theories consider **individuals** sitting within their organisations and/or environment. The theories vary considerably not only in terms of their theoretical underpinnings and construction, but also the extent to which they have been applied to pharmacy practice research (Table 8.1).

8.2.1.1 Social Cognitive Theory

Social cognitive theory is one of the more commonly applied (to pharmacy research) micro-level management theories. Studies of moral disengagement by pharmacists and pharmacists' provision of information to Spanish-speaking patients have been undertaken by the Wisconsin group (Lee et al. 2014; Young et al. 2014).Theoretical positions have also been published about hospital pharmacists and behaviour change related to their doctor colleagues (Mutavdzic 2010). Widening the construct to include self-efficacy (which is founded on social

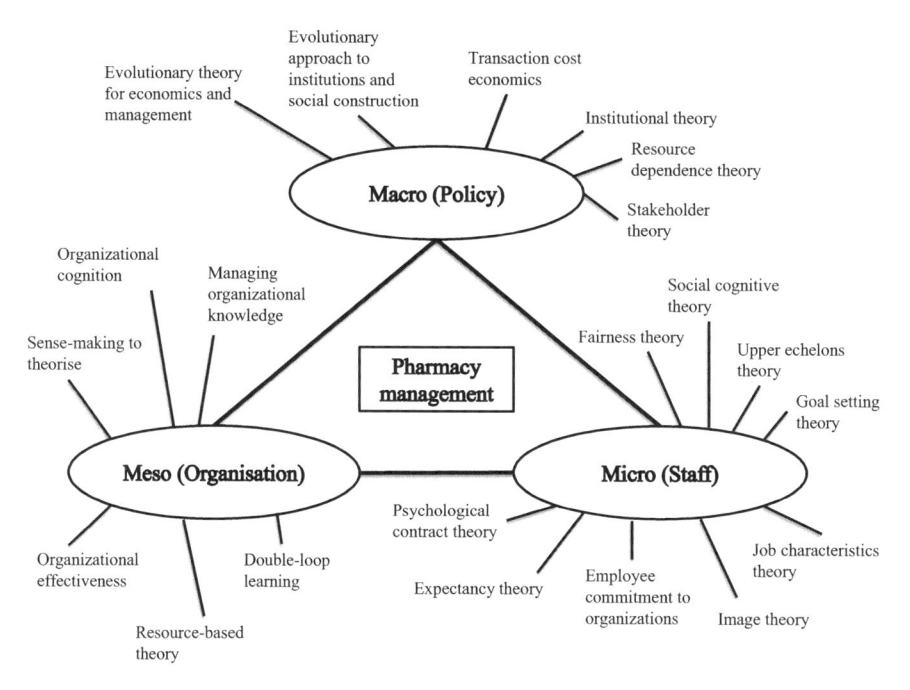

Fig. 8.1 Micro-, meso-, macro-level theories. *Source*: Smith and Hitt (2005)

cognitive theory) highlights work undertaken in pharmacy student patient counselling (Rogers and King 2012), pharmacist communication with Spanish-speaking peoples (Young et al. 2014), pharmacists performing medicines therapy management (Johnson 1996), intention and behaviour in service provision (Farris and Schopflocher 1999) and pharmacy curriculum evaluation and pharmacist preceptor teaching of drug therapy assessment (Metzger et al. 2010).

8.2.1.2 Goal Setting

At the individual level, goal setting has been applied within the community pharmacy context; specifically, collaborative decision-making between patient and pharmacist for the self-management of asthma (Smith et al. 2005). Linked to goal setting is consumer satisfaction. Goals are, at the same time, outcomes to attain but also standards for judging individual accomplishments, and it seems likely that people are more satisfied when they attain goals or make progress towards them. Structural equation modelling (SEM) has been used to understand factors associated with pharmacy technician job satisfaction in relation to goals set (Desselle and Holmes 2007). The role of non-clinician pharmacy assistants (versus pharmacists) in a goal-setting model for management of allergic rhinitis in community pharmacy has been explored (Smith et al. 2011). This study is interesting in that it straddles 'levels of work' within the organisation and highlights the fact that with training,

Table 8.1 Micro-level individual theories

Theory	Tenets	Lead academic(s)
Social cognitive theory	Agentic perspective to self-development, adaptation and change. People are self-organising, proactive, self-regulating and self-reflecting. Intentionality prevails	Albert Bandura
Upper echelons theory	The central idea is that executives act on the basis of their highly personalised interpretations of the situations and opinions they face—experiences, personalities and values shape their behaviour. This behaviour influences strategy and the way they influence others	Donald Hambrick
Active approaches to work	Personal initiative (PI) of employees with self-starting work behaviour; being proactive and overcoming difficulties; being persistent. These aspects reinforce each other, and PI is not always welcomed by supervisors or colleagues in the short term, but is crucial for long-term organisational health and survival	Michael Frese
Goal-setting theory	Goal directedness is an essential attribute of human action and conscious self-regulation of action, though volitional, is the norm. Performance goals lead to the highest level of performance when they are both clear (specific) and difficult. Goals have been found to affect performance at the individual, group, organisational unit and organisational levels	Edwin Locke, Gary Latham
Fairness theory	Roots in justice and equality literatures. Stresses the theme of moral accountability—could (what could have occurred), should (what should have occurred), would (how it would have felt had an alternative action been taken)	Robert Folger
Job characteristics theory	Explains how properties of the organisational tasks people perform affect their work attitudes and behaviour. Helps to identify the conditions under which these effects are likely to be strongest. Informs strategies for redesigning or enriching the properties of jobs intended to enhance both jobholders' performance and their own well-being	Greg Oldham, Richard Hackman
Image theory	The decision-maker is an individual acting alone. This theory does not regard groups or organisations as capable of making decisions per se; they are simply contexts within which individual member decisions become consolidated. The individual	Lee Beach and Terence Mitchell

(continued)

Table 8.1 (continued)

Theory	Tenets	Lead academic(s)
	makes up their own mind, which might change when presented to others. Each decision-maker possesses values that define how things should be and how people ought to behave	
Employee commitment to organisations theory	The relative strength of an individual's identification with, and involvement in, a particular organisation. Characterised by strong belief in goals and values, willingness to exert considerable effort, strong desire to maintain membership in the organisation. Job performance, employee turnover, employee absenteeism and extra-role behaviour are variables influenced by organisational commitment	Lyman Porter, Richard Steers, Richard Mowday, Barry Staw
Psychological contract theory	Comprises the beliefs an individual holds regarding an exchange agreement to which he or she is party, typically between an individual and an employer. The belief is that an agreement exists that is mutual, with a common understanding that binds each party to a particular course of action	Denise Rousseau
Expectancy theory	Underpinned by why people choose the kinds of work they do, the satisfaction that they derive from that work and the quality of their work performance. It has almost exclusively been applied to behaviour work through its initial connection with work and motivation	Victor Vroom

Source: Adapted from Smith and Hitt (2005)

pharmacy assistants can effectively deliver interventions that improve patient self-efficacy and quality of life.

8.2.1.3 Employee Commitment

Commitment is underpinned by strong beliefs and values and the desire to exert considerable effort (Campbell et al. 2013; Perkins et al. 2008). Career and organisational commitment are reasonably well covered in the pharmacy practice literature (Conklin and Desselle 2007; Desselle 2005; Desselle and Holmes 2007; Fink et al. 1989; Kong 1995). The main thrust is that job performance (and therefore organisational effectiveness) is influenced by employees' commitment to their organisation (Gaither 1999; Gaither et al. 2008; Gaither and Nadkarni 2012). What does stand out is the empiric nature by which the employee commitment construct has been studied. Fink and colleagues (1989) have investigated gender differences and commitment to the pharmacy profession by pharmacists. This is an important area because the demographics of the modern-day pharmacist are changing to include more diverse ethnicities and a greater proportion of females (Bissell and Morgall Traulsen 2005).

Job satisfaction and organisational commitment was found to directly affect job turnover intention in US-based studies (Gaither 1999; Gaither et al. 2008). In a later study Gaither and Nadkarni (2012) frame a jobs–demand–resources model with employee commitment as the outcome and explore the interplay for hospital pharmacists between levels of demand of the job and interactions with other healthcare professionals (Gaither and Nadkarni 2012). In Australia, White and Klinner (2012) have taken an organisational-wide approach to investigating quality of service provision in community pharmacy through interviewing both pharmacists and service staff. Organisational commitment among customer service staff was central to delivering quality service. The same type of study could be undertaken in hospital pharmacy where the organisations are larger and the roles more specialised. There seems to be a greater body of literature investigating commitment of students to the pharmacy profession in developed countries such as New Zealand (Perkins et al. 2008), and in developing countries like Ghana (Owusu-Daaku et al. 2008). Conklin and Desselle (2007) have also undertaken an interesting study which demonstrates the moderating effect of support from the Department Chair and organisational commitment on job turnover in pharmacy academia in USA (Conklin and Desselle 2007). In an earlier study, Desselle and Holmes looked at pharmacy technician job satisfaction and through the use of SEM found that uncertainty about their future career plans was lessened through commitment to their current employer (Desselle 2005; Desselle and Holmes 2007). The notion of career commitment is also an interesting one for which more work in community pharmacy could be undertaken (Kong 1995).

Social cognitive, goal-setting and employee commitment theories appear to be well covered by the pharmacy practice literature. On the other hand, very little has been published in areas based on expectancy theory, job characteristics theory and psychological contract theory, all of them areas that are very important internationally for re-professionalisation of pharmacy driven by health policy reform and expectant roles of pharmacists. There is a rich and untapped research agenda in applying these theories.

8.2.2 Meso

Meso-level theories consider organisations sitting within their environment (Table 8.2). Pharmacists work within organisations, whether they are embedded in hospital pharmacies, community pharmacies, the pharmaceutical industry, government or nongovernment organisations, or within general practices; meso-level theories are relevant for framing and analysis. As with micro-level analyses there are a broad array of management theories covering topics relevant to pharmacy.

Table 8.2 Meso-level organisational theories

Theory	Tenets	Lead academic
Double-loop learning	Single-loop learning occurs when errors are detected and corrected without altering the governing values of the master programme. Double-loop learning occurs when, in order to correct an error, it is necessary to alter the governing variables of that strategy	Chris Argyris
Resource-based theory	As a basis for competitive advantage, resources that are either tangible or intangible are at the disposal of the organisation. The competitive advantage lies in the fact that resources are heterogeneous and not mobilised in a straightforward manner	Jay Barney
Organisational effectiveness	The Competing Values Framework (CVF) presented as an integration of five well-known effectiveness models in the literature	Kim Cameron
Managerial and organisational cognition (MOC)	Understanding cognition is required to understand human affairs. Management involves deliberate attempts to influence human behaviour and its outcomes	Anne Huff
Organisational knowledge	Knowledge is created in organisations through the continuous conversion of subjective tacit knowledge and objective explicit knowledge	Ikujiro Nonaka

Source: Adapted from Smith and Hitt (2005)

Pharmacy practice researchers have not capitalised on the application of management/organisational theory to the extent that they could.

8.2.2.1 Organisational Effectiveness

An area that has received attention is organisational effectiveness. It is difficult to conceptualise effectiveness, and therefore it is a challenge to operationalise what an effective community or hospital pharmacy might look like. There is considerable breadth, lack of convergence, untidiness, conceptual disarray and dichotomy within literature streams describing organisational effectiveness (Scahill 2012). There are many proxies used for the term organisational effectiveness (Cameron 1986) and lots of options for the modelling of effectiveness (Mannion and Goddard 2002). The Donabedian model of quality of care has dominated the community pharmacy literature (Jackson et al. 1975; Panyawuthikrai et al. 2005). This model focuses on quality of care as one indicator of high performance, with the impetus on the structures and processes shaping health services delivery and outcomes achieved. Organisational effectiveness can be seen as much broader than this. The question can be asked: 'effectiveness in the eyes of whom—who is setting this effectiveness criteria?' Effectiveness as it relates to pharmacy can best be seen as socially constructed, value laden, politically charged and decidedly judgemental (Scahill 2012). In this way, effectiveness must include the views of all key stakeholders and multi-constituent groups. A model of what constitutes an effective community pharmacy from a multi-constituent viewpoint has been developed (Scahill et al. 2010). Using concept mapping and pattern matching stakeholders from multiple groupings developed a model, and these interesting techniques have been outlined in more detail in another chapter of this book.

8.2.2.2 Knowledge Management

Knowledge management within pharmacy organisations is another significant area for pharmacy practice research. This academic discipline is within its infancy in Schools of Management and is one area that requires a stronger focus within pharmacy practice research. Within the healthcare sector there is a high degree of complexity and significant volumes of information to manage at multiple levels. This applies to pharmacy at the organisational level and to pharmacists and consumers at the individual level. Knowledge creation and transfer within organisations is something that should be central to organisational level pharmacy practice research. Suffice to say, little work has been undertaken in this area. One of the reasons for this is that understanding knowledge creation and transfer cannot be dealt with solely through positivism (Nonaka 2005) which is the dominant stance that pharmacy practice researchers take (Bissell and Morgall Traulsen 2005), even the most sociological of us! Knowledge emerges out of subjective views of the world and to optimise this theoretical construct there is a need to step outside of the positivist realm into more interpretative epistemologies (Crotty 1998). That is, to step back and stop trying to emulate the natural sciences in discovering how organisational level knowledge management might occur within the pharmacy practice world. Equally, this will need to be the case when exploring the undeveloped area of personal knowledge management (PKM) for pharmacist and consumer/patient decision-making.

Nonaka proposes the SECI process (socialisation, externalisation, combination, internalisation), where knowledge is created through the continuous conversion of subjective tacit knowledge and objective explicit knowledge (Nonaka 2005). This theory suggests knowledge creation starts with socialisation—process of converting new tacit knowledge through shared experiences in day-to-day social interaction. This tacit knowledge is then articulated into objective explicit knowledge through externalisation, which Nonaka defines as a dialectic process in thought (Nonaka 2005). The third step involves the combination process whereby explicit knowledge is collected from inside or outside the organisation and then combined, edited and processed to form a more complex and systematic set of explicit knowledge (Nonaka 2005). The final stage is where the knowledge is applied and used in practical situations and becomes the foundation for new routines.

The other important thrust in this field is the importance of leadership as the force to push forward knowledge-creating processes (Smith and Hitt 2005). It is thought that flexible distributed leadership is more likely to propagate knowledge creation and transfer, over leadership, as a fixed control mechanism. Knowledge is created through dynamic interactions among individuals and between individuals and their environments, including between organisations. Flow through the organisation is important and middle management provides the connectivity between upper management and staff. Mapping knowledge creation and transfer and the leadership thereof is applicable and necessary in both community- and hospital-based pharmacy practice research.

8.2.3 Macro

Macro-level theories consider in a broader way the environment within which individuals and organisations are embedded (Table 8.3). Internationally community pharmacy is undergoing considerable change and largely policy driven and calls for increased clinical involvement for the benefit of the patient. Pharmacy professional bodies are also generating vision statements that are expected to underpin the re-professionalisation of community pharmacy through integration with the uptake of new clinical roles and integration within the primary care team.

Community pharmacy has a dual nature being both business retailer and healthcare provider, and there are potential ethical dilemmas associated with this (Scahill 2012). Morals and values in managing a business are therefore important, and so business ethics is a focus within stakeholder theory that could take a more prominent position within the pharmacy practice research agenda. As with ethics, little has been borrowed from transaction cost economics (Williamson 2005), evolutionary theory for economics and management (Winter 2005) or resource dependence theory (Pfeffer 2005). Much more work could be undertaken using macro-organisational theory as a platform to understand community pharmacy and interactions with, influences of and responses to the environment within which it operates.

8.3 Research Design: Theory Building and Testing

8.3.1 Multi-level Considerations

Research design must centre on the nature of the research question (Andrews 2003), although Yin (1994) suggests that the extent of control an investigator has over actual behavioural events and the degree of focus on contemporary as opposed to historical events are also considerations (Yin 1994). Crotty (1998) broadens the requirement to include: theoretical perspective, philosophical stance, epistemology, theory of knowledge, methodology, plan of action and techniques for data collection and analysis (Crotty 1998).

Table 8.3 Macro-level theories

Theory	Tenets	Lead academic
Stakeholder theory	Management considering the interests of internal and external stakeholder groups and taking an active approach. Morals and values in managing a business are important, and so business ethics is a focus within stakeholder theory	Edward Freeman
Resource dependence theory	Organisations as open systems have to obtain resources and, after some transformation, deliver goods or services to customers to provide money to acquire more inputs and continue the cycle	Jeffrey Pfeffer
Institutional theory	Social behaviour and associated resources are anchored in rule systems and cultural schema. Institutions are made up of diverse elements that differ in important ways—different bases of order and compliance, varying mechanisms and logistics, diverse empirical indicators, and alternative rationales for establishing legitimacy claims. Institutions are composed of various combinations, and have been studied through regulative, normative and cultural–cognitive lenses	Richard Scott
Transaction cost economics	Interdisciplinary field in which law, economics, and organisational theory are joined	Oliver Williamson
Evolutionary approach to institutions and social construction (process and structure)	Understanding institution building and institutionalisation includes explaining how action reinforces, maintains or alters structure. Process-based theory stresses action and differentiates kinds of actions that lead to institution building and divergent structures. Structure-based theory stresses the outcome of action in the form of resilient structures: in norms, values, regulations and laws. Process and social construction or social structure and widespread framing of action are the two theoretical approaches, although they overlap	Lynne Zucker, Michael Darby

(continued)

Table 8.3 (continued)

Theory	Tenets	Lead academic
Evolutionary theory for economics and management	Large firms have a major influence on the system as a whole. Managers of large firms make real choices under real uncertainty. Evolutionary economics theory urges that enquiry extends to the inner workings of the firm in understanding the problems they face in dealing with competitive environments	Sidney Winter

Source: Adapted from Smith and Hitt (2005)

There are two juxtaposed positions of research design, on a spectrum from solidly positivist at one end to purely interpretative at the other (Creswell 2003; Denzin and Lincoln 2005; Hussey and Hussey 1997; Liamputtong and Ezzy 2005; Lincoln and Guba 1985; Martin 2002). The terms positivist/objectivist/functionalist on the one hand and interpretative/subjectivist/naturalistic on the other are used interchangeably in the literature to describe each end of the research spectrum. The terms 'quantitative' and 'qualitative' are also used; however, it is important to note that quantitative and qualitative techniques can justifiably be applied to both ends of the research design spectrum (Creswell 2003).

Ontological and epistemological assumptions are what dictate the choice of operational methodology and method. Further, these underpinning assumptions must align with the research question and the position of the researcher based on their world view (Crotty 1998; Hussey and Hussey 1997; Liamputtong and Ezzy 2005; Lincoln and Guba 1985; Martin 2002). Development of the research design can be framed in terms of levels of philosophical thought and operational method (Scahill 2012) (Fig. 8.2).

8.3.2 Level 1: Ontological Assumptions

Ontology is the study of 'being or reality', describing the fundamental 'nature of things' (Lincoln and Guba 1985). As part of the research process, it is necessary to consider whether the world is objective and external to the researcher or whether the world is socially constructed and best understood through examining human perception (Hussey and Hussey 1997). Pure positivists adopt the view that the world is completely objective and the world remains uninfluenced by 'who is looking'. Conversely, pure interpretivists see the world as fluid, and fundamentally shaped by the person who is observing and perceiving (Crotty 1998; Liamputtong and Ezzy 2005; Lincoln and Guba 1985). The positivist and interpretivist views are

```
┌─────────────────┐     ┌──────────────────────────────────────────────────────────────┐
│ Ontological     │─────│ The study of 'being or reality'; the fundamental nature of things │
│ assumptions     │     │ •Positivist – world as objective, uninfluenced by who is looking  │
│                 │     │ •Interpretivist – world is fluid and always changing and fundamentally │
└─────────────────┘     │ shaped by the person who is observing                        │
         │              └──────────────────────────────────────────────────────────────┘
         ▼
┌─────────────────┐     ┌──────────────────────────────────────────────────────────────┐
│ Epistemological │─────│ The study of how people know about 'being or reality'        │
│ stance          │     │ •Positivist – knowledge through objectively gathering facts  │
│                 │     │ •Interpretivist – role of subjective understanding in shaping our knowledge │
└─────────────────┘     └──────────────────────────────────────────────────────────────┘
         │
         ▼
┌─────────────────┐     ┌──────────────────────────────────────────────────────────────┐
│ Paradigm of inquiry │─│ A theoretical framework: A world view, a general perspective, a way of │
│                 │     │ framing and breaking down complexity of the real world       │
└─────────────────┘     └──────────────────────────────────────────────────────────────┘
         │
         ▼
┌─────────────────┐     ┌──────────────────────────────────────────────────────────────┐
│ Methodology     │─────│ The way the plan of action is to be approached: construct development │
│                 │     │ and exploration of relationship between them – development of a theory │
└─────────────────┘     └──────────────────────────────────────────────────────────────┘
         │
         ▼
┌─────────────────┐     ┌──────────────────────────────────────────────────────────────┐
│ Methods         │─────│ The tools by which data are collected and analysed           │
└─────────────────┘     └──────────────────────────────────────────────────────────────┘
```

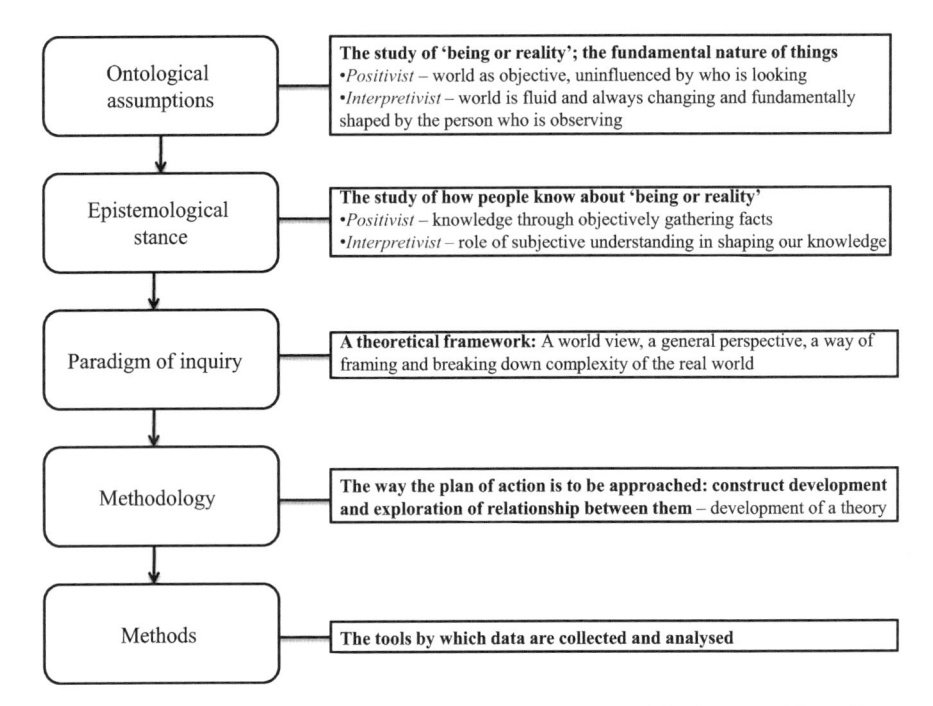

Fig. 8.2 Levels of research design. *Source*: Scahill (2012) thesis originally adapted from Crotty (1998), Hussey and Hussey (1997), Liamputtong and Ezzy (2005), Lincoln and Guba (1985)

at two extremes of the research spectrum and Hussey and Hussey (1997) remind us that:

very few people would operate in their pure forms (Hussey and Hussey 1997, p. 50).

Ontological assumption ranges from reality as a concrete structure where the social world is the same as the physical world, through to reality as a projection of human imagination. At the far right of the spectrum, there is no social world apart from that which is inside the individual's mind (Fig. 8.3) (Hussey and Hussey 1997; Morgan and Smircich 1980). The ontological assumption of a single tangible 'reality' (Lincoln and Guba 1985) viewed exactly the same by all, a reality that is concrete in structure, where the social world is like the physical world, does not sit well with interpretative researchers, but positivists have empathy for this stance (Hussey and Hussey 1997; Morgan and Smircich 1980). As a researcher, it is important to posit what you identify with, for me, reality as a social construction.

When reality is considered to be a social construction (Berger and Luckmann 1967; Crotty 1998), interpretative studies are posited towards the subjectivist end of the continuum (Fig. 8.3). In this instance the following view is adopted:

…all knowledge, and therefore all meaningful reality as such, is contingent upon human practices, being constructed in and out of interaction between human beings and their world, and developed and transmitted within an essentially social context. (Crotty 1998, p. 42)

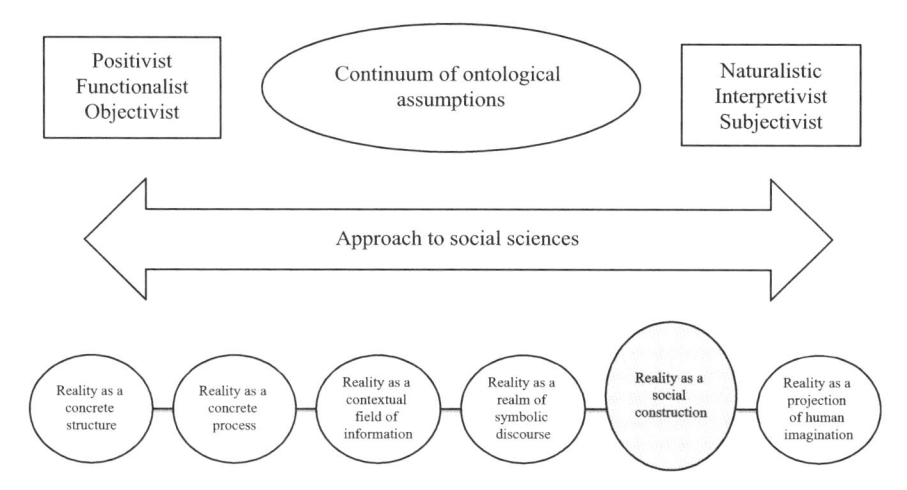

8 Applying Organisational Theory in Pharmacy Practice Research

```
┌─────────────┐      ╭──────────────────╮      ┌─────────────┐
│ Positivist  │     (  Continuum of      )     │ Naturalistic│
│Functionalist│     ( ontological         )    │Interpretivist│
│ Objectivist │      (  assumptions      )     │ Subjectivist│
└─────────────┘      ╰──────────────────╯      └─────────────┘

      ⇐══════════ Approach to social sciences ══════════⇒

  ◯         ◯         ◯         ◯         ◯         ◯
Reality   Reality   Reality   Reality   Reality   Reality
as a      as a      as a      as a      as a      as a
concrete  concrete  contextual realm of  social    projection
structure process   field of   symbolic  construction of human
                    information discourse          imagination
```

Fig. 8.3 Ontological assumptions. *Source*: Scahill (2012) thesis adapted from Hussey and Hussey (1997), Morgan and Smircich (1980)

This stance does not align with the existence of a single tangible reality, lying within a purely objective world, described as 'same' by all. The world is deemed to be bounded by both time and context, with reality being constructed around participants' own definitions (Hussey and Hussey 1997; Lincoln and Guba 1985; Morgan and Smircich 1980). Adopting an ontological position of social constructionism (Berger and Luckmann 1967; Crotty 1998) suggests the need for an interpretative frame for the development of organisational constructs, along with exploring the nature of the relationship between them. For example, the theoretical framework in my own PhD thesis [which explores the influence of organisational culture (OC) on effectiveness (OE)] sets out OC and OE as socially constructed, time dependent, value laden, contextually bound, decidedly judgemental and therefore multi-constituent in nature (Allaire and Firsirotu 1984; Alvesson 2002; Cameron 1985, 1986; Cameron and Whetten 1983; Campbell 1976a, b, 1977; Connolly et al. 1980; Martin 1992, 2002; Michalski and Cousins 2000). The assumption is made that if OC and OE are socially constructed, then the nature of the relationship between them is also socially constructed, which fits with the ontological position of that study.

8.3.3 Level 2: Epistemological Assumptions

Epistemology is the study of how people know about 'being' or 'reality' (Liamputtong and Ezzy 2005). The epistemological stance must flow logically from the ontological assumptions of the researcher, to ensure alignment and robust methodological rigour (Liamputtong and Ezzy 2005; Lincoln and Guba 1985). The positivist researcher gains knowledge through objectively gathering facts, whilst the interpretivist considers the role of subjective understanding in the shaping of knowledge (Denzin and Lincoln 2005; Liamputtong and Ezzy 2005). In order to understand study participants' socially constructed realities when building theory, there is a need to engage in the research process as 'human instrument'. The interpretative approach allows for this, through immersion in data collection, analysis and interpretation to gain deep and rich description of the nature of the relationship between organisational constructs (Lincoln and Guba 1985).

An ontological approach underpinned by social constructionism and an epistemological stance that is interpretative provides the freedom to explore research questions which are rich in complexity, without the pressure of needing to remain entirely 'value-free' (Alvesson 2002; Geertz 1973). Both emic (researcher internal/native) and etic (researcher external) approaches can be used at different stages throughout studies, but within a largely interpretative or positivistic frame (Burchell and Kolb 2003; Martin 1992, 2002; Martin et al. 1985; Michalski and Cousins 2000; Trochim and Kane 2005).

In addition to congruent ontological and epistemological assumptions, Lincoln calls for consideration of three other axioms of interpretative research which wholly apply to theory building: generalisation, causal linkage and the role of values in inquiry (Lincoln and Guba 1985). These need to be considered in terms of the position of any theory-building or theory-testing study.

8.3.3.1 The Concept of 'Generalisability'

The degree of generalisability of the findings that constitute the theory is considered to be of lesser interest within the interpretative frame, where the aim is to develop an idiographic body of knowledge about a particular context (Lincoln and Guba 1985; Martin 1992, 2002). Positivists, however, strive for a much higher degree of generalisability in their work. In my own PhD thesis, the nature of the relationship between organisational culture and organisational effectiveness is conceptualised as socially constructed and by definition cannot be completely context- or value-free (Scahill 2012). Interpretative research is wholly time bound and context specific, and a level of generalisability is only possible through transferability of findings between 'like' contexts as determined by those immersed within such contexts (Lincoln and Guba 1985).

8.3.3.2 Direct Linkages, Causality and the Notion of Linearity

The issue of causality has always fascinated the human race (Lincoln and Guba 1985) and is central to understanding most theory-building endeavours. In my own thesis it was apparent that the popular press and corporate culture literature has developed through direct linear causality and the notion of cultural strength (Deal and Kennedy 1982; Kotter and Heskett 1992; Peters and Waterman 1982; Schein 1985), which has been challenged for its simplicity in dealing with complex phenomena and relationships (Alvesson 2002; Freeman and Peck 2010; Martin 1992, 2002).

Within healthcare, identification of contingent and potentially recursive relationships between OC and performance has supported the contemporary movement away from linearity, with a mandate for a richer and deeper look at the dynamics of the OC–OE relationship (Davies et al. 2007; Mannion et al. 2005, 2010; Scott et al. 2003a, b). This is supported by studies outside of healthcare (Ashkanasy et al. 2000; Schein 1996; Wilderom et al. 2000).

The interpretive frame questions linearity and direct causality as viable concepts. Lincoln and Guba (1985) take an extreme view of the concept of causality:

> ...moving to transform the theory of causality into an attributional theory whereby mutual shaping replaces absolute cause and effect. (Lincoln and Guba 1985, p. 145)

The stance taken in most theory development is more tempered, and rather than excluding causality theory outright, an attempt is usually made to understand the complexity within relationships, whether they be causal or not. The notion is generally adopted that, in some way, individual constructs may influence each other and the researcher sets out to understand what the influences are and explain this as a whole through theory.

8.3.3.3 Naturalistic Enquiry Is Not Value-Free

Interpretive epistemology is underpinned by the recognition that research is not value-free.

> If there is only one objective (real? true?) perspective, then, by definition no others are worth considering. But when values are recognised as being involved, it is imperative that their meaning and implication be sorted out. (Lincoln and Guba 1985, p. 173)

Under the interpretative framework, researchers bring their own values to the work when framing studies and collecting, analysing and interpreting data (Creswell 2003; Crotty 1998; Liamputtong and Ezzy 2005). Further, organisational life is socially constructed, and so it must hold true that perspectives on organisational constructs and their interrelationships are value laden (Scahill 2012).

8.3.4 Level 3: Theoretical Framework as Research Paradigm

Paradigm is loosely referred to in the academic literature and means different things to different authors (Crotty 1998; Hussey and Hussey 1997; Lincoln and Guba 1985). There is some consensus that paradigm constitutes a world view, a general perspective on an issue, a way of breaking down the complexity of the real world (Hussey and Hussey 1997). Consistent with ontological and epistemological assumptions, paradigm is a framework of beliefs, values and theoretical underpinning of concepts under study (Creswell 2003). Hussey and Hussey (1997) suggest that paradigms provide a framework comprising an accepted set of theories, methods and ways of defining both concepts and data (Hussey and Hussey 1997).

The paradigm of the study has been deemed the theoretical framework (Scahill 2012). The research paradigm outlines the conception of organisational constructs—how the relationship between them has been, and is being, viewed. The theoretical framework is central to the research design as it provides linkage between the ontological assumptions, epistemological stance and operational methods for data collection, analysis and interpretation.

8.4 Developing and/or Testing Theory

Development of theory is a central activity in organisational research (Eisenhardt 1989), and advancing the field of management requires more theory building (Smith and Hitt 2005). If, as Smith and Hitt (2005) imply, this is a relatively young field of study in the wider management literature, then it most certainly is in the pharmacy practice literature:

> Theory development is highly important in the discipline of management and organizations as it is a relatively young field of study, in comparison to many other social science disciplines. As a young field of study, new theory provides important and unique insights that can advance the fields of understanding of management phenomena. (Smith and Hitt 2005, p. 1)

There are many definitions of theory, and many ways have been proposed to theorise (Morse 1994). Not all people use the same approach (Zucker and Darby 2005). The development of the theory can be underpinned by a theoretical framework which aligns with the ontological and epistemological stance adopted by the investigators (Huff 2005). Theoretical frameworks help to guide the exploration of relationships between constructs (Ashkanasy et al. 2000; Braithwaite et al. 2010; Davies et al. 2007; Kernick 2004; Scott et al. 2003a, b; Wilderom et al. 2000). However, the theoretical framework is exactly that, a framework for the development of theory, and these frameworks have also been labelled 'preliminary' theories (Mintzberg 2005). Frameworks provide the conceptualisation of constructs and the nature of the relationship between two or more constructs. Frameworks describe part but not all of the theory-building process, and the following section outlines the thought required during the theory-building process.

8.4.1 Philosophical Considerations Regarding Theory Building

Definitions of what theory is range from being structured to being more general in nature. Kerlinger (1979) has described theory as:

'...a set of interrelated constructs (variables), definitions and propositions that presents a systematic view of phenomena by specifying relationships among variables with the purpose of explaining natural phenomena' (Kerlinger 1979, p. 64).

In developing theory about developing theory, Mintzberg (2005) suggests that all theories:

> ... are, after all, just words and symbols on pieces of paper, about the reality they purport to describe; they are not that reality. So they simplify it. This means we must choose our theories according to how useful they are, not how true they are. (Mintzberg 2005, p. 356)

There are two main types of theory development: hypothesis testing and proposition generating (Bacharach 1989; Mintzberg 2005). These two approaches are reflected in the above quotes. Theory building is generally more abstract than theory testing and involves inductively derived theoretical propositions which help to describe relationships between constructs. On the other hand, theory testing is a more deductive–hypothetical approach which involves the development and testing of hypotheses which relate to the relationship between variables, which may or may not come from construct development within a theoretical framework (Bacharach 1989; Eisenhardt 1989; Locke and Latham 2005; Mintzberg 2005; Morse 1994) (Fig. 8.4).

The development of any theory, but in the case of this chapter management-oriented theory, requires the reader to understand some basic terminology along with aspects that help to describe the theory-building process. The terms conceptualisation and operationalisation are integral to understanding theory and its development.

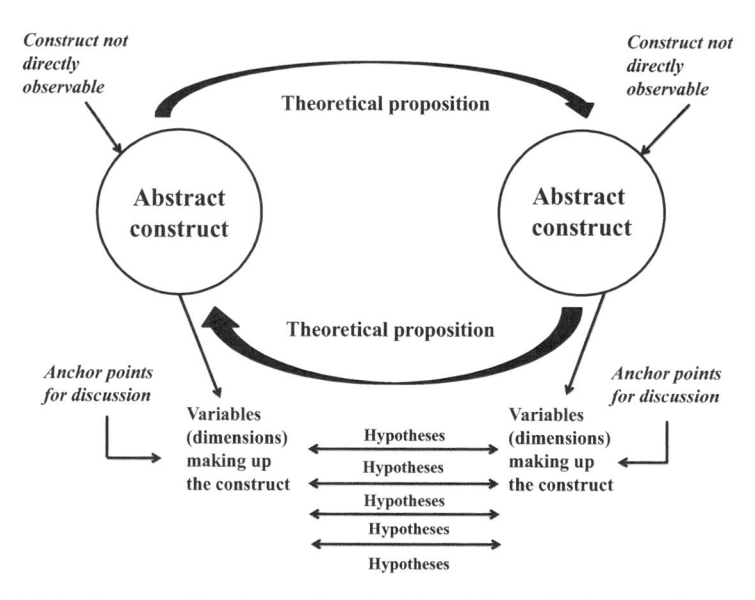

Fig. 8.4 Inductive–propositional versus hypothesis-based theory development. *Source*: Scahill (2012)

8.4.1.1 Conceptualisation

These higher level constructs need to be distilled down into a series of 'bite-sized' dimensions that participants helping develop theory, those building and interpreting and those consuming can understand!

8.4.1.2 Operationalisation

Variables (some call these dimensions) that help describe constructs are often developed as anchor points for discussion with interview participants—the building of these constructs into more tangible elements. The focus on theory building can be on the development of theoretical propositions that describe the dynamic interplays (relationships) between constructs. However, the variables making up the constructs lend themselves to further analysis and empirical approaches to generation and testing of hypotheses.

The approach to theory building should align with the ontological and epistemological stance of the researcher (Smith and Hitt 2005). Early academics exploring the theory development process came largely from a positivist frame (Bacharach 1989; Kuhn 1970; Popper 1959). They were of the belief that the theory development process must include an empiric testing phase. A theory was not a good theory until it was 'falsified' by testing deductions from it (Bacharach 1989; Popper 1959; Whetten 1989).

As management science has matured, some researchers have become frustrated with the dominance of positivism in the field (Smith and Hitt 2005), and the author has suffered through journal rejection on several occasions based on reviewers not being sympathetic to the more subjective approaches but more importantly, not understanding them. There has been the realisation that more and less abstract theories can stand on their own (Locke and Latham 2005; Mintzberg 2005). As with other sociological disciplines, the positivist versus interpretative (inductive–deductive) arguments have occurred, and the approach to be taken is dependent on the purpose of theory development (Locke and Latham 2005; Mintzberg 2005). The need for theory building rests with the need for humans to firstly order and secondly make sense of reality (Dubin 1969). The purpose of theory is to understand and explain the relationship between constructs, and if an inductive approach is taken, then the reasoning is based on the need to understand the 'nature' of the relationship—in what way(s) one construct influences another (Scahill 2012). Theory building often involves exploring processes of institutionalisation, and Zucker and Darby (2005) suggest that:

> Much of the process of institutionalisation is tacit and not open to direct measurement...Constructing institutional theory is much like social construction; it is inherently a social process, and also often has tacit components. (Zucker and Darby 2005, pp. 547, 567–68)

The tacit nature of many organisational constructs and of the theory-building process *per se* presents significant challenge within organisationally focussed research. The major challenge is the 'codification' of abstractions: the summarising, organising and distributing of key arguments into a comprehensive framework (Smith and Hitt 2005). The more abstract the theory, the more difficult the codification process. The socially constructed nature of theory building and the challenges associated with its tacit nature fit with the ontology and epistemology of those researchers at the more subjectivist end of the research spectrum.

If theory-building efforts are *inductive*, then they go from *the particular* to *the general* or from tangible data to general concepts (Mintzberg 2005). This is counter to the *hypothetico-deductive* method where theory development follows a line from *the general* to *the particular*. Those who align with positivism (the more objective end of the research spectrum) take the view that knowledge of reality is impossible (Kuhn 1970; Popper 1959). They believe that theories are not based on observations of reality and so cannot be proven; they can only be falsified by testing deductions from them (Bacharach 1989; Popper 1959). These two processes of inductive and deductive methods feed into each other, but the work is often undertaken by people representing different schools of thought (Mintzberg 2005).

The level at which theory is developed is important. Classification for types of theory have predominantly been that of *grand theories* or *mid-range theories* (Frese 2005; Merriam 1988). Grand theories attempt to understand the 'complete' picture and as a result, tend to be complex and tacit in nature. Grand theories are all encompassing, 'uncertainty reducing' and less precise. Mid-range theories consist of a limited number of variables; they fit between a working hypothesis and an all-inclusive effort of a unified grand theory, are supported by limited assumptions and have high problem specification (Frese 2005; Mintzberg 2005). It is important that those whom are building theory explicitly state at which level their theory is being built. This is for the theory builder to interpret and decide and for the reader to refute and dispel.

8.4.2 The Process of Theory Development

Developing new theory is a creative act (Smith and Hitt 2005). Mintzberg (2005) alludes to the tacit processes associated with this process of theory building, stating:

> I have no clue about how I develop theory. I don't think about it; I just try to do it. Indeed, thinking about it could be dangerous. (Mintzberg 2005, p. 355)

There are many ways to develop *the particular* of the theory, and cognitive mapping processes have been used in inductive theory development where interplays between constructs need to be uncovered, interpreted and described (Scahill 2012). Cognitive mapping is chosen to help make sense of the likely complex and nonlinear interactions between organisational constructs. Theory-building processes are inductive, and there are broad guidelines offered by contemporary management theorists for those that want to follow an inductive approach (Locke and Latham 2005; Smith and Hitt 2005). Theory development requires researchers to identify constructs and/or variables associated with constructs, state relationships and clarify boundary conditions (Smith and Hitt 2005). The approach to theory building of 30 organisational scientists has been summarised into four steps which can be applied to theory development studies within the arena of pharmacy practice research. These steps include: outlining tension/phenomena or an interesting question, development of an initial framework to guide the research, elaboration and the research per se and proclamation and presentation of the theory (Smith and Hitt 2005).

Outlining the tension/phenomena or interesting question. This is an important part of the process of theory development as context is significant in the setting of socially constructed organisational constructs (Crotty 1998; Lincoln and Guba 1985; Mintzberg 2005). Tension often underpins the need to explore issues more deeply and to develop theories about them.

Development of a theoretical framework is part of the conceptualisation process which helps to steer development of the theory going forward. Theoretical frameworks are a necessary part of the hypothesis-based theory development process. In this way, the constructs are able to be defined and the rationale for any stated hypotheses can be outlined in full. Taking the deductive–hypothetical stance there are often multiple constructs to be considered. Relationships between constructs are assumed to be direct and causal, and moderating and mediating effects are often proposed and/or discovered (Bacharach 1989; Whetten 1989).The use of a theoretical framework in these more positivistic studies helps to make the hypotheses more explicit and provides clarity in structure and of the relationships between constructs and variables. Techniques such as SEM are used to describe the theory (Byrne 2013). Taking the interpretative stance and building theory inductively, the theoretical framework provides something quite different to the researcher. The conceptualisation process is not quite so rigid under this framework and allows more focus on developing a sense of the constructs under study, prior to exploring the nature of the relationship between them (Lincoln and Guba 1985).

The elaboration/research part of the process is most often undertaken through interviewing and sense-making thereof. This part of the process includes data gathering, reduction and differentiation and re-integration; identifying causal relationships, interplays and feedback loops; and taking time to generate multiple iterations to ensure a seasoned understanding of how the theory is developing over time (Locke and Latham 2005; Smith and Hitt 2005). This is able to be undertaken through the use of cognitive mapping of the dialogue from interviews, as the dynamic interplays can be outlined in this way (Scahill 2012). When exploring relationships between constructs (which is the whole idea of theory), participants need to be provided with definitions of the constructs and also need to be given time to read the profiles of these constructs and to understand in their own minds what these constructs are made up of in terms of dimensions.

8.4.2.1 Data Management and Transcribing

The sound files from each interview need to be downloaded from a digital recording device and saved onto a password-protected personal computer (PC). Transcription is not simply a technical procedure, but is an opportunity for further immersion in the data (Denzin and Lincoln 2005). Based on this reasoning, those researchers involved in theory development should undertake the transcribing themselves, and this task should not be out-sourced. Once transcribed, the interview transcripts can be formatted in a uniform manner to allow uploading into NVivo™. The verbatim text should clearly identify researcher and respondent voice and ideally be at least 1.5 spaced for ease of reading and note-taking.

8.4.2.2 Analysis of Interview Dialogue

As is often the case with interpretative research, clear and complete delineation between data management, analysis and interpretation is not possible (Kvale 1996, 2007; Liamputtong and Ezzy 2005; Miles and Huberman 1999). Kvale (1996) defines analysis in three stages: structuring, clarification and analysis proper. Structuring involves systematic formatting of transcripts to manage large and complex interview materials. Clarification involves making the material amenable to analysis through:

> eliminating superfluous material such as digressions and repetitions, distinguishing between the essential and the non-essential (Kvale 1996, p. 191).

Kvale's account of the analytic process appears to end at data analysis, whilst other researchers suggest the importance of the interpretation of analytic findings and attempt to highlight the importance of the interpretative stage in making sense of the data (Crotty 1998; Denzin and Lincoln 2005; Miles and Huberman 1999; Morgan and Smircich 1980; Silverman 2001). An attempt should be made to highlight the contributions of both the analytic process and interpretation in order to develop theory.

Cognitive mapping can be used as a primary analytic method and sense-making schema/technique. It reflects the data, with the opportunity to take participants' language into the maps. Cognitive mapping is a powerful way to represent dialogue from raw data in order to assist analysis, through questioning and understanding of the data (Miles and Huberman 1999). Maps can be generated for the questions being asked of each construct (or even each of the dimensions within a construct) and the relationships between them. Although interpretation through cognitive mapping may sound relatively straightforward, prolonged periods of time can be spent managing the transition from data reduction and storage to the process of mapping, and this should not be underestimated.

There is a need to understand the complexity of the interplays and the process is generally emergent, although there is a need to depict data analysis in this manner. It often takes much longer than expected to transition into the full cognitive mapping process. The emergent nature of theory does not suggest a lack of rigour; it often takes much longer to get to the end point of analysis and interpretation than one would expect. The main considerations for the adoption of cognitive mapping as data reduction and sense-making steps are both theoretical and operational (Hussey and Hussey 1997; Miles and Huberman 1999). Theoretical considerations include alignment with the ontological and epistemological stances adopted in order to conduct studies and the theoretical basis for cognitive mapping techniques *per se*. Operational considerations include: preparation and reduction of the source data, the mapping process, analysis and sense-making (also labelled interpretation). The subsequent theory development is outlined in a separate section, as it relies on other analytic and interpretative processes in addition to the use of cognitive mapping data.

8.4.2.3 Theoretical Basis for Cognitive Mapping

Cognitive mapping is not simply a mechanical drawing tool or process; it is also bounded by theory itself. Cognitive maps contain raw field data and are used to construct meaning and allow the development of theoretical accounts of phenomena. Based on Kelly's (1955) Theory of Personal Constructs, cognitive mapping is a method of data representation and analysis used to structure and make sense of written or verbal accounts of phenomena (Hussey and Hussey 1997; Kelly 1955).

Ackerman et al. (1990) note that Kelly's Theory of Personal Constructs suggests:

> ...we make sense of the world in order to predict how, all things being equal, the world will be in the future, and to decide how we might act or intervene in order to achieve what we prefer within that world—a predict-and-control view of problem solving. (Ackerman et al. 1990, p. 1)

Personal Construct Theory aligns with the ontology of social constructionism and the interpretative epistemology adopted in inductive theory building through the need for making sense of the participant's world, that is, from their perspective. The notion within cognitive mapping theory of a 'predict and control view' (to some extent) supports a cause and effect theory when exploring the relationship between two constructs. However, there is no major misalignment in inductive theory building, as cognitive mapping allows for and accommodates nonlinear and dynamic interplay, through the linking of distinct influences (Ackerman et al. 1990). In this way, its use is extended beyond the direct cause and effect mentality seen with deductive–hypothetical theories.

8.4.2.4 Data Reduction and Management

Data cleaning processes involve an initial first read of transcripts to look for sections of text that don't make sense or for where there are omissions.

Amendments should be made prior to upload of the transcripts into NVivo™ software. A standard format should be used. Tree nodes can be developed to reflect the structure of the interview schema. In this way, NVivo™ software can be used as a data reduction tool. Within each of the NVivo™ nodes, descriptions of influence are represented by phrases of about ten words which retain the language of the participant. These snippets of language are treated as distinct influences, and the interplays between them can be mapped out. Long sentences need to be separated into shorter sentences and mapped.

8.4.2.5 Analytic Mapping Processes and Data Presentation

Cognitive maps can be developed that depict the influence of dimensions of one or more constructs on others. The language of participants is used, and distinct phrases can be linked in a hierarchical flow of dialogue of influence and endpoint. The flow of mapping is not assumed to be linear or causal when developing inductive theory about complex constructs and the interplays between them. It is necessary, though, to provide the explanations leading to consequences. All attempts need to be made at retaining ownership of participant language, by not abbreviating words and phrases used by them. Meaning also needs to be retained as constructed and not lost in translation when moving from raw dialogue to cognitive map.

The mapping process can be manual, with phrases being mapped by hand or through the early use of technology. The manual approach involves quotes and phrases being physically cut out from paper printouts of the NVivo™ tree nodes, sellotaped and mapped onto A3 sheets of paper. A cognitive map can then be developed for the key streams of dialogue generated by each participant and then amalgamated at the level of the individual dimensions of the constructs under study. A manual approach allows further immersion in the data. The NVivo™ software can provide the platform for data reduction, and Visio (Microsoft Office™) can provide a tool to move from manual mapping to electronic presentation of the maps on a single sheet of A4 paper. In this way, influences and interplays can be depicted and are able to be interpreted in a single view.

Hierarchy of interplays and influences can then be built up by following through the flow of dialogue. Influences and interplays are summarised in small rectangle text boxes rather than as continuous lines (see Fig. 8.5). The starting point for the map is often the bottom of the page depicting the cultural orientation. The beginning of each interview should provide a description of the construct, and then the interplays that influence the outcomes expected by participants can be mapped from this. This map follows the flow of dialogue in the interview. Alternatively the dialogue can be mapped from left to right, depending on how the theoretical framework is constructed (i.e. influence of one construct on another from left to right, right to left or in both directions).

The page can also be split in half for the mapping exercise and different scenarios represented, e.g. the bottom half of the map depicting the organisation being effective, the bottom half not.

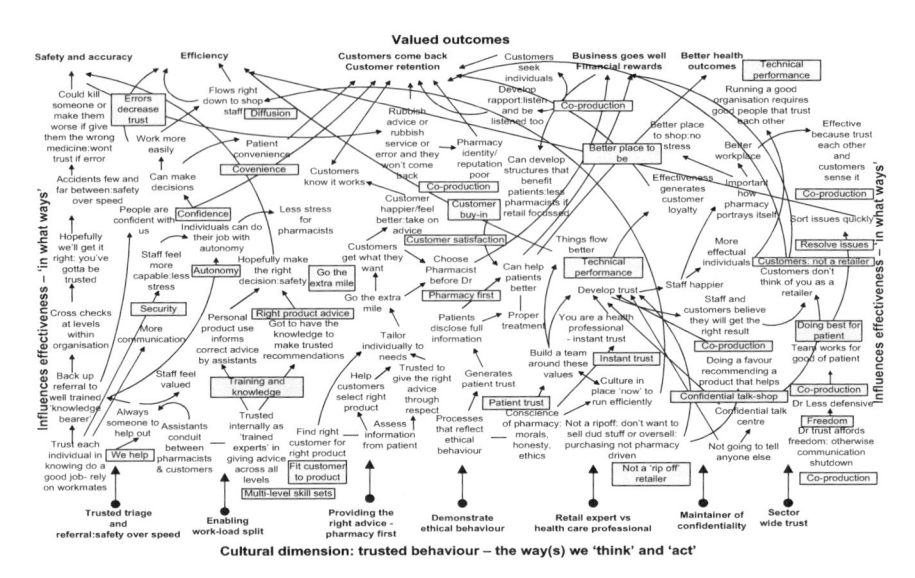

Fig. 8.5 Example of a cognitive map: influence of trusted behaviour on outcomes that are valued. *Source*: Scahill (2012)

The opposite poles of the maps are deemed important for clarification regarding start and end points, not only of discussion in the interview, but also of influences and of that being influenced. Sense-making can also be aided by placing influences in the imperative form, including actors and actions as possible and appropriate. The patterns of interplay and dominant relationships can be made superordinate to specific items that contribute to them, and the mapping can include explanation. Without reducing complexity and losing the link to raw data, a 'tidy-up' of maps generated allows a complete and clear depiction of the influences and interplays that occur within each one.

8.4.2.6 Interpretation: The Sense-Making Process

Mapping reveals the patterns or reasonings about influences of one construct on another in a way that a stream of linear text cannot. The influence of one construct relative to another can be thought about whilst mapping, and during subsequent interpretation of the maps collectively. Descriptive narratives of each map can be developed as part of the analytic process, to assist with the interpretation and sense-making processes 'of the whole'. Narratives used to build these maps can be extensive and lengthy—they serve as a working analysis and a platform for reflexive thinking by those developing the theory. Common patterns of influence across the various dimensions of constructs can be identified and explored through the maps, the narratives and also summary tabulation resulting from the narrative analysis. Patterns of influence and interplay that participants may see as a primary idea can be identified by the researcher and described (Miles and Huberman 1999).

It is important to realise that theories do not emerge 'all at once—in a flash of insight' and this has been well described by Oldham and Hackman (2005):

> We suspect that no theory, and certainly not ours, emerges all at once in a flash of insight. Instead, theory development can seem as if it is an endless iterative process, moving back and forth between choice of variables and specification of the links among them, hoping that eventually the small, grudgingly achieved advances will outnumber the forced retreats. (Oldham and Hackman, p. 161)

Rather, development is an ongoing iterative process, moving back and forth between constructs and the variables that make up these constructs and the relationships between them. Theory development is often undertaken over a prolonged period of time, and some of the key management theories have been worked on for 20 years and longer (Miles 2014; Smith and Hitt 2005). This is usually through a process of continual refinement via peer review and mutual collaboration (Miles 2014; Mintzberg 2005; Smith and Hitt 2005).

8.5 Techniques for Ensuring Rigour

Researchers taking a pure naturalistic route have endured much scepticism from their positivist colleagues about the 'trustworthiness' of taking such approaches (Freeman and Peck 2010; Lincoln and Guba 1985). It can feel like a continuous battle; the development of organisational theory, in particular, has come up against a barrage of evaluative criteria, generally set within a positivistic frame (Smith and Hitt 2005). As pharmacists we are trained as 'hard scientists', and yet every day we deal with other humans as part of our organisations or in dealing with consumers and patients. It is the minority of pharmacists that turn to the social sciences in an attempt to obtain a deeper, richer understanding of phenomenon. Cautioning against inflexibility and scientific rigidity, the issue of theory evaluation is sensitive and the application of rigid criteria cautioned:

> To dangle criteria (for the evaluation of theory) above the head of a theorist like the Sword of Damocles may stifle creativity. In most of our work, flaws in theoretical logic can be found. However, during the early stages of theory building, there may be a fine line between satisfying the criteria of the internal logic of theory and achieving a creative contribution. A good theorist walks this line carefully. (Bacharach 1989, p. 513)

Theory building is a process of social construction, and Mintzberg (2005) highlights that what theories are not is 'true' (Mintzberg 2005). Theory building is founded on interpretative epistemologies where validity and reliability hold no credence. It seems that considering different forms of rigour is a more acceptable approach even than applying Lincoln and Guba's (1985) well-known categories of trustworthiness: credibility, transferability, dependability and confirmability. Liamputtong and Ezzy (2005) provide a framework with categories of rigour, including: theoretical, procedural, interpretative, triangulation, evaluative and rigour reflexivity. This approach is more pertinent to theory building (Liamputtong and Ezzy 2005).

8.5.1 Theoretical Rigour

Theoretical rigour is demonstrated by a study that integrates the research question into the study design—that integrates and aligns a theoretical frame with operational method (Crotty 1998; Liamputtong and Ezzy 2005; Smith and Hitt 2005). Considerable time and energy must be spent developing a research design which reflects this. Ontological assumptions are generally founded on social constructionism when developing inductive theory. The constructs are framed in this way, as is the relationship between them—meaning is constructed not discovered (Crotty 1998). Theories that are built through cognitive mapping of dialogue retaining the language of participants and are founded on Personal Construct Theory present a strong theoretical rigour (Kelly 1955). This aligns with the socially constructed nature of most organisational constructs. This is an accepted analytic method when taking an interpretative approach.

8.5.2 Procedural Rigour

An explicit account of how the research was conducted provides operational rigour (Silverman 2001). The aim is to carefully document the development of theoretical propositions. From sample selection through data collection, analysis, interpretation and theory development, procedures need to be documented, and there needs to be alignment between the different parts of the study. Methodological and analytic decisions made need to be documented so that an end of study audit can be undertaken. Tracking back beyond original source data to the respondents needs to be made possible, thereby enhancing the dependability and credibility of the study (Lincoln and Guba 1985).

Procedural rigour also includes aspects of courteous and ethical conduct such as negotiation of access, approach towards participants, the development of trust and rapport, how surprises were dealt with and feedback to participants of findings. Due process needs to be followed to ensure the study is conducted ethically.

8.5.3 Interpretative Rigour

Liamputtong and Ezzy (2005) highlight that many researchers encounter crises of confidence about the validity of their own interpretations (Liamputtong and Ezzy 2005). However, Lincoln and Guba (1985) suggest that the notion of validity is foreign to true interpretative research, and assessing credibility is more appropriate (Lincoln and Guba 1985). Rejection of modernist positivist assumptions that there is one true objective interpretation does not mean that research rigour should be discarded. Postmodernists have argued that there are no final grounds for accepting all interpretations as 'accurate' (Grbich 2004). To reiterate again in this chapter, often inductive theory building is founded on the ontology of social constructionism. In this way meaning is constructed, not discovered, and therefore the interpretation is dependent on who constructs the meaning. Multiple interpretations of the same phenomena by different individuals is possible—in fact highly likely and overwhelmingly acceptable (Berger and Luckmann 1967; Crotty 1998; Huff 2005; Liamputtong and Ezzy 2005; Lincoln and Guba 1985; Weick 1995, 2005)! An interpretative stance is therefore appropriate under an ontological frame of social constructionism, as long as rigorous process is demonstrated and outlined (Crotty 1998; Hussey and Hussey 1997; Lincoln and Guba 1985). Liamputtong and Ezzy suggest that interpretative rigour is afforded if a study accurately represents the understandings of events and actions within the worldview of the people engaged with it and the broader framework of the study. Interpretative rigour is assisted by maintaining the language of the respondents in the cognitive maps as data, alongside analysis and subsequent interpretation. The participant voice is carried through.

8.5.4 Triangulation

Triangulation allows the researcher to develop a complex picture of the phenomenon being studied, which might otherwise be unavailable if only one method were utilised (Kotter 1995; Patton 1980, 1990; Silverman 2001). Triangulation is an important feature of establishing trustworthiness of data with use of multi-methods (Denison and Mishra 1995; Hofstede et al. 1990; Jick 1979; Martin 2002; Siehl and Martin 1990). Pure positivist researchers appear not to incorporate triangulation into their research designs, with the focus being on validity and reliability of the typology used (Cameron and Quinn 1999) in contrast to human as research instrument; more of an agency focus (Lincoln and Guba 1985).

Multi-methods including qualitative and quantitative techniques are acceptable within an interpretative framework, although qualitative processes tend to dominate (Lincoln and Guba 1985). If the nub of the research question is wholly interpretative, mixed methods approaches can still be used. The constructs can be formulated into a series of dimensions, and this data can be used as anchor points for discussion rather than as data cross-check. Over time, theories can morph in their development to become more or less dimensional and therefore more or less 'empiric'. As a consequence, the mixed methods techniques can be used more for construct operationalisation and less for triangulation purposes. Triangulation is largely a positivist phenomenon, and interpretative rigour and rigorous reflexivity are more important to inductive theory building under interpretativist epistemologies.

8.5.5 Evaluative Rigour: Ethics, Politics and Exposure Through Publication

Simply completing the operational tasks required by procedural ethics does not address the more general issue of considering the political and social consequences of research (Liamputtong and Ezzy 2005; Lincoln and Guba 1985). Editorials, commentary and data-driven publications should be derived from all work, and there is an ethical and moral obligation to publish findings. The papers derived from studies may challenge particular professions, academia, policy-makers and professional groups, along with the literature. Evaluation of projects results from this process.

8.5.6 Rigorous Reflexivity

Inductive theory is often founded on the ontological assumptions of social constructionism. In this way, knowledge is not discovered, knowledge is constructed as people go about their daily lives (Crotty 1998). The theory-building process is a form of social construction and so the researcher is often a firmly entrenched instrument of the research (Grbich 2004). The reflexivity within this process plays out at both the conceptual and the operational level. At the conceptual level, the discussion sections of reports about study limitations and future research must examine the position of project and researcher on the positivist–interpretivist research spectrum. The other activity that ensures reflexivity (of a verbal nature) is rigorous debate within research and/or supervisory teams about emerging data and the developing narratives of cognitive maps, defence of any theoretical frameworks, the methods adopted and the more tacit aspects of the theory. Often the entire journey of theory development is an exercise in rigorous reflexivity.

8.6 Concluding Statements

This chapter set out to achieve three things. The first aim is to introduce pharmacy practice researchers to the myriad of management theories available for research at multiple levels—from individual through organisational to the environmental level. In summary form the aim is to highlight theories that have, and have not been adopted by pharmacy practice researchers. Clearly there are areas that are well covered by the literature, including social cognitive, organisational effectiveness and employee commitment, and areas that haven't, mainly the macro-level environmental theories. Second, the aim is to introduce some of the assumptions that need to be considered and decisions made when building and testing organisational theory as pharmacy practice researchers and to also understand what theory is, and what it is not! Theory building needs to be founded on ontology and epistemologies that align with a subjective approach. The methods must also follow on from this. The third aim is to outline the processes of theory building and testing in some detail. Theory building is an iterative process that is no less rigorous than more empiric theory testing. Theory building is inductive and founded on four main processes; the identification of a need/tension and phenomena, search through motivation to solve a problem, elaboration/research and proclamation/presentation.

The final aim is to outline how in our fields of pharmacy practice research we can ensure the rigour of our theory development processes and deny pure positivists an impression that theory building is any less rigorous than theory testing or any other empirically based research for that matter. Rigour involves consideration of theoretical, procedural, interpretative, triangulation, evaluative facets and aspects of reflexivity which is an all-encompassing approach to managing robust research processes.

References

Ackerman F, Eden C, Cropper S (1990) Cognitive mapping: a user guide, working paper No. 12. Strathclyde University, Glasgow
Allaire Y, Firsirotu ME (1984) Theories of organizational culture. Organ Stud 5(3):193–226. doi:10.1177/017084068400500301
Alvesson M (2002) Understanding organizational culture. Sage, London
Andrews R (2003) Research questions. Continuum, London
Ashkanasy NM, Wilderom CPM, Peterson MF (2000) Handbook of organizational culture and climate. Sage, Thousand Oaks, CA
Bacharach SB (1989) Organizational theories: some criteria for evaluation. Acad Manage Rev 14(4):496–515
Berger PL, Luckmann T (1967) The social construction of reality. Penguin University Books, London
Bissell P, Morgall Traulsen J (2005) Sociology and pharmacy practice, 1st edn. Pharmaceutical Press, London
Braithwaite J, Hyde P, Pope C (eds) (2010) Culture and climate in health care organizations. Palgrave Macmillan, London
Burchell N, Kolb D (2003) Pattern matching organisational cultures. J Aust New Zeal Acad Manage 9(3):50
Byrne BM (2013) Structural equation modeling with AMOS: basic concepts, applications, and programming. Routledge, London
Cameron KS (1985) Institutional effectiveness in higher education: an introduction. Rev High Educ 9(1):1
Cameron KS (1986) Effectiveness as paradox: consensus and conflict in conceptions of organizational effectiveness. Manage Sci 32(5):539–553
Cameron KS, Quinn RE (1999) Diagnosing and changing organisational culture: based on the competing values framework, 1st edn. Addison Wesley, USA
Cameron KS, Whetten DA (1983) Some conclusions about organizational effectiveness. In: Cameron KS, Whetten DA (eds) Organizational effectiveness: a comparison of multiple models. Academic Press, New York, NY
Campbell JP (1976a) Contributions research can make in understanding organisational effectiveness. In: Spray SL (ed) Organisational effectiveness: theory, research and utilization. Kent State University Press, Kent, OH, pp 29–45

Campbell JP (1976b) Contributions research can make in understanding organizational effectiveness. Organ Adm Sci 7(1/2):29

Campbell JP (1977) On the nature of organizational effectiveness. In: Goodman PS, Pennings JM (eds) New perspective on organizational effectiveness. Jossey–Bass, San Francisco, CA

Campbell U, Arrowood S, Kelm M (2013) Positive work culture: a catalyst for improving employee commitment. Am J Health Syst Pharm 70(19)

Conklin MH, Desselle SP (2007) Job turnover intentions among pharmacy faculty. Am J Pharm Educ 71(4):62

Connolly T, Conlon EJ, Deutsch SJ (1980) Organizational effectiveness: a multiple-constituency approach. Acad Manage Rev 5(2):211

Creswell JW (2003) Research design: qualitative, quantitative, and mixed methods approaches, 2nd edn. Sage, Thousand Oaks, CA

Crotty M (1998) The foundations of social research: meaning and perspective in the research process. Sage, London

Davies HTO, Mannion R, Jacobs R, Powell AE, Marshall MN (2007) Exploring the relationship between senior management team culture and hospital performance. Med Care Res Rev 64 (1):46–65

Deal TE, Kennedy AA (1982) Corporate cultures. Addison–Wesley, Reading, MA

Denison DR, Mishra AK (1995) Toward a theory of organisational culture and effectiveness. Organ Sci 6(2):204–223

Denzin NK, Lincoln YS (eds) (2005) The Sage handbook of qualitative research, 3rd edn. Sage, Thousand Oaks, CA

Desselle SP (2005) Job turnover intentions among Certified Pharmacy Technicians. J Am Pharm Assoc (2003) 45(6):676–683

Desselle SP, Holmes ER (2007) Structural model of Certified Pharmacy Technicians' job satisfaction. J Am Pharm Assoc (2003) 47(1):58–72

Dubin R (1969) Theory building. Free Press, New York, NY

Eisenhardt KM (1989) Building theories from case study research. Acad Manage Rev 14 (4):532–550

Farris KB, Schopflocher DP (1999) Between intention and behavior: an application of community pharmacists' assessment of pharmaceutical care. Soc Sci Med 49(1):55–66

Fink RJ, Draugalis J, McGhan WF (1989) Commitment to the profession of pharmacy: are there sex differences? Am Pharm NS29(1):28–34

Freeman T, Peck E (2010) Culture made flesh: discourse, performativity and materiality. In: Braithwaite J, Hyde P, Pope C (eds) Culture and climate in health care organizations. Palgrave Macmillan, London

Frese M (2005) Grand theories and mid-range theories: cultural effects on theorising and the attempt to understand active approaches to work. In: Smith KG, Hitt MA (eds) Great minds in management: the process of theory development. Oxford University Press, Oxford

Gaither CA (1999) Career commitment: a mediator of the effects of job stress on pharmacists' work-related attitudes. J Am Pharm Assoc 39(3):353–361

Gaither CA, Kahaleh AA, Doucette WR, Mott DA, Pederson CA, Schommer JC (2008) A modified model of pharmacists' job stress: the role of organizational, extra-role, and individual factors on work-related outcomes. Res Social Adm Pharm 4(3):231–243. doi:10.1016/j.sapharm.2008.04.001

Gaither CA, Nadkarni A (2012) Interpersonal interactions, job demands and work-related outcomes in pharmacy. Int J Pharm Pract 20(2):80–89. doi:10.1111/j.2042-7174.2011.00165.x

Geertz C (1973) The interpretation of cultures. Basic Books, New York, NY

Grbich CF (2004) New approaches in social research. Sage, London

Hofstede G, Neuijen B, Ohayv D, Sanders G (1990) Measuring organizational cultures: a qualitative and quantitative study across twenty cases. Adm Sci Q 35(2):286

Huff AS (2005) Managerial and organisational cognition: islands of coherence. In: Smith KG, Hitt MA (eds) Great minds in management: the process of theory development. Oxford University Press, Oxford

Hussey J, Hussey R (1997) Business research: a practical guide for undergraduate and postgraduate students, 1st edn. Palgrave Macmillan, New York, NY

Jackson RA, Smith MC, Mikeal RL (1975) Quality of pharmaceutical services: structure, process and state board requirements. Drugs Health Care 2(1):39–48

Jick TD (1979) Mixing qualitative and quantitative methods: triangulation in action. Adm Sci Q 24:602–611

Johnson JA (1996) Self-efficacy theory as a framework for community pharmacy-based diabetes education programs. Diabetes Educ 22(3):237–241

Kelly GA (1955) The psychology of personal constructs. Norton, New York, NY

Kerlinger FN (1979) Behavioural research: a conceptual approach. Rinehart & Winston, New York, NY

Kernick D (2004) Organisational culture and complexity. In: Kernick D (ed) Complexity and healthcare organisation: a view from the street. Radcliffe Medical Press, Oxford

Kong SX (1995) Predictors of organizational and career commitment among Illinois pharmacists. Am J Health Syst Pharm 52(18):2005–2011

Kotter J (1995) Leading change: why transformation efforts fail. Harv Bus Rev 73(2):59–67

Kotter J, Heskett J (1992) Corporate culture and performance. Free Press, New York, NY

Kuhn TS (1970) The structure of scientific revolutions. Chicago University Press, Chicago, IL

Kvale S (1996) InterViews: an introduction to qualitative research interviewing. Sage, Thousand Oaks, CA

Kvale S (2007) Doing interviews. Sage, London

Lee C, Segal R, Kimberlin C, Smith WT, Weiler RM (2014) Reliability and validity for the measurement of moral disengagement in pharmacists. Res Social Adm Pharm 10(2):297–312

Liamputtong P, Ezzy D (2005) Qualitative research methods, 2nd edn. Oxford University Press, Melbourne

Lincoln YS, Guba EG (1985) Naturalistic inquiry, 1st edn. Sage, Newbury Park, CA

Locke EA, Latham GP (2005) Goal setting theory: theory building by induction. In: Smith KG, Hitt MA (eds) Great minds in management: the process of theory development. Oxford University Press, Oxford

Mannion R, Davies HTO, Harrison S, Konteh FH, Greener I, McDonald R, Hyde P (2010) Changing management cultures and organisational performance in the NHS (OC2). National Institute for Health Research, London

Mannion R, Davies HTO, Marshall MN (2005) Cultural characteristics of "high" and "low" performing hospitals. J Health Organ Manag 19(6):431–439

Mannion R, Goddard M (2002) Performance measurement and improvement in health care. Appl Health Econ Health Policy 1(1):13–23

Martin J (1992) Cultures in organisations: three perspectives, 1st edn. Oxford University Press, New York, NY

Martin J (2002) Organisational culture: mapping the terrain, 1st edn. Sage, Thousand Oaks, CA

Martin J, Sitkin S, Boehm M (1985) Founders and the elusiveness of a cultural legacy. In: Frost P, Moore L, Louis M, Lundberg C, Martin J (eds) Organisational culture. Sage, Beverly Hills, CA

Merriam SB (1988) Case study research in education: a qualitative approach. Jossey–Bass, San Francisco, CA

Metzger AH, Finley KN, Ulbrich TR, McAuley JW (2010) Pharmacy faculty members' perspectives on the student/faculty relationship in online social networks. Am J Pharm Educ 74(10):188

Michalski GV, Cousins JB (2000) Differences in stakeholder perceptions about training evaluation: a concept mapping/pattern matching investigation. Eval Program Plann 23(2):211–230

Miles J (ed) (2014) New directions in management and organization theory. Cambridge Scholars, Newcastle Upon Tyne

Miles MB, Huberman M (1999) Qualitative data analysis: an expanded sourcebook, 2nd edn. Sage, Thousand Oaks, CA

Mintzberg H (2005) Developing theory about the development of theory. In: Smith KG, Hitt MA (eds) Great minds in management: the process of theory development. Oxford University Press, Oxford

Morgan G, Smircich L (1980) The case for qualitative research. Acad Manage J 5(4):491–500

Morse JM (1994) Emerging from the data: the cognitive processes of analysis in qualitative inquiry. In: Morse JM (ed) Critical issues in qualitative research methods. Sage, Thousand Oaks, CA

Mutavdzic A (2010) Hospital pharmacists and behavioural change theory: who, why and how? J Pharm Pract Res 40(1):43–45

Nonaka I (2005) Managing organizational knowledge: theoretical and methodological foundations. In: Smith K, Hitt M (eds) Great minds in management: the process of theory development. Oxford University Press, Oxford

Oldham GR, Hackman RJ (2005) How job characteristics theory happened. In: Smith KG, Hitt MA (eds) Great minds in management: the process of theory development. Oxford University Press, Oxford, pp 151–170

Owusu-Daaku F, Smith F, Shah R (2008) Addressing the workforce crisis: the professional aspirations of pharmacy students in Ghana. Pharm World Sci 30(5):577–583. doi:10.1007/s11096-008-9214-7

Panyawuthikrai P, Sakulbumrungsil R, Wongwiwatthananukit S, Pitaknitinan K (2005) Development of perceived community pharmacy service quality scale in client perspective for Thai community pharmacy accreditation. Thai J Hosp Pharm 15(2):151–161

Patton MQ (1980) Qualitative evaluation methods. Sage, Beverly Hills, CA

Patton MQ (1990) Qualitative evaluation and research methods. Sage, Newbury Park, CA

Perkins RJ, Horsburgh M, Coyle B (2008) Attitudes, beliefs and values of students in undergraduate medical, nursing and pharmacy programs. Aust Health Rev 32(2):252–255

Peters T, Waterman RH (1982) In search of excellence. Harper Collins, New York, NY

Pfeffer J (2005) Developing resource dependence theory: how theory is affected by its environment. In: Smith K, Hitt MA (eds) Great minds in management: the process of theory development. Oxford University Press, Oxford

Popper KR (1959) The logic of scientific discovery. Basic Books, New York, NY

Rogers ER, King SR (2012) The influence of a patient-counselling course on the communication apprehension, outcomes expectations and self-efficacy of first-year pharmacy students. Am J Pharm Educ 76(8):63–69

Scahill SL (2012) Exploring the nature of the relationship between organisational culture and organisational effectiveness within six New-Zealand community-based pharmacies. University of Auckland, Auckland

Scahill SL, Harrison J, Carswell P (2010) What constitutes an effective community pharmacy? Development of a preliminary model of organizational effectiveness through concept mapping with multiple stakeholders. Int J Qual Health Care 22(4):324–332. doi:10.1093/intqhc/mzq033

Schein EH (1985) Organisational culture and leadership, 1st edn. Jossey–Bass, San Francisco, CA

Schein EH (1996) Culture: the missing concept in organization studies. Adm Sci Q 41(2):229–240

Scott T, Mannion R, Davies HTO, Marshall MN (2003a) Healthcare performance and organisational culture, 1st edn. Radcliffe Medical Press, Oxford

Scott T, Mannion R, Marshall MN, Davies HTO (2003b) Does organisational culture influence health care performance? A review of the evidence. J Health Serv Res Policy 8(2):105–117

Siehl C, Martin J (1990) Organizational culture: a key to financial performance? In: Schneider B (ed) Organisational climate and culture. Jossey–Bass, San Francisco, CA

Silverman D (2001) Interpreting qualitative data: methods for analysing talk, text and interaction. Sage, London

Smith KG, Hitt MA (eds) (2005) Great minds in management: the process of theory development. Oxford University Press, Oxford

Smith L, Bosnic-Anticevich S, Mitchell B, Saini B, Krass I, Armour C (2005) Collaborative goal setting in community pharmacy: towards the effective self-management of asthma. Aust J Psychol 57:255

Smith L, Nguyen T, Seeto C, Saini B, Brown L (2011) The role of non-clinicians in a goal setting model for the management of allergic rhinitis in community pharmacy settings. Patient Educ Couns 85(2):e26–e32. doi:10.1016/j.pec.2010.10.003

Trochim WMK, Kane M (2005) Concept mapping: an introduction to structured conceptualization in health care. Int J Qual Health Care 17(3):187–191

Weick KE (1995) Sensemaking in organizations. Sage, Thousand Oaks, CA

Weick KE (2005) The experience of theorising. In: Smith KG, Hitt MA (eds) Great minds in management: the process of theory development. Oxford University Press, Oxford

Whetten DA (1989) What constitutes a theoretical contribution? Acad Manage Rev 13:490–495

White L, Klinner C (2012) Service quality in community pharmacy: an exploration of determinants. Res Social Adm Pharm 8(2):122–132. doi:10.1016/j.sapharm.2011.01.002

Wilderom CPM, Glunk U, Maslowski R (2000) Organisational culture as a predictor of organisational performance. In: Ashkanasy NM, Wilderom CPM, Peterson MF (eds) Handbook of organizational culture and climate. Sage, Thousand Oaks, CA, 629 pp

Williamson O (2005) Transaction cost economics: the process of theory development. In: Smith K, Hitt M (eds) Great minds in management: the process of theory development. Oxford University Press, Oxford

Winter S (2005) Developing evolutionary theory for economics and management. In: Smith K, Hitt M (eds) Great minds in management: the process of theory development. Oxford University Press, Oxford

Yin RK (1994) Case study research: design and methods, vol 5, 1st edn. Sage, Thousand Oaks, CA

Young HN, Dilworth TJ, Mott DA, Cox ED, Moreno MA, Brown RL (2013) Pharmacists' provision of information to Spanish-speaking patients: a social cognitive approach. Res Social Adm Pharm 9(1):4–12

Zucker LG, Darby MR (2005) An evolutionary approach to institutions and social construction: process and structure. In: Smith KG, Hitt MA (eds) Great minds in management: the process of theory development. Oxford University Press, Oxford

Chapter 9
Applying Pharmacoeconomics in Community and Hospital Pharmacy Research

Syed Tabish Razi Zaidi and Zaheer-Ud-Din Babar

Abstract Increasing pressure on maximising the output from limited resources has forced health-care policy makers to use health economic evaluation tools to evaluate the efficacy and efficiency of pharmacy services. Increasingly to evaluate these services, pharmacoeconomic evaluation is being used. This chapter introduces the concept of pharmacoeconomics and discusses different pharmacoeconomic methodologies. It also traverses literature covering economic evaluation studies in community and hospital pharmacy setting. The chapter discusses conducting economic evaluations and debates issues related to data sources, perspectives, costs, outcomes measures, sensitivity analysis and strengths, weaknesses and opportunities related to this research.

9.1 Introduction

Medicine expenditure is growing globally. This is well reflected by the fact that the prescription drug expenditures in the United States have more than doubled over the last decade; the US spent $120 billion on prescription medicines in the year 2000 compared with $263 billion in 2011 (CDC 2014). Similar trends have been observed across the world where pharmaceutical expenditures per capita in Organisation for Economic Co-operation and Development (OECD) countries have consistently increased over the period of 2008–2013 (OECD 2014).

S.T.R. Zaidi (✉)
Department of Pharmacy, School of Medicine, University of Tasmania, Private Bag 26, Hobart 7001, Tasmania, Australia
e-mail: Tabish.RaziZaidi@utas.edu.au

Z.-U.-D. Babar
Faculty of Medical and Health Sciences, School of Pharmacy, University of Auckland, Private Mail Bag 92019, Auckland, New Zealand
e-mail: z.babar@auckland.ac.nz

Given the growing pressures of cost-containment initiatives, funding decisions are increasingly based on objective data. Funding bodies in the United Kingdom (UK) (Rawlins et al. 2010) and Australia (Committee PBA 2014) require pharmacoeconomic and budget impact analysis at the time of submission for new Health Technology applications. The majority of pharmacy practice research activities are geared towards new pharmacy services and aim to introduce the research as a routine professional practice (Martinez et al. 2013; Ottenbros et al. 2014). Nevertheless, new pharmacy services should demonstrate the value for money when competing with initiatives proposed by other disciplines such as medicine, nursing and allied health (Chan and Wang 2004). In this context, pharmacoeconomics (PE) research can be a useful tool for practising pharmacists, pharmacy managers and those who are involved in pharmacy practice research and in quality improvement projects.

9.2 Pharmacoeconomics

Pharmacoeconomics (PE) is an established discipline of Health Economics. It is a scientific discipline that compares the value of one pharmaceutical agent, service or program to another in an attempt to make conclusion about the preferred choice from payer, society or an individual perspective. Table 9.1 briefly describes the types of pharmacoeconomic analysis; however, a detailed description of the types and methodologies is beyond the scope of this chapter and has been described elsewhere (Drummond et al. 2005). The subsequent sections of this chapter will discuss the available PE research methods, drawing on examples from the existing literature and possible applications to the practice of pharmacy.

9.3 Relevance of Pharmacoeconomics to Pharmacy Practice Research

There are many applications of pharmacoeconomics in pharmacy practice research. Economic analysis of medicines prior to inclusion in hospital formulary, evaluation of unique pharmacy services, estimating willingness to pay for pharmacy services by consumers and cost consequence of various pharmacy models are few examples in this area. The most frequent application of pharmacoeconomics methodology in the pharmacy discipline is the evaluation of medicines to determine their relative cost-effectiveness to similar agents that are already available in the market. This is partly because such evaluations are often required by payers of pharmaceutical services (Rawlins et al. 2010; Committee PBA 2014). While a number of studies reporting pharmacy practice research have included costs associated with pharmacy services (Branham et al. 2013; Lucca et al. 2012; Desborough et al. 2012; Kopp

Table 9.1 Types of Pharmacoeconomics analyses and relevant examples

Type of analysis	Brief description	Unique practical applications
Cost-minimisation analysis (CMA)	Analysis to identify the most economical option when efficacy of comparison is similar	Choosing generics of a same medicine; selecting medicine from the same class; selecting dispensing software for pharmacy
Cost-effectiveness analysis (CEA)	Analysis to identify the most economical option when efficacy is not similar. Outcomes are measure as increase effectiveness delivered for each $ invested	Choosing model of care such as hospital admissions vs. day care admissions; service delivery such as Pharmacist vs. nurse run asthma clinic; choosing medicine with same outcome: Atorvastatin vs. Rosuvastatin
Cost–benefit analysis (CBA)	Analysis to identify the most economical option when efficacy is not similar like CEA. Outcomes are measure as net $ benefit	Above mentioned examples are CEA if outcomes are presented as incremental effectiveness per $ invested OR CBA if outcomes are presented as net $ benefit
Cost–utility analysis (CUA)	Analysis to identify the particular option that will deliver the best utilisation of existing resources. Outcomes are measured in terms of utility measures such as Quality Adjusted Life Years (QALYs) for each $ invested	Allocation of resources across various clinical areas such as funding a smoking cessation program or allocating resources for staff lounge. Choosing an antiemetic for hospital formulary for cancer patients or a new analgesic for chronic pain

et al. 2007; Hilleman et al. 2004; Zaidi et al. 2003; Crowson et al. 2002; Devlin et al. 1997; Dranitsaris et al. 1995), the robust use of pharmacoeconomic analysis is limited (Saokaew et al. 2013; Rubio-Valera et al. 2013; Aspinall et al. 2013; Weant et al. 2009; Chisholm et al. 2000).

9.3.1 Economic Evaluations of Pharmacy Practice Research

A number of pharmacy practice studies have reported economic evaluations as a part of their methodology. Applying economic evaluation to pharmacists' interventions was common in early studies (Kopp et al. 2007; Zaidi et al. 2003; Crowson et al. 2002; Devlin et al. 1997; Chuang et al. 1994; Cooper 1997; Cowper et al. 1998), whereas recent studies focus more on disease-specific contribution of the pharmacists' role (Rubio-Valera et al. 2013; Aspinall et al. 2013; Weant et al. 2009; Cies and Varlotta 2013; Gray et al. 2007; van Boven et al. 2014; Johnson 2009; Klepser et al. 2012; Perraudin et al. 2013; Thavorn and Chaiyakunapruk 2008). A bulk of published economic evaluations of pharmacists' interventions have been conducted within hospital settings (Kopp et al. 2007; Zaidi et al. 2003; Crowson et al. 2002; Devlin et al. 1997; Chuang et al. 1994; Cooper

1997; Cowper et al. 1998) as opposed to community settings (Branham et al. 2013; Desborough et al. 2012; Marciante et al. 2001; Avery et al. 2012). A brief discussion of available studies according to the area of investigations will be presented in the following section.

9.3.1.1 Economic Evaluations of Pharmacists' Interventions

A number of studies have evaluated the cost impact of pharmacist's interventions in critical (Lucca et al. 2012; Kopp et al. 2007; Zaidi et al. 2003; Devlin et al. 1997; Chuang et al. 1994) and noncritical care settings (Crowson et al. 2002; Cooper 1997). Most of the critical care setting studies have focused on direct cost savings associated with a pharmacist's intervention to justify the additional cost of having a clinical pharmacist on board (Zaidi et al. 2003; Devlin et al. 1997; Chuang et al. 1994). These studies are of shorter duration, ranging from 4 to 13 weeks. An important aspect of pharmacist's presence in critical care settings is related to educating prescribers and nurses about medicines use. This fact is highlighted by a Malaysian study that demonstrated a relative decrease in the number of interventions over a four-week study period (Zaidi et al. 2003).

Studies evaluating pharmacists' interventions in non-critical and community settings are of a comparatively longer duration (Branham et al. 2013; Desborough et al. 2012; Cooper 1997; Cowper et al. 1998; Avery et al. 2012; Wallerstedt et al. 2012). Furthermore, studies from community settings are mostly multi-centred and often have large number of patients. This gives them sufficient power for data analysis and also makes findings generalizable (Branham et al. 2013; Desborough et al. 2012; Avery et al. 2012). Following the trend from critical care-related studies, most studies of pharmacists' interventions in community settings have focused on direct cost savings. These studies also have placed little emphasis on the cost impact of patients as well as on process-related outcomes such as length of hospital stay, quality of life, educational impact and prevention of Adverse Drug Events (ADEs).

Other than the direct cost savings resulting from pharmacists' interventions, there are also benefits in patient health outcomes. These are important for two reasons: first, cost savings resulting from such heath outcomes are often greater than the direct cost savings from medicines use and, therefore, omitting such outcomes can significantly underestimate the economic impact of pharmacists' interventions. Second, such outcomes can contribute to administrative decision making and help convince decision makers about the importance of pharmacists' role in a given area. Adverse drug events are often associated with an increase in a patient's length of stay and morbidity and mortality (Gyllensten et al. 2014; Kane-Gill et al. 2010). It has been estimated that the cost of managing ADEs can be as high as around 10 % of the total health-care cost (Gyllensten et al. 2014). One particular study of interventions made by clinical pharmacist in surgical ICU reported cost avoidance of more than US$200,000 over a 5-month period (Kopp et al. 2007).

9.3.1.2 Economic Evaluations of Disease Management by Pharmacists

Earlier reports of economic evaluations of pharmacists' role in the management of a disease or condition can be found as early as 50 years ago (Mutchie et al. 1979). However, most older studies were focused on a particular aspect of disease management instead of on the pharmacist solely managing a disease or condition (Dranitsaris et al. 1995; Mutchie et al. 1979). A number of recent studies have investigated the cost-effectiveness of pharmacist-managed care for a variety of disease states such as pharmacist-managed smoking-cessation clinics (Thavorn and Chaiyakunapruk 2008), asthma program (Chan and Wang 2004), diabetes and heart disease (Branham et al. 2013), depression clinics (Rubio-Valera et al. 2013) and anaemia management in end stage renal disease (Aspinall et al. 2013).

Compared to the economic evaluations of pharmacists' interventions, most recent studies evaluating pharmacists' impact on disease management have employed formal pharmacoeconomic analysis including sensitivity analysis (Rubio-Valera et al. 2013; Aspinall et al. 2013; Thavorn and Chaiyakunapruk 2008). Sensitivity analysis is where researchers modify the cost of different study variables to assess the cost-effectiveness of a particular intervention under different scenarios (Drummond et al. 2005). This allows policy makers to assess risks involved in funding a particular service or health technology. This is because as individual costs and the probability of attaining intended outcomes may vary from one practice settings to other or from one health-system to another.

Another feature of published pharmacoeconomic studies in pharmacist-managed disease states is the detailed description of cost-effectiveness modelling and associated costs and consequences estimations (Rubio-Valera et al. 2013; Aspinall et al. 2013; Thavorn and Chaiyakunapruk 2008). An overarching aim of publishing scientific research is to contribute to the existing scientific literature so others can benefit from the literature. Unfortunately, apart from few well-conducted pharmacoeconomic studies, the majority of studies have methodological limitations thus making it difficult for other investigators to either adopt the reported methodology or to compare their own results with that of published literature (Elliott et al. 2014). Future studies evaluating the economic impact of pharmacist's interventions and pharmacist-based care models should focus on direct and indirect costs associated with patients' and process-based outcomes. This would then be helpful to assess the true nature of pharmacist contributions.

The discussion so far has been focused on introducing readers to the various types of pharmacoeconomic analyses, their application in pharmacy practice research and the limitations of the existing literature. The following section will briefly discuss some key considerations in designing a pharmacoeconomic analysis.

9.3.2 Designing a Pharmacoeconomic Analysis

A detailed description of a step-wise approach to designing a pharmacoeconomic analysis is beyond the scope of this chapter. Guidance on designing PE studies is available from the experts in the field (Drummond et al. 2005). Furthermore, World Health Organisation (WHO) has developed guidelines on generalised cost-effectiveness analyses that provide excellent commentary on some of the methodological issues on the subject (Tan Torres Edejer et al. 2003). The purpose of this particular section is rather to introduce readers to some of the considerations and background work required for designing and conducting a pharmacoeconomic analysis. Although most of this will be applicable to general economic analysis, the discussion will focus on pharmacy practice research. In order to keep this discussion relevant to the practice of pharmacy, two distinct case studies are chosen, one from hospital pharmacy and the other from community pharmacy settings (Box 9.1).

9.3.3 Scope of the Study

Defining the scope of a study is one of the first key steps. The scope of the study needs to be realistic and should feed into one's own practice setting.

Being realistic means conducting the study within the context of available data sources. For example, it might be desirable to measure long term patient-related outcomes such as mortality, morbidity and hospitalisations while measuring the cost-effectiveness of a pharmacist managed Chronic Obstructive Pulmonary Disease (COPD) clinic. However, this may not be realistic as these are long term outcomes requiring substantial time to show improvements. Hence, the researchers in this particular case may want to focus on direct cost savings, length of stay and concordance data, for example. Though the data may still be collected on long term outcomes from hospital medical records, any association found would be most likely unreliable where the duration of intervention is shorter. Contrarily, if the proposed intervention is planned to be delivered over at least 6–12 months, to not include clinical outcomes data would be inappropriate.

Box 9.1. Case Studies of Hospital and Community Pharmacy Settings
Hospital case study:
Poor compliance to antibiotic prescribing guidelines at your hospital is a chronic problem. As such, there is a plan to implement an electronic decision support system to streamline restricted antibiotics approval prior to prescribing in an attempt to improve physician's compliance to the prescribing guidelines. You are the project pharmacist and the hospital administrator

(continued)

Box 9.1 (continued)

wants to know if the cost of implementing an electronic decision support is justifiable?
  Community case study:
  You are the newly appointed strategic planning manager of a company that manages a brand of chains of pharmacies. Under increasing competition, the board of directors is considering better engagement with patients to ensure their loyalty to the company. There is a plan to roll out a memo-care program that will incorporate prescription reminders, active communication with patients at each repeat dispensing and monitoring of compliance and adverse effects by pharmacists, so as to ensure patients experience a visible difference that may translate into long term loyalty with the pharmacy brand. The board wants you to evaluate the cost-effectiveness of this strategy.

Considerations to the relevant practice settings are also vital, as the scope for both community and hospital settings would be different. This is due to differences in the operations and priorities of each health-care setting as well as the way in which these services are funded. Hospital-based interventions are likely to have complex indirect costs such as loss of productivity due to illness, opportunity cost due to funding of the studied intervention, expensive diagnostic procedures, to name a few (Locatelli and Marazzi 2013; Jackson 2000). Whereas in community-based economic evaluations, it is likely to be less complex as fewer indirect costs need to be incorporated.

Using the hospital case study from Box 9.1, the overall aim of the intervention is to improve a physician's concordance to the prescribing guidelines and therefore the scope is focused on concordance rather than clinical outcomes. However, the community case (Box 9.1) will be broader in scope as it aims to implement multiple interventions such as prescription reminders, close communication, monitoring of compliance and adverse effects. While such complexity will play an important role in measuring costs and deciding which variables to include in the economic evaluation, the scope of this evaluation is reasonably straightforward. The primary aim of this intervention is to increase customer loyalty, and therefore the scope of the intervention focuses on customer satisfaction, proportion of repeat dispensing and long term loyalty. It does not take in account other meaningful but irrelevant outcomes (in context of the evaluation) such as hospitalisation attainment of target clinical measures and health-related quality of life.

9.3.4 Choosing Perspective

Pharmacoeconomic analysis can be carried out from a variety of perspectives such as patient's perspective, insurer's perspective, government perspective or societal perspective. Perspective refers to the funder of a particular intervention or service in question. While the choice of perspective appears to be simplistic, in reality choosing a perspective can be a complex process (Tan Torres Edejer et al. 2003).

The societal perspective is the preferred perspective within WHO guidelines (Tan Torres Edejer et al. 2003) and experts in the field support its use as well (Byford and Raftery 1998). Nevertheless, the societal perspective has its own limitations. First, the concept that society (or tax payers at large) is paying for health-care services or the intervention in question may only be applicable in public health-care system and it is challenging to apply the same concept to private insurance system or in developing countries where patients often pay for their own health expenses. Second, an estimation of all possible costs related to the societal perspective can be challenging and may not always be quantifiable (Mason and Mason 2006). Third, a societal perspective may not be applicable to some economic analysis. This third limitation is quite relevant to pharmacy practice research specifically during the initial phase of the studies.

Pharmacy practice research often proposes models of care that are collaborative in nature, where pharmacists are offering their services in collaboration with other health-care professionals such as nurses or doctors (Zaidi et al. 2003; Cooper 1997; Avery et al. 2012). Having said that, a number of pharmacist-based patient care interventions can and should be evaluated from a societal perspective, especially while being considered for a wider implementation. Particular examples of such services are pharmacists undertaking government-subsidised home and residential aged care medicine reviews in Australia (Sorensen et al. 2004) and similar program known as Meds-Check in Canada (Grindrod et al. 2013).

Most single site hospital-based or small scale community-based economic evaluations can choose a non-societal perspective. However, in large scale intervention studies, using societal perspective may be a better option. Referring back to Box 9.1, the specific aim of the electronic decision support is reasonably narrow and a societal perspective may not be suitable for this evaluation regardless whether the hospital is funded from public or from private resources. However, if the same system is found to be economically feasible and there is a will to expand the system to a number of public hospitals, then a societal perspective will be worth exploring. Given the obvious commercial nature of the community pharmacy example (Box 9.1), a company or payer perspective will be perhaps the most reasonable choice.

9.4 Choosing Particular Analysis

Most economic analyses are applicable to pharmacy practice research. Cost-minimisation analysis is more applicable to in-house projects where pharmacy departments within hospitals or community pharmacy organisations can look into different service delivery models, for example, or choosing generics for a given drug. Cost-effectiveness analysis is more likely to be used for intervention studies (Branham et al. 2013; Avery et al. 2012) and studies evaluating pharmacist-based care model for chronic diseases such as asthma (Chan and Wang 2004) and smoking-cessation programs (Thavorn and Chaiyakunapruk 2008). The limited use of cost–benefit analysis compared with cost-effectiveness analysis can be explained in the context of technical challenges in defining the cost of clinical outcomes. As shown in Table 9.1, cost–benefit analysis (CBA) requires all consequences of a particular intervention to be translated into monetary value and there are ethical concerns in putting a monetary figure on certain humanistic and clinical outcomes (Drummond et al. 2005; Mason and Mason 2006). Nevertheless, CBA can be reasonably applied for most interventions especially while evaluating a new pharmacy model (Desborough et al. 2012; Zaidi et al. 2003; Chisholm et al. 2000), while cost–utility analysis (CUA) can be applied for different intervention in isolation to another (Drummond et al. 2005). However, this is rare in pharmacy practice research as mostly a direct comparator is available.

Considering the example of electronic decision support from Box 9.1, CEA as well as CBA are equally applicable in this scenario. Nevertheless, CBA will simply provide the net benefit ratio of the intervention and will not be able to summarise the relative increase in guideline adoption. Conversely, CEA will be able to provide the relative increase in guideline adoption as incremental cost-effectiveness ratio with varying degrees of physicians' concordance with the guidelines, and hence this would be more applicable.

With regard to the community pharmacy intervention (Box 9.1), CBA is preferred. This is because CBA will provide a clear indication of return on investment in terms of relative financial gains. Though CEA will provide information on customer-retention rates and may be considered a suitable method, it will not provide information about the net financial benefit. Given the payer's perspective in the scope of Memo-Care program, to retain and grow business in the competing environment, CBA will be preferred over CEA in this particular example.

9.4.1 Estimating Costs

Costs and outcomes are the essential part of any pharmacoeconomic analysis. A number of factors are related to the estimation of direct and indirect costs of the particular intervention being evaluated. The direct cost of delivering a health-care intervention include the cost of intervention and indirect cost may include the cost of delivering, accessing, maintaining and any associated opportunity cost (which is being lost due to providing the intervention in question) (Drummond et al. 2005; Tan Torres Edejer et al. 2003). As described earlier, most studies evaluating the economic impact of a pharmacist's interventions have not used formal pharmacoeconomic methods and therefore have not included a number of relevant costs in their analyses (Elliott et al. 2014). However, there are few formal pharmacy practice pharmacoeconomic studies in which direct and indirect costs-associated interventions have been studied (Rubio-Valera et al. 2013; Aspinall et al. 2013).

Most notable is the cost-effectiveness analysis of pharmacist's intervention in depression (Rubio-Valera et al. 2013). Authors of this particular study have considered all relevant costs related to not only implementing the intervention but also indirect costs associated with service utilisation, training health-care professionals, resource utilisation and lost productivity (Rubio-Valera et al. 2013). An important issue in estimating costs is that some costs overlap between different categories. A practical and easy to understand example could be the cost of preparing training materials for the delivery of intervention. Although training may differ for different health-care professionals, allocating material preparation costs repetitively will overestimate costs associated with training. Therefore, it is important to avoid such duplication wherever possible. WHO guidelines on generalised CEA clearly recommend avoiding such mistakes (Tan Torres Edejer et al. 2003).

Referring to our examples from Box 9.1, cost estimates for decision support should not only consider cost of procuring and initial implementation of the system but should also include costs for ongoing maintenance and for staff training. Other costs worth considering are costs related to ongoing training of new staff, cost of updating the decision support knowledge base, cost of integration with other system and cost of measuring outcomes of interest to demonstrate its value. Another rather difficult to measure cost will be the cost of proportional share of using existing technology infrastructure. Equally important are the costs of comparator in this example. Clinical governance framework in modern health-care requires that all health-care institutions have appropriate systems in place to provide guidance to clinicians about the standard of care. As such, the cost of implementing antibiotic-prescribing guidelines as well as initial implementation and monitoring should be measured. Similarly, the cost of updating such guidelines and ongoing dissemination and monitoring of concordance are important considerations. Contrary to the matters discussed earlier in this chapter, decisions regarding costs are often complicated and are often made according to the availability of existing data sources available to researchers. Costs such as opportunity cost are beyond the scope of this particular example but may be applicable if a broader perspective such as societal perspective has been adopted (Drummond et al. 2005).

Common costs across community pharmacy and hospital examples (Box 9.1) will be costs of training and initial rollout of the 'Memo-Care' program, ongoing training of staff, ongoing monitoring to assess pharmacists' compliance and costs associated with measuring outcomes of interest.

9.4.2 Estimating Benefits or Outcome Measures

Estimating outcome measures and benefits associated with a particular intervention can be tedious. With the exception of pharmacist's based care models of disease management, outcome measures for most pharmacy practice research projects can be measured directly from the existing data sources. For example, studies evaluating specific pharmacist's interventions can measure direct cost savings associated with accepted recommendations (Zaidi et al. 2003). Benefits such as cost of preventing ADEs can not only be complicated but can also be measured from the probability of resultant harm and cost resulting from preventing such harm (Gyllensten et al. 2014). Studies on disease management models require patient-specific outcome measures such as Disease Adjusted Life Years (DALYs) or Quality Adjusted Life Years (QALYs) as well as estimation of years of life saved due to improvement in mortality where applicable (Drummond et al. 2005). A detailed description of these measures is beyond the scope of this chapter; nevertheless, DALYs and QALYs are time-based measures of health that assess the effect of intervention on years of life (Tan Torres Edejer et al. 2003).

In our hospital example, the outcome measure of interest would be antibiotic expenditures, physician's concordance rates with guidelines and physician's acceptance of interventions. Clinical outcomes relevant to the diagnosis being treated can also be considered with some limitations. This is because the intervention here is only changing the mode of guidelines delivery and not the contents of the guidelines per se. However, a case can be made because the intervention is likely to increase the concordance rates with antibiotic prescribing guidelines and perhaps evidence suggests that guideline based care can improve clinical outcomes (McBride et al. 2014). Outcome measures related to community pharmacy would be customer retention, repeat business, patient compliance and customer satisfaction.

9.4.3 Sources of Data

Data on costs and benefits related to an intervention can be collected in a number of ways. Data sources can be classified as routinely collected data and data that require collection for the study purpose. Most medium-to-large organisations are required to record and report financial data based on regulatory requirements. Countries with welfare approach to public health such as Australia, the United Kingdom and a number of European countries often have substantial contribution of public funding to health care. In these countries, financial reporting on each clinical activity is often mandated by the government. Health-care expenses for OECD countries are easily accessible from the organisation's website (OECD 2014) and such data is often created from individual reports from each institution within a particular country.

It is important to review the existing dataset available while conducting an innovative service delivery project in community pharmacies. Measuring and recording baseline data are also pertinent, given in the context that the outcome measures will most likely be affected by the intervention. Apart from individual data sources, researchers can also rely on published model to conduct economic analysis. A number of published pharmacoeconomic studies are available and if the topic of research is similar to a published study then adaptation of an existing model can not only save time but also can provide validity to the research (Sanchez and Lee 2000). Also, in cases where researchers have to estimate their own costs, it is important to define cost as total acquisition cost rather than the unit cost of a particular item.

The examples from Box 9.1 can further explain the use of existing vs. non-existing data sources. Considering the case of electronic decision support, cost will need to be calculated for this intervention. The relevant information technology and finance departments may also be able to provide practical insights on this cost calculation. The costing data may also be available about training of staff from other projects. In the first instance, researchers undertaking economic analysis like the one in the hospital example (Box 9.1) should contact their safety and quality office to see if an existing dataset may be available and is relevant to their study. Hospitals in most countries are accredited by various quality-related organisations. Typical examples are Joint Commission in the US, Care Quality Commission in the UK and Australian Commission on Safety and Quality in Healthcare in Australia. Hence, there is a possibility that some relevant data might be available.

Given the commercial nature of the project related to community pharmacy (Box 9.1), most data related to cost and benefit will already be available in pharmacy records. The bulk of this project cost lies within the project manager whose salary is already taken into account. The time costs of individual pharmacist across the network can also be accessible through human resource department of the organisation. Health benefits of patient compliance are the most difficult outcome to measure if the project has adopted a societal perspective. Nevertheless, published literature on pharmacist's role in disease management can provide useful insights in this area (van Boven et al. 2014; Johnson 2009).

9.5 Discounting and Sensitivity Analysis

Discounting and sensitivity analysis are two different yet inter-related concepts in pharmacoeconomics. Discounting is when researchers adjust for underlying inflation in economy by increasing the cost of a project by certain percentage. This is often correlated to the inflation rate. Sensitivity analysis is when researchers modify the values of costs and benefits in a given economic model to test the performance of the intervention under study. Sensitivity analysis is carried out because of the presence of the uncertainty with economic modelling. Prices can go up or down depending upon the demand of a particular intervention; same is true for the values of a particular benefit as factors other than the interventions may affect the associated benefits. Typical examples can be the availability of superior dispensing software, poor patient compliance or emergence of new adverse effects.

Traditionally, discounting is applied when the intervention under study is implemented over more than a year (Rubio-Valera et al. 2013; Aspinall et al. 2013); nevertheless, WHO guidelines on generalized cost-effectiveness analysis recommend to include discounting in all studies. This is to make them more applicable to practice settings (Tan Torres Edejer et al. 2003). As often publications of results take time, this also helps those considering similar intervention in their own practice settings. Various methods of discounting are available but the most common approach is to use a fixed rate across several years in the proposed economic model (Chan and Wang 2004; Hilleman et al. 2004; Chisholm et al. 2000; Avery et al. 2012). WHO guidelines recommend a fixed rate of 3 % as a baseline for CEA and 6 % for sensitivity analysis. Often discounting is not as universally applied to health outcomes/benefits as it is applied to costs (Chan and Wang 2004; Hilleman et al. 2004; Chisholm et al. 2000; Avery et al. 2012; Tan Torres Edejer et al. 2003)

Sensitivity analysis provides much needed information for decision makers about an intervention in the presence of uncertainty. The other significant reason to conduct a sensitivity analysis includes differences in population studied and population of interest (for a particular intervention), uncertainty in the values of variables in the economic model and uncertainty in study variables (costs as well as benefits) (Tan Torres Edejer et al. 2003).

Researchers undertaking a pharmacoeconomic analysis within pharmacy practice research perform sensitivity analysis by modifying one (one-way) or multiple variables (multi-way) at a time. Existing pharmacoeconomic studies on pharmacy practice research lacks specific sensitivity analysis and where sensitivity analysis has been performed, it lacks appropriate details about the methodology (Elliott et al. 2014). Advanced methods are available for the estimation of sensitivity analyses, and pharmacy practice researchers should pay more attention to such methods to make their research more meaningful (Tan Torres Edejer et al. 2003).

Given the limited scope of both of our practicing examples from Box 9.1, the WHO recommendations on discounting and sensitivity analysis can be used for both projects (Tan Torres Edejer et al. 2003). This means a discounting rate of 3 % for all the costs and a variable rate of 0–3 % for benefits. Sensitivity analysis can use a range of 3–6 % for costs and 0–3 % for benefits.

9.5.1 Reporting Pharmacoeconomic Analysis

Despite the availability of clear recommendations and checklists related to the reporting of pharmacoeconomic analysis (Drummond et al. 2005; Tan Torres Edejer et al. 2003), published reports have been criticized due to limitations in the conduct, analysis and reporting of results (Elliott et al. 2014). There are few plausible explanations for this observation. First, studies reporting pharmacoeconomic evaluations are often published in non-specialty journals, and reviewers available to a particular journal may not have relevant expertise to critically evaluate pharmacoeconomic evaluation. Second, there is a scarcity of economic evaluations of pharmacy practice research and therefore any study reporting pharmacoeconomic evaluation is being looked at favourably. Lastly, the scope of pharmacy practice research carried out in an individual institution is more of a local nature, they are not aimed at global audience hence they are open for criticism.

Fortunately, International Society of Pharmacoeconomics and Outcomes Research (ISPOR) had commissioned a taskforce on developing a consolidated statement on the reporting of pharmacoeconomic evaluations. The taskforce has recently developed and published a statement on the reporting of pharmacoeconomic evaluations. The Consolidated Health Economic Evaluation Reporting Standards (CHEERS) statement is a 24 items checklist and is freely available from the ISPOR website. The checklist provides clear descriptions about each step of a pharmacoeconomic evaluation (http://www.ispor.org/TaskForces/EconomicPubGuidelines.asp) (Husereau et al. 2013).This statement has been endorsed by 12 leading health-care journals including British Medical Journal (Husereau et al. 2013). Researchers interested in publishing the results of their economic evaluations are highly recommended to follow this statement to ensure the quality of their reports as well as maximising the chances of publication.

9.6 Summary

Health-care policy makers require clear information about the relevant costs and benefits associated with new pharmacy services, and pharmacoeconomic evaluations provide the much needed information. However, most studies evaluating the economic impact of pharmacist's interventions have not used formal pharmacoeconomic methods. This chapter aims to improve the understanding about the use of pharmacoeconomics and has attempted to elaborate some of the practical issues surrounding pharmacoeconomic evaluations.

References

Aspinall SL, Smith KJ, Good CB et al (2013) Incremental cost effectiveness of pharmacist-managed erythropoiesis-stimulating agent clinics for non-dialysis-dependent chronic kidney disease patients. Appl Health Econ Health Policy 11(6):653–660

Avery AJ, Rodgers S, Cantrill JA et al (2012) A pharmacist-led information technology intervention for medication errors (PINCER): a multicentre, cluster randomised, controlled trial and cost-effectiveness analysis. Lancet 379(9823):1310–1319

Branham AR, Katz AJ, Moose JS, Ferreri SP, Farley JF, Marciniak MW (2013) Retrospective analysis of estimated cost avoidance following pharmacist-provided medication therapy management services. J Pharm Pract 26(4):420–427

Byford S, Raftery J (1998) Perspectives in economic evaluation. BMJ 316(7143):1529–1530

CDC (2014) Fast stats-health expenditures. http://www.cdc.gov/nchs/fastats/health-expenditures.htm Accessed 16 October 2014

Chan AL, Wang HY (2004) Pharmacoeconomic assessment of clinical pharmacist interventions for patients with moderate to severe asthma in outpatient clinics: experience in Taiwan. Clin Drug Investig 24(10):603–609

Chisholm MA, Vollenweider LJ, Mulloy LL, Wynn JJ, Wade WE, DiPiro JT (2000) Cost-benefit analysis of a clinical pharmacist-managed medication assistance program in a renal transplant clinic. Clin Transplant 14(4 Pt 1):304–307

Chuang LC, Sutton JD, Henderson GT (1994) Impact of a clinical pharmacist on cost saving and cost avoidance in drug therapy in an intensive care unit. Hosp Pharm 29(3):215–218, 221

Cies JJ, Varlotta L (2013) Clinical pharmacist impact on care, length of stay, and cost in pediatric cystic fibrosis (CF) patients. Pediatr Pulmonol 48(12):1190–1194

Committee PBA (2014) Guidelines for preparing submissions to the Pharmaceutical Benefits Advisory Committee. http://www.pbac.pbs.gov.au/. Accessed 16 October 2014

Cooper JW Jr (1997) Consultant pharmacist drug therapy recommendations from monthly drug regimen reviews in a geriatric nursing facility: a two-year study and cost analysis. J Nutr Health Aging 1(3):181–184

Cowper PA, Weinberger M, Hanlon JT et al (1998) The cost-effectiveness of a clinical pharmacist intervention among elderly outpatients. Pharmacotherapy 18(2):327–332

Crowson K, Collette D, Dang M, Rittase N (2002) Transformation of a pharmacy department: impact on pharmacist interventions, error prevention, and cost. Jt Comm J Qual Improv 28 (6):324–330

Desborough JA, Sach T, Bhattacharya D, Holland RC, Wright DJ (2012) A cost-consequences analysis of an adherence focused pharmacist-led medication review service. Int J Pharm Pract 20(1):41–49

Devlin JW, Holbrook AM, Fuller HD (1997) The effect of ICU sedation guidelines and pharmacist interventions on clinical outcomes and drug cost. Ann Pharmacother 31(6):689–695

Dranitsaris G, Warr D, Puodziunas A (1995) A randomized trial of the effects of pharmacist intervention on the cost of antiemetic therapy with ondansetron. Support Care Cancer 3 (3):183–189

Drummond MFSM, Torrance GW, O'Brien BJ, Stoddart GL (2005) Methods for the economic evaluation of health care programmes, 3rd edn. Oxford University Press, Oxford

Elliott RA, Putman K, Davies J, Annemans L (2014) A review of the methodological challenges in assessing the cost effectiveness of pharmacist Interventions. Pharmacoeconomics 32 (12):1185–1199

Gray DR, Garabedian-Ruffalo SM, Chretien SD (2007) Cost-justification of a clinical pharmacist-managed anticoagulation clinic. Ann Pharmacother 41(3):496–501

Grindrod K, Sanghera N, Rahmaan I, Roy M, Tritt M (2013) Living MedsCheck: Learning how to deliver MedsCheck in community practice in Ontario. Can Pharm J (Ott) 146(1):33–38

Gyllensten H, Hakkarainen KM, Hagg S et al (2014) Economic impact of adverse drug events–a retrospective population-based cohort study of 4970 adults. PLoS One 9(3):e92061

Hilleman DE, Faulkner MA, Monaghan MS (2004) Cost of a pharmacist-directed intervention to increase treatment of hypercholesterolemia. Pharmacotherapy 24(8):1077–1083

Husereau D, Drummond M, Petrou S et al (2013a) Consolidated Health Economic Evaluation Reporting Standards (CHEERS) statement. BMJ 346:f1049

Husereau D, Drummond M, Petrou S et al (2013b) Consolidated Health Economic Evaluation Reporting Standards (CHEERS)–explanation and elaboration: a report of the ISPOR Health Economic Evaluation Publication Guidelines Good Reporting Practices Task Force. Value Health 16(2):231–250

Jackson T (2000) Cost estimates for hospital inpatient care in Australia: evaluation of alternative sources. Aust N Z J Public Health 24(3):234–241

Johnson SG (2009) Improving cost-effectiveness of and outcomes from drug therapy in patients with atrial fibrillation in managed care: role of the pharmacist. J Manag Care Pharm 15(6 Suppl B):S19–25

Kane-Gill SL, Jacobi J, Rothschild JM (2010) Adverse drug events in intensive care units: risk factors, impact, and the role of team care. Crit Care Med 38(6 Suppl):S83–89

Klepser DG, Bisanz SE, Klepser ME (2012) Cost-effectiveness of pharmacist-provided treatment of adult pharyngitis. Am J Manag Care 18(4):e145–154

Kopp BJ, Mrsan M, Erstad BL, Duby JJ (2007) Cost implications of and potential adverse events prevented by interventions of a critical care pharmacist. Am J Health Syst Pharm 64(23):2483–2487

Locatelli I, Marazzi A (2013) Robust parametric indirect estimates of the expected cost of a hospital stay with covariates and censored data. Stat Med 32(14):2457–2466

Lucca JM, Ramesh M, Narahari GM, Minaz N (2012) Impact of clinical pharmacist interventions on the cost of drug therapy in intensive care units of a tertiary care teaching hospital. J Pharmacol Pharmacother 3(3):242–247

Marciante KD, Gardner JS, Veenstra DL, Sullivan SD (2001) Modeling the cost and outcomes of pharmacist-prescribed emergency contraception. Am J Public Health 91(9):1443–1445

Martinez AS, Saef J, Paszczuk A, Bhatt-Chugani H (2013) Implementation of a pharmacist-managed heart failure medication titration clinic. Am J Health Syst Pharm 70(12):1070–1076

Mason JM, Mason AR (2006) The generalisability of pharmacoeconomic studies: issues and challenges ahead. Pharmacoeconomics 24(10):937–945

McBride P, Stone NJ, Blum CB (2014) Should family physicians follow the new ACC/AHA cholesterol treatment guideline? Yes: implementing the new ACC/AHA cholesterol guideline will improve cardiovascular Outcomes. Am Fam Physician 90(4):212–216

Mutchie KD, Smith KA, MacKay MW, Marsh C, Juluson D (1979) Pharmacist monitoring of parenteral nutrition: clinical and cost effectiveness. Am J Hosp Pharm 36(6):785–787

OECD (2014) Pharmaceutical expenditure per capita. http://www.oecd-ilibrary.org/social-issues-migration-health/pharmaceutical-expenditure-per-capita_pharmexpcap-table-en. Accessed 16 October 2014

Ottenbros S, Teichert M, de Groot R et al (2014) Pharmacist-led intervention study to improve drug therapy in asthma and COPD patients. Int J Clin Pharm 36(2):336–344

Perraudin C, Le Vaillant M, Pelletier-Fleury N (2013) Cost-Effectiveness of a Community Pharmacist-Led Sleep Apnea Screening Program - A Markov Model. PLoS One 8(6):e63894

Rawlins M, Barnett D, Stevens A (2010) Pharmacoeconomics: NICE's approach to decision-making. Br J Clin Pharmacol 70(3):346–349

Rubio-Valera M, Bosmans J, Fernandez A et al (2013) Cost-effectiveness of a community pharmacist intervention in patients with depression: a randomized controlled trial (PRODEFAR Study). PLoS One 8(8):e70588

Sanchez LA, Lee JT (2000) Applied pharmacoeconomics: modeling data from internal and external sources. Am J Health Syst Pharm 57(2):146–155, quiz 155-146

Saokaew S, Permsuwan U, Chaiyakunapruk N, Nathisuwan S, Sukonthasarn A, Jeanpeerapong N (2013) Cost-effectiveness of pharmacist-participated warfarin therapy management in Thailand. Thromb Res 132(4):437–443

Sorensen L, Stokes JA, Purdie DM, Woodward M, Elliott R, Roberts MS (2004) Medication reviews in the community: results of a randomized, controlled effectiveness trial. Br J Clin Pharmacol 58(6):648–664

Tan Torres Edejer T, Baltussen R, Adam T et al (2003) Making Choices in Health: WHO guide to cost-effectiveness analysis. World Health Organisation, Geneva

Thavorn K, Chaiyakunapruk N (2008) A cost-effectiveness analysis of a community pharmacist-based smoking cessation programme in Thailand. Tob Control 17(3):177–182 van Boven JF, Stuurman-Bieze AG, Hiddink EG, Postma MJ, Vegter S (2014) Medication monitoring and optimization: a targeted pharmacist program for effective and cost-effective improvement of chronic therapy adherence. J Manag Care Pharm 20(8):786–792

Wallerstedt SM, Bladh L, Ramsberg J (2012) A cost-effectiveness analysis of an in-hospital clinical pharmacist service. BMJ Open 2:e000329

Weant KA, Armitstead JA, Ladha AM, Sasaki-Adams D, Hadar EJ, Ewend MG (2009) Cost effectiveness of a clinical pharmacist on a neurosurgical team. Neurosurgery 65(5):946–950, discussion 950-941

Zaidi ST, Hassan Y, Postma MJ, Ng SH (2003) Impact of pharmacist recommendations on the cost of drug therapy in ICU patients at a Malaysian hospital. Pharm World Sci 25(6):299–302

Chapter 10
Concept Mapping and Pattern Matching in Pharmacy Practice Research

Shane L. Scahill

Abstract This chapter aims to introduce techniques to the pharmacy practice research community that have been applied to the wider health services research sector. The health-care environment is busy, complex and ever-changing, and clear and structured thinking about the future is a challenging task. This is an international problem for the health-care sector, and pharmacy has not escaped this challenge. Pharmacists don't have an adequate voice and have been found not to think enough about the future. "Concept mapping" is a generic term that describes any process which helps to represent ideas as pictures or maps. There are many types of concept-mapping techniques, and variants have been used mostly to aid individual creativity in problem solving. Usually this occurs through synthesis of maps by a single person who is endeavouring to conceptualise complex issues within health and find solutions to them. Trochim's Concept-Mapping technique is underpinned by the need for group creativity; it uses mixed methods, is participatory and predominantly interpretative. This means that it is a meld of robust statistical process and subjective interpretation, based on the researcher(s) understanding of study context. The focus of this chapter is to introduce concept mapping and pattern matching and to outline the application of these techniques within the context of community pharmacy practice. A future research agenda is posed.

Keywords Concept mapping • Pattern matching • Pharmaceutical health services research • Structured conceptualisation • Structured thinking in pharmacy

10.1 Introduction

This chapter aims to introduce techniques to the pharmacy practice research community that have been applied to the wider health services research sector. The health-care environment is busy, complex and ever-changing, where clear and

---

S.L. Scahill (✉)
School of Management, Massey Business School, Massey University, Albany, Auckland, New Zealand
e-mail: s.scahill@massey.ac.nz

structured thinking about the future is a challenging task. This is an international problem for the health-care sector, which impacts at multiple levels including: policymakers, funding and planning organisations, individual clinicians and their professional bodies. Some of the issues which are applicable to multiple health-care sectors include how to: define and assess quality of care and quality of life; plan and evaluate services; define and implement safety procedures and utilise evolving technologies effectively (Trochim and Kane 2005). The health sector is complex and more so for pharmacy when individuals pass from one sector of care to another (such as between primary and secondary care) (Maxwell et al. 2013). The challenges described are compounded by increasing pressure on the health-care sector, in order to plan and deliver high performing services in transparent, efficient, effective and sustainable ways through human engagement, to improve performance (Scott et al. 2003).

This is implicit for pharmacy in New Zealand health-care policy, where there is the expectation of improved health outcomes and patient experiences through integration of a broad range of services and along with multi-disciplinary teamwork (Scahill et al. 2010d). Developing solutions to these challenges requires structured and systematic thinking through integration of perspectives from multiple stakeholders and is important in managing the health sector going forward. In addition, all levels of the system (macro, meso and micro) need to be thought about through policy development, service planning and delivery and improvements in individual professional practice (Ferlie and Shortell 2001).

Community pharmacy is a health-care hub (McMillan et al. 2013) that has a central place and important functions within primary care. It has not escaped the pressures of other health-care providers and itself faces a broad array of challenges. Consumers visiting pharmacies that do so for medical reasons range from those seeking over-the-counter (OTC) medicines and advice to those transitioning between hospital and home (or vice versa) who have complex medicines-related problems (MRP) (Maxwell et al. 2013). The community pharmacy sector is going through significant change, and there is a need to think about a number of complex issues micro through macro (Scahill and Babar 2010; Scahill et al. 2010d). The sector as a whole would benefit from policymakers, professional bodies, academics and practitioners focussing on thinking about key issues specific to community pharmacy and planning/evaluating interventions in systematic ways (Scahill et al. 2010d). Over time, community pharmacy has adopted dual identities as business retailer and health-care provider (Scahill 2012a, Scahill SL, Babar ZU (2010)). Considering this potential tension, it is reasonable to suggest that strategic thinking has been dominated by a focus on pharmacy as "retailer" (Scahill and Babar 2010). This is in part due to historic funding mechanisms, but there is also international evidence to suggest that pharmacists may not think enough about "their environment", current issues associated with it and future models of care (Rosenthal et al. 2010; Scahill et al. 2009b).

In fact, pharmacists may be their own worst enemies with respect to the way they "think and act", being inward and negative about the primary care environment, having poor relationships with funders and lacklustre response to integration with the rest of the primary care team Scahill Harrison Sheridan 2009b (Adamcik et al. 1986; Anderson et al. 2003, 2008; Bryant 2006; Bush et al. 2006, 2009; Edmunds and Calnan 2001; Rosenthal et al. 2010; Walker 2000). Truly collaborative service provision requires an active voice, leadership and integrated governance, all of which seem to be missing from the community pharmacy sector in some countries (Rosenthal et al. 2010; Scahill et al. 2009b). Pharmacists don't have an adequate voice and have been found not to think enough about the future (Scahill et al. 2009b). It is important to consider stakeholders when moving forward and to integrate their demands, of which policymakers are a good example. Operations which require at least cooperation and preferably collaboration between community pharmacists and other health care providers [mainly General Practitioners (GPs) and Primary Care Nurses (PCN)] are necessary for moving forward (Scahill 2011; Scahill et al. 2010d). Significant interaction with funders and planners such as District Health Boards (DHBs) and Primary Health Organisations (PHOs—in New Zealand, for example) will also be required in order to achieve strategic "whole of District" shifts in the way service delivery is thought about (Scahill et al. 2009b). This is a trend which echoes internationally, particularly within several Commonwealth countries (Roberts et al. 2006, 2007; Rosenthal et al. 2010; Scahill et al. 2009b).

In New Zealand as with other Commonwealth countries, long-term vision documents generated by professional pharmacy bodies have called for *reprofessionalisation* (Pharmaceutical Society of New Zealand 2004). This is expected to occur through the uptake of enhanced clinical roles and services. Government health policy followed the impetus of professional bodies in New Zealand; in other countries such as the United Kingdom, policy from Government and professional leaders has been developed in tandem (Anderson et al. 2008). The drivers of New Zealand heath policy appear to be two-pronged for improved patient outcomes and to assist the integration of community pharmacy within the rest of the primary health-care team (Scahill 2012a, b). The *reprofessionalisation* agenda, integration within the sector, potential for role restructure, new models of care and service provision and an understanding of what constitutes a high performing community pharmacy under current health policy are complex and significant concepts for the sector to deal with. Understanding and managing complexity is best approached in systematic ways, using change management techniques founded on evidence from robust quantitative and qualitative research (Graetz et al. 2002). There is difficulty in conceptualising pharmacy issues, although increasingly pharmacy practice researchers are adopting organisational behaviour theory in practice and research (Scahill 2008, 2012a, b).

Organisational scientists and health services researchers working in other healthcare sectors have developed a technique dubbed "structured conceptualisation" (Trochim and Kane 2005) for dealing with issues similar to those faced by the community pharmacy sector. This chapter provides an overview of the theory underpinning one form of structured conceptualisation—Trochim's "Concept Mapping" (Trochim and Kane 2005). Pattern matching is a technique derived from concept mapping, and this chapter provides examples of how the principle of structured conceptualisation can be applied (Burchell and Kolb 2003). The focus of this chapter is to introduce concept mapping and pattern matching and to outline the application of these techniques within the context of community pharmacy practice. A brief research agenda underpinned by these techniques is posed for the wider pharmacy sector.

10.2 Structured Conceptualisation

This area of research and planning/evaluation has developed significantly over the last three decades. Since its introduction, Concept Mapping methodology has been used in the health care context in over 20 project areas. It is a well-established technique which has only recently been applied to exploring organisational culture and effectiveness in community pharmacy (Scahill 2012a, b; Scahill et al. 2009a, 2010a, b, c).Concept mapping is a generic term which describes any process that helps to represent ideas as pictures or maps. There are many types of concept mapping techniques, and variants have been used mostly to aid individual creativity in problem solving (Trochim 1989a). Usually, this occurs through synthesis of maps by a single person who is endeavouring to conceptualise complex issues within health and find solutions to them (Trochim and Kane 2005).

The greatest proponent is Professor Bill Trochim (Cornell University) who outlines four notable characteristics that are helpful in addressing the health-care challenges previously outlined (Trochim and Kane 2005). First, concept mapping is purposely designed to integrate input from multiple sources. This is important for the pharmacy sector as it attempts to break down the silos within which it works and to improve policymaker and funder–stakeholder relationships (in some countries). Second, rigorous and sophisticated multi-variate data analyses are used to generate structured outputs. In this way, the process is robust and the pharmacy sector benefits from dealing with challenges in a research savvy manner. Third, the outputs are a visual depiction of a composite group. This is important and useful for future discussion of pharmacy-related matters. Finally, and perhaps most importantly, outputs provide a structure that is immediately available to guide planning and action or evaluation and measurement. This is important for the pharmacy sector and particularly community pharmacy, which internationally is at a policy-inflicted cross-roads (Mossialos et al. 2013; Scahill 2012a, b; Scahill et al. 2010d). There is a great need for the evaluation of ongoing policy and action/interventions relating to this. The pharmacy sector and its key stakeholders should find concept mapping and pattern matching helpful for structured thought about complex issues and action required to remediate these.

10.3 Trochim's Concept Mapping

Trochim's Concept Mapping technique is underpinned by the need for group creativity; it adopts mixed methods philosophies, is participatory but is predominantly interpretative (Trochim 1989a). This means that it is a meld of robust statistical process and subjective interpretation based on the researcher (s) understanding of study context. There is a significant literature on the theoretical underpinning of Trochim's technique. The reader is directed to this for a deeper and richer explanation of the theory, as well as its practical applications (Trochim 1989a, b; Trochim and Kane 2005; Trochim and Linton 1986). Within health care, there appears to be less of a focus on the use of these techniques than in other sectors (Nabitz et al. 2005; Roeg et al. 2005).

The pattern matching technique is an extension of concept mapping. That technique allows comparison of rating scales across two or more variables to elucidate patterns for change, which is fundamental to understanding past, present and future in a complex environment. There are very few studies published which utilise pattern matching in health care, and this method should be considered more often by pharmacy practice researchers (Scahill et al. 2010a).

10.3.1 Steps of Trochim's Concept Mapping

Trochim's concept mapping technique is divided into discrete steps (Fig. 10.1) (Trochim 1989b; Trochim and Kane 2005):

10.3.2 Preparation

Aspects of preparation involve sampling, selection and engagement, outlining the process and providing the brainstorm meeting aims and context of the study. The method allows for development of constructs from the viewpoint of multiple stakeholders through sampling criteria of case sites and individuals (Michalski and Cousins 2000). The aims and background of the concept mapping meeting (s) need to be outlined to the participant groups by the facilitator at the face-to-face meeting or via the internet with the web-based option. Often boundaries need to be placed around the project so that all of the stakeholder groups that are represented are equally informed and able to contribute. The preamble most often involves setting the scene and providing background to any policy drivers or environmental factors that participants (or the sector they work in) are facing.

Fig. 10.1 Concept mapping process Source Scahill (2012b)

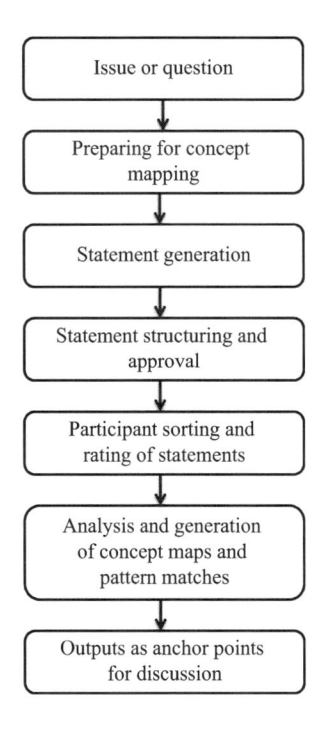

```
Issue or question
      ↓
Preparing for concept
      mapping
      ↓
Statement generation
      ↓
Statement structuring and
       approval
      ↓
Participant sorting and
  rating of statements
      ↓
Analysis and generation
  of concept maps and
    pattern matches
      ↓
Outputs as anchor points
      for discussion
```

10.3.3 Statement Generation

A 2-h face-to-face brainstorm session is usually long enough to generate approximately 100 statements about a predetermined concept. The session needs to be moderated by a facilitator (often the main study researcher) who has completed a training programme prior to project initiation and is familiar with the technique. Training with Concept Systems^{TM} staff (face to face, Webinar or via the telephone) involves project set-up, meeting facilitation techniques and use of the Concept Systems^{TM} software for data collection and analysis. Based on theoretical underpinnings, a focus statement is generated by the researchers prior to the meeting and is used to stimulate discussion within the concept mapping session. This is also able to be undertaken online with the use of Concept Systems^{TM} Global software. The standard focus statement structure is generally:

Please generate statements (short phrases or sentences of less than 15 words) that in your opinion describe...

The statement will make sense if preceded by:

An (construct) is one that...

Participants should be free to articulate whatever they deem to be relevant to the focus statement. Participants should feel they are able to share their knowledge through structured group process. To achieve this, discussion requires moderation in a logical fashion. Participants should be given 15 min to write down statements which provide a starting point and stimulation of further discussion. By going around the table in turn, each participant may contribute a statement to begin the process. The discussion then generally flows from this, until all ideas have been captured and the concept is saturated.

The statements generated are added to a whiteboard, and participants are free to disagree with the individual statements generated by the group. However, disagreement is not a precedent for excluding individual statements in the listing. No criticism is allowed regarding whether individual statements are right or wrong (Roeg et al. 2005; Trochim and Kane 2005). However, it is a requirement that all members understand each statement before it is added to the list. Statements are not able to be added to the list if they are an exact duplication of previously added statements. The facilitator needs to ensure that all individuals are given an equal opportunity to speak, so as not to have a dominant cohort.

10.3.4 Statement Structuring, Statement Validation

Following the face-to-face brainstorming (or online through the web portal), the statements are taken from the printable whiteboard and edited in a uniform manner, so they can be systematically reviewed by participants and later approved. Using Concept Systems™ software, the statements are randomly assigned numbers by the researcher to reduce bias in the sorting stage. Following the methodology suggested by Trochim, participants receive the edited statement list and are given the opportunity to reduce the original statement list further. The lists can be forwarded by email to participants who are asked to identify any duplicated statements. They should also be asked to suggest an alternative statement which in their view would address any duplication. Participants need to be asked to carefully review individual statements and to outline if the researcher's editing has resulted in any misrepresentation. If not, participants need to be asked to formally approve the statements as the "pre-pilot" listing. Once the statement lists are approved, they can be uploaded into the web-based Concept Systems™ software, so participants can sort and rate them.

10.3.5 Statement Sorting and Rating

The process of sorting and rating can be undertaken by participants through the web-based portal. Participants involved in the brainstorm activity should be forwarded an email with a final set of instructions, provided with a hyperlink, login and password and asked to complete the sorting and rating steps. Sorting the statements requires the participant to think about the individual statements as they relate to each other. The instruction for the sorting stage is to "sort the statements into clusters in a way that makes sense to you" (Nabitz et al. 2005).

This is able to be completed by the participants through a drop and drag function within the Concept Systems™ software.

Statements are rated on a Likert scale based on predetermined criteria, commonly—importance, relevance or how typical the statement is of that construct. The rating of statements is not limited to participants who attend the brainstorm sessions. The instrument can be used to rate the statements with a wider audience. The instructions are generally laid out as follows: "rate the statements in terms of how (selected criteria) each statement is to your idea of (named construct) using the electronic dot-click Likert scale ranging from $1 =$ least to $5 =$ most important". Throughout the entire process the researcher has administrator status of the Concept Systems™ software and can view progress of individuals completing different stages of the project. This is helpful for tracking and monitoring the progress of the project.

10.3.6 Data Analysis

Trochim and colleagues have published the rationale and analytic theory supporting their approach to concept mapping. For more detail than this chapter provides, the reader is referred to a bibliography of their work (Trochim 1989a, b, c; Trochim and Kane 2005; Trochim and Linton 1986).

The major calculations performed by the Concept Systems™ software includes: data sorting aggregation, multidimensional scaling, cluster analysis, bridging analysis and sort pile label analysis. The two main statistical techniques used to develop the concept maps are multi-dimensional scaling (MDS) and hierarchical cluster analysis (HCA). Descriptive statistical analyses such as mean ratings of each cluster making up the final solutions are able to be calculated. Statistical analysis does not need to be undertaken to compare the different cluster solutions for selection, as that phase is interpretative. MDS differs from factor analysis, the former being determined by the participants, the latter by the researcher (Scahill 2012a, b).

Following the sorting stage, data from the concept mapping exercise are subjected to MDS. This is an exploratory statistical technique that allows the visualisation of similarities or differences between lists of statements sorted by groups of individuals. MDS takes (dis)simlarity data and represents them as distances in Euclidean space which describes the relationships between distances and angles. In this way, MDS places the statements on a two-dimensional framework and provides the size and shape of each cluster of statements within this frame, dependent on the number of clusters selected when generating the concept maps (Trochim 1989b; Trochim and Linton 1986). An MDS algorithm starts with a matrix of item–item similarities, assigns a location of each item in a dimensional space and is suitable for graphing or 3D visualisation. For each statement, the MDS analysis yields an x and y value which in a bivariate plot constitutes the basic point map form of the concept map. The x, y values are the input for HCA using Ward's algorithm, which has the effect of partitioning the MDS statement map hierarchically into non-overlapping clusters (Trochim and Kane 2005). The solution is restricted to two dimensions and the size and shape of each cluster within this two-dimensional frame are dependent on the number of clusters selected when generating the concept maps. Kolb and Shepherd (1997) highlight that individual points do not change position on a concept map, but the clustering of points can be manipulated by the researcher to yield a map in which statements within the cluster relate to a common theme, and that each cluster is distinctive from other clusters and can be interpreted as such (Kolb and Shepherd 1997).

Being a predominantly interpretative technique, the selection process for the number of dimensions is by necessity subjective (Kolb and Shepherd 1997; Trochim 1989a, b; Trochim and Kane 2005). Cluster maps can be printed out, usually ranging from 5 to 12 cluster solutions for the mapped constructs. Using an iterative process, solutions are eliminated leaving a final solution that best aligns with the context of the study (Burchell and Kolb 2003; Kolb and Shepherd 1997).

10.3.7 Outputs Available from Trochim's Processes

There are a number of outputs which can be made available from concept mapping activities, and the outputs that are most appropriate depend on the individual project.

10.3.7.1 Statement Lists and Tabular Statistical Results

Statement lists can be tabulated to include the cluster number, cluster definition, mean importance of cluster (or some other criteria, usually rated via a Likert scale), number of items making up the cluster and the statements per se (Scahill et al. 2010a, b, c). Representation of the construct(s) in this way allows the reader to gain a sense of the content of each cluster (sometimes denoted dimensions) in addition to the labels and positions of clusters as labelled.

A full profile of the construct can be generated from the cluster statements and a summary profile developed for future use interviews or for discussion in focus groups or strategic planning sessions/action research meetings.

10.3.7.2 Concept Maps: Point and Cluster Maps

Point maps show the frequency of similarity or dissimilarity among statements. Cluster maps aggregate different groupings of adjacent statements from the point maps, generally 7–12 clusters (Burchell and Kolb 2003; Kolb and Shepherd 1997). MDS allows for integration of additional information from cluster and rating analyses. When the point cluster maps are combined with the criteria ratings they form three-dimensional maps. The layers of thickness represent the relative importance of each cluster with respect to the predetermined rating (often importance). The pictorial representation provides the beginnings of emerging models of the construct under study. The outputs from concept mapping exercises include a list of dimensions from which a profile can be developed as anchor points for discussion in the interviews.

10.3.7.3 Go-Zone Graph

The Go-zone graphs are a pictorial output from the rating process. These graphs compliment the Pattern Matching graphs. The Go-zone graphs are a bivariate plot of two patterns of ratings at the statement level. The bivariate space is divided into quadrants based on the average x and y values. For example construct 1 (e.g. importance) and construct 2 (e.g. feasibility) rating of the statements, the go-zone is the quadrant showing the statements as simultaneously rated above average in both importance and feasibility (see Trochim and Kane 2005). While pattern matching is especially useful for high-level pattern assessment, go-zones are particularly valuable for detailed use of the maps for planning or evaluation at the statement level.

10.3.7.4 Pattern Matches

A rating tool also allows the generation of pattern matches, which can be discussed in interviews or used as part of action research. Pattern matching can be undertaken to provide an anchor for discussion in the interview setting about organisational change as it relates to cultural dimensions, as well as the potential for interplay between dimensions. The following sub-section outlines the pattern matching method as an extension of concept mapping.

10.3.8 *Development of a Rating Instrument for Pattern Matching*

A process of piloting is undertaken as a part of the development of rating surveys of the list of statements generated in the face-to-face or web session. The range of individuals selected for piloting needs to align with those who are likely to participate in the full study. The people invited should be representative of but not work in the organisation(s) under study.

The focus of the pilot for developing rating instruments should be to determine whether the instructions are understood and feedback can be requested on the following:

- Whether draft email for the survey ratings is clear regarding the software login process?

- Whether modifications are needed to invitation emails to ensure participants understand that there are two or three ratings to complete?
- That it is clear that participants have a set time in which to complete questionnaires?
- That it is clear to participants that when completing ratings, it is their perception of what they see as important.
- That any summary profiles generated are understood.
- That any statements that are not understood are identified and explanation given about how they should be best rewritten to ensure clarity.
- That the language used in the survey is appropriate to all levels of staff in the organisations under study?

Improvements can be made to email invitations after feedback from each pilot interview, especially to ensure wording is not too complex. Any instructions that are not relevant to the completion of the survey should be removed. A statement around confidentiality must be included and the tone must demonstrate the research team's appreciation of individual participation. Request for participants' own perceptions when completing rating scales must also be made clear.

In terms of the statements, each one needs to be clarified with respondents and against pilot notes made by the research team when this process is being undertaken. Grammatical changes may need to be made on the recommendation of pilot feedback; however, the tenets of the statements are not expected to change, and so they may not need to be forwarded to the original concept mapping groups for approval.

10.3.9 The Method of Pattern Matching

Pattern matching involves the specification of a theoretical pattern, the acquisition of an observed pattern and an attempt to match these two (Trochim 1989c; Trochim and Kane 2005). As such, pattern matching allows for the combination of any two measures (e.g. typical and beneficial ratings of cultural statements within or between groups).

10.3.10 The Rating Phase

Following the piloting process, the final survey can be uploaded and activated within the web-based system. Relevant participants are invited electronically and post-consent can be forwarded a login and password (for the Concept Systems^{TM} software) by email. They can be asked to complete two survey ratings (e.g. typical and beneficial organisational culture) via an online web-based Concept System^{TM} software package (Copyright 2004–2008, all rights reserved, Concept Systems Inc, Ithaca, USA).

This technique has been employed in a study of organisational culture (OC) in a large New Zealand firm (Burchell 2003; Burchell and Kolb 2003). Pattern matching provides a visual comparison of patterns among the clusters of variables within statements (Burchell and Kolb 2003). These ladder graphs are useful for quickly spotting disconnects between two measures (Michalski and Cousins 2000). The results of a pattern match are represented both graphically (as a ladder graph) and numerically, as a correlation coefficient (Burchell and Kolb 2003; Michalski and Cousins 2000). The ladder graph is comprised of two vertical scales—one for each measure, joined by variably sloping lines, each corresponding to a labelled concept map cluster (e.g. a labelled cultural dimension) (Scahill et al. 2010a). If the match is perfect, all lines will be horizontal and the resulting graph resembles a ladder with the lines connecting the clusters having a zero gradient. In terms of numerical representation, the correlation coefficient associated with each pattern match can range between −1 and +1. The level of correlation is represented through a standard Pearson r (product-moment correlation) between the average ratings of the two variables (Burchell and Kolb 2003; Field 2005; Michalski and Cousins 2000). The Pearson r is useful to describe the strength of relationship between two ratings, for example, between typical and beneficial ratings for the same cultural statements in each cluster between the scales (Michalski and Cousins 2000; Scahill et al. 2010a). The diagram on the left signifies a high level of match between clusters, on the right a mismatch, with a likely low-correlation coefficient (Fig. 10.2).

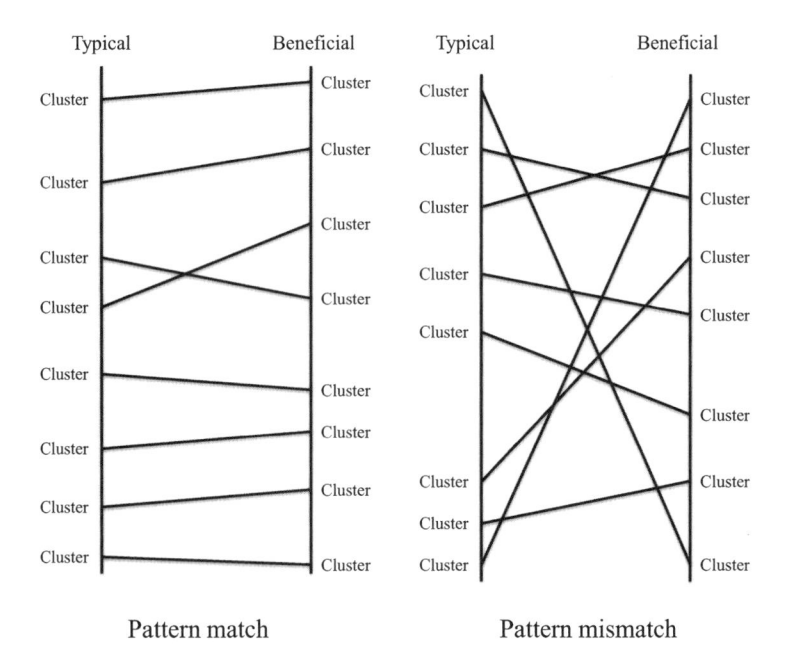

Fig. 10.2 Pattern matching Source: Scahill et (2012b)

Table 10.1 The benefits of concept mapping and relevance to pharmacy

Characteristic	Relevance to pharmacy
Integrate input from multiple sources with differing content expertise or interest	Policymakers, pharmacists, technicians, etc. and other health-care professionals
Group brainstorming combined with multivariate analyses	Systematic gathering of thoughts related to pharmacy and analysis through robust means
Visual depiction of concepts through maps and graphs	Used in meetings for visual impact and rapid understanding
Guide action and planning	Pharmacy can be assisted with moving forward

Source: Adapted from Trochim and Kane (2005)

10.4 Advantages of Adopting Trochim's Methods

The notable characteristics of Trochim's concept mapping which are relevant for addressing the problems of contemporary health care are applicable to pharmaceutical health services research (Trochim 1989a, b; Trochim and Kane 2005). Table 10.1 outlines the characteristics of concept mapping and its relevance to the pharmacy sector. The ability to integrate input from multiple sources with differing content expertise, interest and views means policymakers, pharmacists, technicians, retail staff and other health-care professionals who have a stake in what community does have input. Importantly, consensus is not a requirement which differentiates this method from others such as Delphi and is helpful in the scenario where agreement is very unlikely, as is the case in multi-stakeholder-based studies (Scahill 2012a, b).

10.5 Application in Pharmaceutical Health Services Research

Despite increasing levels of complexity, relative chaos and rapid pace of change within the health sector, concept mapping techniques remain underutilised in the pharmacy practice arena (Scahill 2012a, b). This technique has been successfully applied to sectors outside of health care (Burchell 2003; Burchell and Kolb 2003). Concept mapping and pattern matching have been used to "conceptualise" and "operationalise" organisational culture and organisational effectiveness in New Zealand community pharmacy (Scahill et al. 2009a, 2010a, b, c). These constructs were developed as part of a PhD program exploring the nature of the relationship between organisational culture and effectiveness (Scahill 2012a, b). Two examples of previously published works are provided which highlight the use of Trochim's mapping techniques within pharmacy practice research (Scahill et al. 2010a, b, c).

10.5.1 Example 1: Concept Mapping Organisational Effectiveness

Organisational culture influences how organisations function (Deal and Kennedy 1982; Schein 2004) and therefore effectiveness and this applies to community pharmacy (Scahill 2008, 2012a, b; Scahill et al. 2009a). In order to better understand the relationship between organisational culture and effectiveness in community pharmacy, a profile of what constitutes an effective community pharmacy had to be developed. Concept mapping has been used to model what constitutes an effective community pharmacy (Scahill et al. 2010c).

An eight cluster solution provided a concept map that was formulated into a quadrant model of organisational effectiveness (Fig. 10.3). The vertical axis of the OE model was labelled "stakeholder focus" with poles "internal capacity and efficiency" and "social utility". The horizontal axis was labelled "role development" with poles "traditional safety role" and "integration and innovation". The ratings of importance were depicted as increasing layers. They signify that human resources (skilled staff) management and leadership, safe and effective workflow and contribution to the safe use of medicines were seen by participants as the most important clusters. Less importance was placed on innovation, integration, having a community focus, providing health promotion and preventative care and advocating for patients and communicating amongst this multi-constituent group.

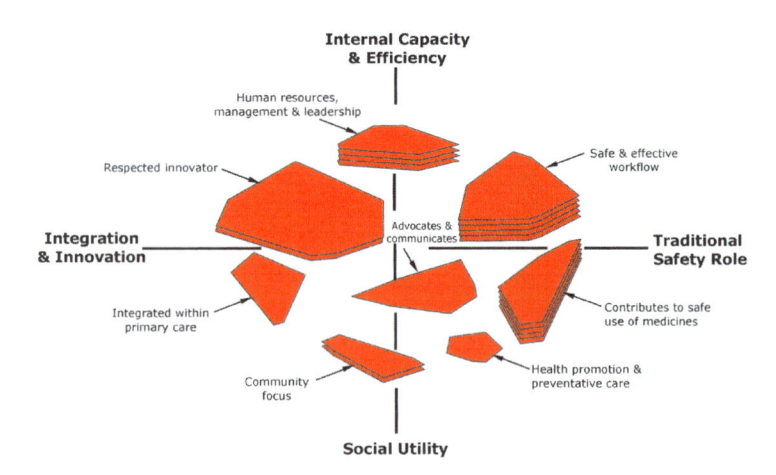

Fig. 10.3 Concept map: organisational effectiveness. *Source*: Scahill et al. (2010c) Reprinted with permission from Oxford University Press

A full descriptive profile of OE was developed (Panel 10.1) for use in interviews.

Panel 10.1 Full profile of the dimensions of organisational effectiveness

Below are clusters of activity that describe an effective community pharmacy from the viewpoint of multiple stakeholders.

Cluster 1: Has a community focus
Description: Is an advocate who stands in the shoes of patients and is aware of their needs. Provides a friendly welcoming environment where confidentiality is maintained. Identifies gaps in service provision for patients. Is an integral part of the community being culturally adapted to that community.

Cluster 2: Communicates and advocates
Description: Is an advocate for the benefit of medicines, role models healthy lifestyles, explains health policy and lobby for patients. Is a gateway to the health care system, assessing and referring patients and has the ability to recognise health crises and respond. Works collaboratively with health screening, works with prescribers to improve prescribing and undertakes tasks that will reduce their workload. Provides counselling at the time of dispensing.

Cluster 3: Involved with health promotion and preventative care
Description: Involves itself in primary care preventative medicine and has positive impact on health outcomes. Identifies health risk, promotes healthy lifestyles, supports patients in public health and recovery programmes and empowers them to manage their health and wellness. Takes a holistic approach to health care, particularly chronic care. Provides confidential advice in an appropriate environment and carries a range of OTC products that enhance health and well-being in a holistic sense.

Cluster 4: Has safe and effective workflows
Description: Has a workplace environment that supports efficient workflow and safe and accurate dispensing. Has procedures in place and picks up errors inherent in the prescription system, holds adequate stock and manages stock levels. Keeps accurate records of medicines dispensing, dispenses in a timely and safe manner. Works within the law and belongs to appropriate professional bodies.

Cluster 5: Contributes to the safe use of medicines
Description: Safeguards the public from medicines related harm, with medicines safety as its primary concern. Acts as a safety net for prescription medicine errors and inaccurate lay advice. Assesses and helps to manage people with complex medication regimens. Recognises and provides management strategies for adherence and compliance issues. Is a repository for medicines advice, providing evidence-based medicines advice and counselling. Is a health translator who sources unusual or difficult requests.

Cluster 6: Has skilled workers, effective management and leadership
Description: Staffed by skilled people who are trained for the job and accessible to provide advice and intervention. Makes good use of the skill sets of its employees, values staff and is a positive working environment for staff. Has pharmacists working collegially, provides for staff development and is aware of clinical limitations and contracts staff appropriately. Demonstrates good business management, undertakes ongoing business and service assessment and maintains a level of financial sustainability.

Cluster 7: A respected innovator that takes opportunities and prepares for change
Description: Is cognisant of new developments, an early adopter, an embracer of change and always seeking new opportunities. Being innovative, it looks outside the square, adapts to external pressures and drives its own destiny to advance the profession of pharmacy. It responds to new service requirements and uses technology to make life easier. An understanding of the New Zealand Primary Health Care Strategy and Pharmacy has captured the confidence of its funders and is adequately funded to provide appropriate high-level pharmacy services. Being an ethical business, advocating continuing professional development (CPD), it is respected both professionally and as part of the community. It has the confidence of other health professions.

Cluster 8: Is integrated within the rest of primary care
Description: Has active relationships and works collegially with other health-care providers, understands broader health relationships and proactively engages with other health sectors. Understands government health-care policy, involves itself with Primary Health Organisation (PHO) developments and is actively involved in health service development. Is appropriately located relative to the community and medical practices and is interconnected with the rest of the health-care system.

Source: Scahill et al. (2010c) Reprinted with permission from Oxford University Press

10.5.2 Example 2: Pattern Matching Organisational Culture

Pattern matching is a technique which allows the culture of an organisation to be rated according to two or more criteria. In this study, pattern matching was successfully employed to compare typical and beneficial aspects of culture for achieving a profile of an effective community pharmacy (Scahill et al. 2010a). It has been observed that cultural change involving increased focus on integrating within primary care and embracing innovation may be needed in the case site pharmacies under study. Unfortunately, individual pattern matches were used to discuss culture ratings, rather than interpretations of a shared phenomenon such as the overall pattern match. The individual matches did provide an anchor point for discussion, but the analysis and sense-making at a dimensional level became difficult when conceptualising culture as a shared phenomenon. It would have been more appropriate and useful to have all staff talk about the pharmacy level pattern match and to discern whether there were different views. The approach taken has limited the use of the pattern match data at an organisational level and in hindsight was a less useful approach. This is a limitation as well as a learning process.

In terms of the culture construct, staff from all levels of work within the pharmacies were also invited to the concept mapping exercises based on Martin's notion of subculture (Martin 1992; Meyerson and Martin 1987). With culture posited as "the way we do things around here and the way(s) we think and act"; dimensions of organisational culture were developed through a mapping exercise (Scahill et al. 2010b). In this study, a total of 61 pattern matches were performed at multiple levels across the case sites including: individuals, collective cases, pharmacists, technicians, and pharmacy assistants/retail staff. Pattern matches at the individual participant level were utilised within interviews to facilitate discussion, as per an interview schema. The rationale for this approach was based on personal construct theory (Kelly 1955) and a discussion with participants about their lived world (Crotty 1998). The pattern match diagrams (Fig. 10.4) show the difference between typical and beneficial ratings for each cultural cluster, as the aggregated responses of all participants within each pharmacy, using the method outlined previously. Figure 10.4 is an example from one of the six case sites under study. The mean Likert scale scores for the typical and beneficial ratings are all above 3.0.

10 Concept Mapping and Pattern Matching in Pharmacy Practice Research

```
              Typical                              Beneficial

Trusted behaviour  4.59                    4.67   Trusted behaviour

                                                  Leadership and staff management
                                                  Providing systematic advice
Free thinking, fun & open to challenge            Focus on external integration

Focus on external integration                     Free thinking, fun & open to challenge
Leadership and staff management                   Customer relations

Providing systematic advice
      Customer relations
Valuing each other and the team

                                                  Embracing innovation


Embracing innovation  4.1                   4.14
                            r = .74               Valuing each other and the team
```

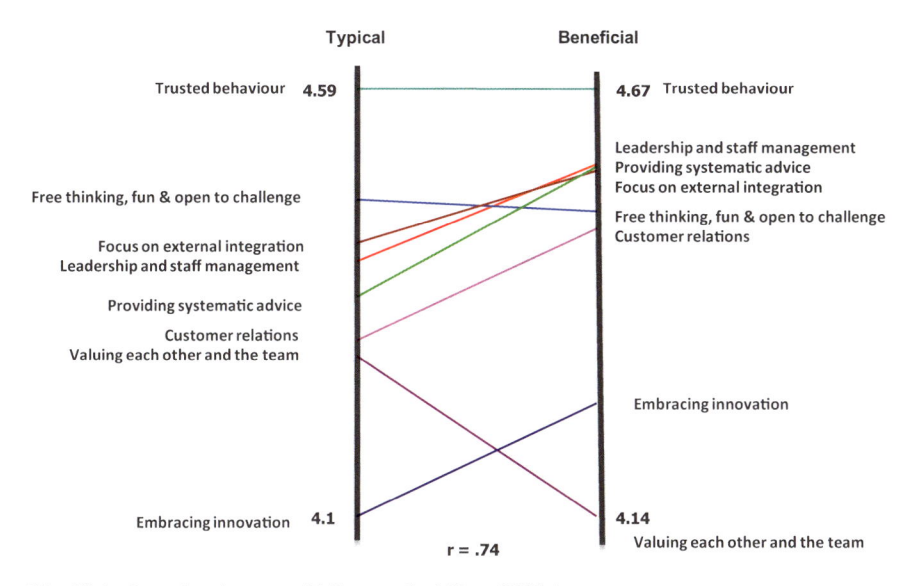

Fig. 10.4 Case site pharmacy #1 Source: Scahill et (2010a)

For the typical rating, this suggests that all clusters are at least somewhat typical. The mean beneficial rating scales are all above 3.0 which infers that all cultural clusters are perceived at the very least to be somewhat beneficial for achieving effectiveness within all case sites. The Pearson r coefficients from the six pattern matches range from 0.71 to 0.90 within the case sites, suggesting a high level of correlation between the means of the two ratings (typical and beneficial) across all eight cultural clusters. This provides a summary of the "gap" in cultural clusters across the six pharmacies (Table 10.2).

Cultural dimensions that have slopes with gradients represent a mismatch between what is typically observed in that pharmacy and what needs to occur for that pharmacy to be effective. These mismatches describe cultural gaps with a positive gradient, suggesting that the cultural dimension is less typical than it need to be for the pharmacy to be effective. Table 10.2 highlights a broad range in the number of cultural clusters with gaps. The culture gaps range from two out of eight in one pharmacy (Case site 5) to seven out of eight in another (Case site 3).

The pattern match for five of six pharmacies highlights the need for "focus on external integration" and "providing systematic advice" to be more typical, which requires further exploration. This trend is closely followed by "leadership and staff management" and "free thinking, fun and open to challenge" with four of the six pharmacies being less typical than they should be to achieve the level of effectiveness. With respect to embracing innovation, the pattern matches for three case site pharmacies (Case site 1, 2, and 4) require this to become more typical (an upward gradient in the pattern match slope). In the three pharmacies with no cultural gap, staff rated embracing innovation is relatively low on the beneficial scale compared with other cultural dimensions, which also warrants consideration.

Table 10.2 Cultural "gap" by cluster and pharmacy case site

Culture cluster	Case site 1	2	3	4	5	6	Total number of pharmacies with gaps by cluster
Leadership and staff management	√	X	√	√	X	√	4
Valuing each other and the team	X	X	√	X	X	X	1
Free thinking, fun and open to challenge	X	X	√	√	√	√	4
Trusted behaviour	X	X	√	X	X	X	1
Customer relations	√	X	X	X	X	√	2
Focus on external integration	√	√	√	√	Xa	√	5
Providing systematic advice	√	√	√	√	√	X	5
Embracing innovation	√	√	a	√	a	a	3
Total number of clusters reporting gaps by pharmacy	5	3	6	5	2	4	

Source: Scahill et al. (2010a) Printed with permission from Elsevier
Notes: √, gap; X, no gap; a, low beneficial rating

10.6 Further Applications: A Research Agenda

There has been a dearth of studies using concept mapping and pattern matching in pharmacy practice research, and there is potential application in the wider field of pharmaceutical health services research. Replication of the aforementioned community pharmacy-based studies could be undertaken within the hospital pharmacy sector (Scahill 2012a, b). Although some work has been undertaken to determine performance indicators for clinical pharmacy services (Ng and Harrison 2010), little work has been undertaken to demonstrate what an effective hospital pharmacy might look like, from a multi-stakeholder viewpoint. Little work has also been done to explore the organisational culture of hospital pharmacy (Scahill 2012a, b) and how different patterns of culture might influence the functioning and therefore the performance of different hospital pharmacies. The extent to which pharmacies (both hospital and community) are innovative can be determined through Concept Mapping and Pattern Matching.

10.7 Caveats and Limitations

As with any methodology, there are limitations, and concept mapping and pattern matching study findings should always be considered in light of these (Scahill 2012a, b). This is a robust mixed methods technique; however, it is very time consuming for both researcher and participants, and the participants must be informed of this prior to or as part of engagement in the study. Well "worked-up" focus statements are critical to project success. They need to be founded on the literature and research questions and be simple yet specific. Trochim suggests wording of the individual statements generated is also important and must be in positive or neutral tones; there should be one idea per statement (Trochim 1989a, b; Trochim and Linton 1986). Note that the wording of each statement is particularly critical for the rating of statements which is undertaken relatively. The facilitator needs to have some expertise in facilitating group exercises and needs to be adequately trained in the use of the software.

10.8 Conclusion

Improvements in methodologies are required which allow for conceptualisation of complex processes relating to health service configuration, integration and delivery. Systematic yet flexible approaches need to be adopted in order to accommodate multi-stakeholder views, where consensus is neither likely nor required in order to progress. Concept mapping and pattern matching are two such techniques which can be applied to pharmaceutical health services research. To date, these techniques remain underutilised. Overall, structured group concept mapping is a promising technique which can be applied to future research agendas in the field of pharmaceutical health services research.

References

Adamcik BA, Ransford HE, Oppenheimer PR, Brown JF, Eagan PA (1986) New clinical roles for pharmacists: study of role expansion. Soc Sci Med 23(11):1187–1200

Anderson C, Blenkinsopp A, Armstrong M (2003) Pharmacists' perceptions regarding their contribution to improving the public's health: a systematic review of the United Kingdom and international literature 1990–2001. Int J Pharm Pract 11(2):111–120

Anderson C, Blenkinsopp A, Armstrong M (2008) The contribution of community pharmacy to improving the public's health: literature review update 2004–2007. London. http://www.pharmacyhealthlink.org.uk. PharmacyHealthLink and Royal Pharmaceutical Society of Great Britain

Bryant L (2006) Evaluation of the barriers to and implementation of comprehensive pharmaceutical care in New Zealand. PhD, University of Auckland, Auckland

Burchell N (2003) Patterns of stability and change orientations in organisational culture: a case study. PhD, University of Auckland, Auckland

Burchell N, Kolb D (2003) Pattern matching organisational cultures. J Aust New Zeal Acad Manage 9(3):50

Bush J, Langley CA, Jesson JK, Wilson KA (2006) Perceived barriers to the development of community pharmacy's public health function: a survey of the attitudes of directors of public health and chief pharmacists in UK primary care organisations. Int J Pharm Pract Suppl 2:B68–B69

Bush J, Langley CA, Wilson KA (2009) The corporatization of community pharmacy: implications for service provision, the public health function, and pharmacy's claims to professional status in the United Kingdom. Res Soc Adm Pharm 5(4):305–318

Crotty M (1998) The foundations of social research: meaning and perspective in the research process. Sage, London

Deal TE, Kennedy AA (1982) Corporate cultures. Addison-Wesley, Reading, MA

Edmunds J, Calnan MW (2001) The reprofessionalisation of community pharmacy: an exploration of attitudes to extended roles for community pharmacists amongst pharmacists and general practitioners in the United Kingdom. Soc Sci Med 53(7):943–955

Ferlie EB, Shortell SM (2001) Improving the quality of health care in the United Kingdom and the United States: a framework for change. Milbank Q 79(2):281–315

Field A (2005) Discovering statistics using SPSS, 2nd edn. Sage, London

Graetz F, Rimmer M, Lawrence A, Smith A (2002) Managing organisational change. Wiley, Sydney

Kelly GA (1955) The psychology of personal constructs. Norton, New York, NY

Kolb D, Shepherd DM (1997) Concept mapping organizational cultures. J Manage Inq 6(4):282–295

Martin J (1992) Cultures in organisations: three perspectives, 1st edn. Oxford University Press, New York, NY

Maxwell K, Harrison J, Scahill S, Braund R (2013) Identifying drug-related problems during transition between secondary and primary care in New Zealand. Int J Pharm Pract 21(5):333–336

McMillan SS, Wheeler AJ, Sav A, King MA, Whitty JA, Kendall E, Kelly F (2013) Community pharmacy in Australia: a health hub destination of the future. Res Soc Adm Pharm 9(6):863–875. doi:10.1016/j.sapharm.2012.11.003

Meyerson D, Martin J (1987) Cultural change: an integration of three different views. J Manage Stud 24(6):623–647. doi:10.1111/j.1467-6486.1987.tb00466.x

Michalski GV, Cousins JB (2000) Differences in stakeholder perceptions about training evaluation: a concept mapping/pattern matching investigation. Eval Program Plann 23(2):211–230

Mossialos E, Naci H, Courtin E (2013) Expanding the role of community pharmacists: policymaking in the absence of policy-relevant evidence? Health Policy 111(2):135–148

Nabitz U, Van den Brink W, Jansen P (2005) Using concept mapping to design an indicator framework for addiction treatment centres. Int J Qual Health Care 17(3):193–201

Ng J, Harrison J (2010) Key performance indicators for clinical pharmacy services in New Zealand public hospitals: stakeholder perspectives. J Pharmaceut Health Serv Res 1(2):75–84. doi:10.1111/j.1759-8893.2010.00001.x

Pharmaceutical Society of New Zealand (2004) Focus on the future: ten year vision for pharmacists: 2004–2014. Pharmaceutical Society of New Zealand, Wellington, New Zealand

Roberts AS, Benrimoj SI, Chen TF, Williams KA, Aslani P (2006) Implementing cognitive services in community pharmacy: a review of facilitators used in practice change. Int J Pharm Pract 14(3):163–170

Roberts AS, Benrimoj SI, Dunphy D, Palmer I (2007) Community pharmacy: strategic change management. McGraw-Hill, Sydney

Roeg D, Van de Goor I, Garretsen H (2005) Towards quality indicators for assertive outreach programmes for severely impaired substance abusers: concept mapping with Dutch experts. Int J Qual Health Care 17(3):203–208

Rosenthal M, Austin Z, Tsuyuki RT (2010) Are pharmacists the ultimate barrier to pharmacy practice change? Can Pharm J 143(1):37–42

Scahill SL (2008) Improving community pharmacy services by studying organizational theory. Southern Med Rev 1(1):18–20

Scahill SL (2011) Community pharmacy doesn't appear as part of the collaboration discourse within New Zealand primary care. J Prim Health Care 3(3):244–247

Scahill SL (2012a) Applying organisation theory to hospital pharmacy research: the case of 'culture' down under! J Pharm Pract Res 42(3):175

Scahill SL (2012b) Exploring the nature of the relationship between organisational culture and organisational effectiveness within six New Zealand community-based pharmacies. PhD University of Auckland, Auckland

Scahill SL, Babar ZU (2010) Community pharmacy practice in high and low income countries: commonalities, differences and the tension of being "retailer" versus "primary health care provider". Southern Med Rev 3(2):1–2

Scahill SL, Harrison J, Carswell P, Babar ZU (2009a) Organisational culture: an important concept for pharmacy practice research. Pharm World Sci 31:517–521

Scahill SL, Harrison J, Sheridan J (2009b) The ABC of New Zealand's ten year vision for pharmacists: awareness, barriers and consultation. Int J Pharm Pract 17:135–142

Scahill SL, Carswell P, Harrison J (2010a) An organizational culture gap analysis in 6 New Zealand community pharmacies. Res Soc Adm Pharm 7(3):211–223

Scahill SL, Harrison J, Carswell P (2010b) Describing the organizational culture of a selection of community pharmacies using a tool borrowed from social science. Pharm World Sci 32(1):73–80

Scahill SL, Harrison J, Carswell P (2010c) What constitutes an effective community pharmacy? Development of a preliminary model of organizational effectiveness through concept mapping with multiple stakeholders. Int J Qual Health Care 22(4):324–332. doi:10.1093/intqhc/mzq033

Scahill SL, Harrison J, Carswell P, Shaw J (2010d) Health care policy and community pharmacy: implications for the New Zealand primary health care sector. New Zeal Med J 123 (1317):41–51

Schein EH (2004) Organisational culture and leadership, 3rd edn. Jossey-Bass, San Francisco, CA

Scott T, Mannion R, Marshall MN, Davies HTO (2003) Does organisational culture influence health care performance? A review of the evidence. J Health Serv Res Policy 8(2):105–117

Trochim WMK (1989a) Concept mapping: soft science or hard art? Eval Program Plann 12(1):87–110

Trochim WMK (1989b) An introduction to concept mapping for planning and evaluation. Eval Program Plann 12(1):1–16

Trochim WMK (1989c) Outcome pattern matching and program theory. Eval Program Plann 12 (4):355–366

Trochim WMK, Kane M (2005) Concept mapping: an introduction to structured conceptualization in health care. Int J Qual Health Care 17(3):187–191

Trochim WMK, Linton R (1986) Conceptualization for planning and evaluation. Eval Program Plann 9(4):289–308

Walker R (2000) Pharmaceutical public health: the end of pharmaceutical care? Pharmaceut J 264:340–341

Chapter 11
Pharmacoepidemiological Approaches in Health Care

Christine Y. Lu

Abstract Pharmacoepidemiology studies patterns of medicines use—also known as drug utilization research—which is an important component of pharmacy practice research. Pharmacoepidemiology also studies the relationship between treatment or exposure and outcomes in large populations under nonexperimental situations over time. This chapter provides an introduction to pharmacoepidemiology. It discusses the key concepts involved in studying the association between medicines and outcomes. These include forming a research question, considering sources of data, defining the study population, and defining drug exposures and outcomes. This chapter also discusses a range of study designs used in pharmacoepidemiological research including cohort studies, case-control design, within-subject methods, cross-sectional studies, ecological studies, and quasi-experimental designs. Frequently used metrics to understand drug utilization and medication adherence are also introduced. This chapter also draws on key challenges such as selection bias as well as commonly used analytical techniques to overcome these challenges.

11.1 Pharmacoepidemiology and the Need for Pharmacoepidemiological Research

Medicines are a major component of modern medicine. The birth of pharmacoepidemiology may be dated to the early 1960s (Wettermark 2013). Initially pharmacoepidemiologic investigations focused on adverse drug reactions (ADRs) but recent decades also include studies of the beneficial effects of medicines. Pharmacoepidemiology is a discipline that uses similar methods to epidemiological studies but focuses on the area of clinical pharmacology. Pharmacoepidemiology studies patterns of medicines use and the relationship between treatment or

---

C.Y. Lu (✉)
Department of Population Medicine, Harvard Medical School and Harvard Pilgrim Health Care Institute, 133 Brookline Ave., 6th Floor, Boston, MA 02215, USA
e-mail: christine_lu@harvardpilgrim.org

© Springer International Publishing Switzerland 2015
Z.-U.-D. Babar (ed.), *Pharmacy Practice Research Methods*,
DOI 10.1007/978-3-319-14672-0_11

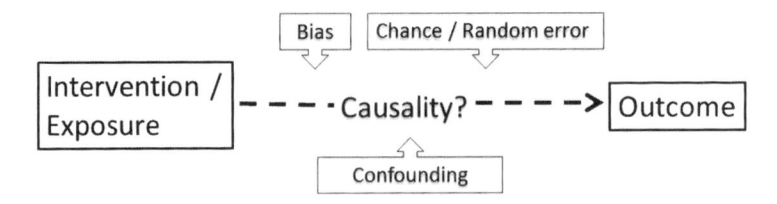

Fig. 11.1 Cause–effect relationship between an intervention and an outcome

exposure and outcomes (good and bad)—see Fig. 11.1—in large, heterogeneous populations under nonexperimental situations over long periods (Avorn 2004). The driving forces behind the development of pharmacoepidemiology are the growing awareness that health outcomes of medicines use in the rigorous setting of randomized controlled trials are not necessarily the same as health outcomes of medicines use in everyday practice and the increasing attention on the safety and effectiveness of medicines.

Randomized controlled trials (RCTs) are seen as the gold standard for assessing the efficacy and safety of an intervention or exposure. Randomization is the most important feature of this study design in determining causality (see Fig. 11.1), which ensures that the groups formed are similar, except for chance difference, in all aspects. This method maximizes the internal validity by minimizing biases and confounding. The internal validity of a study is the extent to which the observed difference in outcomes between the study groups can be attributed to the intervention rather than other factors. However, RCTs have several important limitations. RCTs are resource intensive and focus on effects of an intervention among a small population of carefully selected patients, who are treated and followed up for a relatively short period of time in strictly controlled conditions. RCTs typically have strict inclusion and exclusion criteria that underrepresent vulnerable patient groups (e.g., children, the elderly, individuals with multimorbidity). Because of these limitations, the external validity of RCTs is limited. External validity (also known as generalizability or applicability) refers to whether the causal relationship holds beyond the people included in the study (e.g., other settings or populations). RCTs only provide results of the average patients and do not provide a true reflection of how drug use will impact health outcomes in patients seen in the real-world setting. RCTs are also not feasible to answer many questions of importance such as rare outcomes. Therefore, clinicians, patients, and policymakers must turn to pharmacoepidemiological studies for best available evidence.

Pharmacoepidemiological research has an important role in supporting the rational and cost-effective use of drugs thereby improving health outcomes. Specifically, pharmacoepidemiological investigations can contribute by several ways (Avorn 2004; Lu 2009). Pharmacoepidemiology can define medication needs by defining the prevalence and burden of a particular clinical problem to identify the clinical place for the new therapeutic agent. It assesses patterns of medicines use (also referred to as drug utilization research) and issues such as medication adherence (also known as compliance). Importantly, pharmacoepidemiology examines the safety and *effectiveness* of medicines in large, heterogeneous populations. Effectiveness describes how well a medicine performs in the real-world setting, that is, when it is used by doctors treating typical patients over a prolonged period of time and in comparison with other available therapeutic alternatives. In contrast, efficacy describes how well a medicine performs in RCT settings. Pharmacoepidemiology also includes drug safety surveillance by quantifying the frequency and severity of adverse effects of a drug or drug class.

11.2 Drug Utilization Research

Drug utilization research is an essential part of pharmacoepidemiology and pharmacy practice as it describes the extent, nature, and determinants of drug exposure (World Health Organisation 2003). Drug utilization research provides insights into several aspects of drug prescribing and use. It can estimate the numbers of patients exposed to drugs within a given time period. We can estimate all drug users, regardless of when they started to use the drug (prevalence) or patients who started to use the drug within a given time period (incidence). It also describes the extent and profiles of medicines use at a certain time point and/or in a certain region (e.g., country, state, hospital), and trends in medicines use and costs over time. On the basis of epidemiological data on a disease, drug utilization research can estimate the extent of appropriate use, overuse, or underuse of medicines. It describes the utilization pattern of a group of drugs and their relative market share for a certain disease. By examining utilization patterns by patient or prescriber characteristics (e.g., sociodemographic factors, provider specialty), drug utilization research can help to identify target population for educational interventions to improve medicines use. Drug utilization research also compares observed patterns of medicines use with clinical guidelines for the treatment of a certain disease or local drug formularies. This can help to generate hypotheses whether discrepancies represent less than optimal practice, determine whether educational or other type of interventions are required, or identify if clinical guidelines need to be reviewed in the light of actual practice. In addition, drug utilization research compares utilization patterns and costs of medicines between different regions or time periods. Such comparisons can generate hypotheses to further investigate reasons for, and health implications of, the differences found. Geographical variations and changes over time in medicines use may have medical, social, and/or economic implications both for the individual patient and for society and are thus important to identify, explain, and intervene, if necessary.

Drug utilization research often uses cross-sectional or longitudinal data. Cross-sectional studies provide a snapshot of medicines use at a certain time (e.g., year 2014). Such studies may use similar data to compare medicines use between countries, different regions in a country, or different hospitals. Longitudinal data are often used to describe trends in medicines use (Vitry et al. 2011; Kelly et al. 2014; Chung et al. 2008; Lu et al. 2007a, b). Longitudinal data for drug utilization research can be obtained through health-care claims databases, based on a statistically valid sample of pharmacies or medical practices, or obtained from repeated cross-sectional surveys (data collection is continuous, but the patients or providers surveyed are continually changing. Thus, such data can reflect overall trends, but cannot provide information about prescribing trends for individual practitioners or practices). Data sources are discussed below.

11.3 Defining the Research Question

In pharmacoepidemiology, a prior specification of the research question (and study design and data analysis plan) is recommended to minimize the risk of "cherry-picking" interesting findings and spurious findings because of multiple hypothesis testing (Austin et al. 2006). The rationale for the study should be explicitly stated, and what a new study can add to existing knowledge. The research question should be concise and clearly state the intervention (exposure) and outcome(s) of interest. The research question should be formulated considering the strengths and limitations of the available data.

11.4 Sources of Data in Pharmacoepidemiology

The research question should dictate the choice of data sources and whether the question can be appropriately addressed with a particular database.

Pharmacoepidemiology has grown rapidly as large-scale computer-based databases have become increasingly available over the last two decades. There are three main types of data sources for pharmacoepidemiologic research: administrative health-care databases, electronic medical records (EMR) databases, and patient registries. Administrative databases contain information about the delivery of services or records of events, collected primarily for payment purposes (e.g., dispensing data). EMR data are recorded during the process of clinical care. While administrative and EMR databases are valuable resources, they are not designed for research (Motheral and Fairman 1997; Schneeweiss 2007). Patient registries (disease-based or drug-based) are established for the specific reporting of clinical information and management of certain diseases and procedures.

Administrative databases (Lu 2009) with millions of observations on the use of drugs, biologics, devices, and medical procedures along with health outcomes are valuable sources for drug safety studies (Gram et al. 2000). Rigorous longitudinal, observational studies using large health-care databases can complement results from RCTs by assessing treatment effectiveness in patients encountered in daily clinical practice. Comparisons of observational studies with RCTs have shown that these studies often produce similar results and that well-designed observational studies do not systematically over-estimate the magnitude of treatment effects and do provide valid additional information (Benson and Hartz 2000; Concato et al. 2000). Furthermore, observational studies overcome the limitations found with current pharmacovigilance systems, many rely on voluntary reporting that do not allow estimation of incidence of adverse events.

Administrative health-care databases have several strengths (Lu 2009). There is a good level of compliance with reporting, and the accuracy of data submitted is usually high because the data are collected for payment purposes. These databases contain information on patient demography, some clinical diagnoses, use of medical procedures and drugs, and detailed information on charges. Data can be used to answer a variety of research questions at low-cost in a relatively short time span. In addition, routine health-care data reflect drug effectiveness and safety in patients encountered in real-world practice. Moreover, large populations of patients can be followed over long time periods, allowing better identification of clinically important, rare adverse events as compared with RCTs.

There has been an enormous growth in the use of large health-care databases for pharmacoepidemiology. Examples of health-care databases used in pharmacoepidemiology are listed in Table 11.1.

Electronic Medical Records databases contain rich clinical information on patients that are often lacking in administrative databases (e.g., smoking status, body mass index, vital signs, and laboratory data). EMR data can provide information for better confounding adjustment, particularly for studies that may be susceptible to selection bias. However, EMR data do not record all prescribed medications taken by patients and are generally not considered as a valid source for identifying drug exposure. Another major challenge is the variation in available data fields and data standards across EMR databases (Kush et al. 2008), which may limit data linkage and, therefore, study sample sizes.

Patient registries are also valuable sources for tracking relevant clinical, economic, and humanistic (patient health-related quality of life, patient satisfaction) outcomes of medical treatments, including medicines. They are prospective

Table 11.1 Examples of large health-care databases

Country	Name	Website
US	HMO Research Network	http://www.hmoresearchnetwork.org/
	Health-care Cost and Utilization Project (HCUP)	http://www.hcup-us.ahrq.gov/databases.jsp
	SEER-Medicare Linked Database	http://appliedresearch.cancer.gov/seermedicare/
	Veterans Administration Databases	http://www.virec.research.va.gov/
Canada	Population Health Research Unit	http://metadata.phru.dal.ca/
	Population Data BC	https://www.popdata.bc.ca/researchers
UK	The Clinical Practice Research Datalink	http://www.cprd.com/intro.asp
Netherlands	PHARMO Record Linkage System	http://www.pharmo.nl/
Australia	Medicare Benefits Scheme data, Pharmaceutical Benefits Scheme data	http://www.humanservices.gov.au/corporate/statistical-information-and-data/?utm_id=9

observational studies of patients with certain shared characteristics and collect ongoing and supporting data on well-defined outcomes of interest over time. Given patient registries are designed specifically for a purpose, they may not have data to answer a wide range of questions.

Merging administrative and EMR datasets and data from patient registries can provide the opportunity to leverage the strengths of each type of data. However, such practice must consider privacy issues, data quality and transferability, and feasibility of merging datasets. Data linkage is discussed in the next section. Ultimately, the choice of data sources depends on the research question and whether the question can be appropriately addressed with a particular database. It is important to note that databases do not have all the answers researchers seek in measuring drug exposure and outcomes. In selecting a data source, one must at least consider the breadth and depth of the data in the database, quality of the database itself, quality of the data, the patient population that contributes data, and duration of information contained in the database.

For drug utilization research, household surveys are another data source to examine drug utilization and related issues such as adherence and access to medicines (Paniz et al. 2010; Bertoldi et al. 2008). Medicines available in households have either been prescribed or dispensed at health facilities, purchased at a pharmacy (with or without a prescription), or are over-the-counter medications. They may be for the treatment of a current illness or are left over from a previous illness. Thus, dispensing data and utilization data are not necessarily equivalent because they have not been corrected for nonadherence, which is a common issue. Drug utilization can be assessed by performing household surveys, counting leftover pills, or using special devices that allow electronic counting of the number of times a particular drug is administered.

11.4.1 Data Linkage

A pharmacoepidemiological study may require data from more than one source either to enhance data available through linkage of disparate sources or to expand the size of the population through combination of similar data sources.

Person-level linkage of disparate databases can allow a more robust evaluation by providing a more complete picture of patient care and characteristics (Lu 2009). Common linkages include the combination of inpatient, outpatient, or pharmacy data or linking cancer or death registries to medical records and may be within or across institutions. In the best scenario, each dataset will include several common relevant patient descriptors to allow a high-probability match (e.g., based on medical record number or other standardized person-level identifier, date of birth, residence); the more linkage variables available the better. For common information across sources, rules for handling potentially duplicate information must also be specified (e.g., which to be kept). Linking data from different sources typically require a probabilistic or deterministic linkage algorithm to account for ambiguity, for instance, slightly different spelling of names or addresses. The choice of linking method should be based on expertise in the approach used, previous linkage of the databases (if any), and the acceptable balance of false positives and false negatives, recognizing that some linkages will be incorrect and some will be missed. Furthermore, it is important to assess the overlap in populations because low linkage will affect sample size. Sensitivity analyses should be considered to evaluate potential linkage errors. Patient privacy is a concern when conducting linkages. Approaches have been developed for anonymous linkage (e.g., secure hashing algorithms) (Agency for Healthcare Research and Quality 2013), which are beyond the scope of this chapter.

Linkage of data sources containing similar information on different patients aims to expand the size of the study population (Brown et al. 2010). Many pharmacoepidemiological studies require very large populations. Examples include questions that involve small population of interest (e.g., hypereosinophilic syndrome or chronic eosinophilic leukemia), uncommon exposures (e.g., safety surveillance of new treatments), and/or rare outcomes (e.g., rhabdomyolysis). Multiple sources, for instance, data from more than one health insurer, will be valuable and needed to identify an adequate study population when no single database is large enough to address such research questions in a timely and adequate way. Examples include the Mini-Sentinel program (http://mini-sentinel.org/) and Vaccine Safety Datalink Project (http://www.cdc.gov/vaccinesafety/Activities/VSD.html).

Comparability of data sources refers to the way in which the data are captured and recorded so that the data can be reasonably combined with respect to data capture and terminology. Comparability should be assessed qualitatively through detailed understanding of the data source and quantitatively across all relevant variables to ensure that information from the different sources can be combined. For example, claims databases of different health insurers may be comparable allowing same definition of study populations, the data may be captured via a standardized reimbursement system, and the information is recorded using standardized coding schema (e.g., Anatomical Therapeutic Chemical Classification System for medicines). For multi-institutional studies through a distributed model (Brown et al. 2010, 2013), data owners maintain physical control of their data in adherence to their privacy and security rules instead of owners transferring data to a single site for analysis in a centralized model, thereby giving up control. Comprehensive analysis to characterize data should be conducted to evaluate variability across data partners with respect to overall cohort metrics (e.g., age and sex distribution) and study-specific metrics (e.g., exposure and outcome rates by age, sex, and year).

11.5 Study Population

The design of study population in pharmacoepidemiological studies is critically important because confounding bias is a particular concern in nonexperimental research. Study cohorts in pharmacoepidemiological studies typically include a study group of patients who have the drug exposure and a control group of patients who have *not* had the same drug exposure (but may be exposed to a comparison drug). Study cohorts should be restricted to patients who are homogeneous regarding their indication for the drug exposure, which will provide a better balance of patient characteristics that predict the outcome (Perrio et al. 2007; Schneeweiss et al. 2007). This will reduce but not eliminate confounding because it is likely that there are variables that influence prescribing decisions but are not recorded in the data system.

There are two major exclusion criteria to consider in pharmacoepidemiology to maximize internal validity by reducing confounding. First, exclusion of patients with a history of the outcome of interest; patients may have an increased risk for the outcome and at the same time may be more likely to take a study medication. It would be better to exclude these patients instead of adjustment in the analysis, particularly, if the condition is a strong risk factor for future events (and thus a confounder). Second, studies may restrict to incident medication users. Incident users are those starting on a study medication without evidence of prior dispensings of study drugs during a predefined time interval (i.e., no drug exposure; also known as a wash-out period—see Fig. 11.2). An often used wash-out period is 6 months. However, for some patients it may not be the first time they take the study drug, i.e., they are not really naÿve to the drug. Longer wash-out period increases the certainty that patients are truly incident users. However, it reduces the number of patients eligible for the study and thus reduces precision. Prevalent users are those taking a study medication for some time. Prevalent users are likely to be those who tolerate the drug well, perceive some therapeutic benefit, and may lead to healthy user bias (Glynn et al. 2001). Restricting study cohorts to all patients in a defined population who start a course of treatment with the study medication ("new-user design") may reduce confounding (Johnson et al. 2012). The main advantages of new-user design are that it avoids the problem of adjusting for characteristics that may be in the causal pathway, and that it captures events that occurred after the start of the therapy.

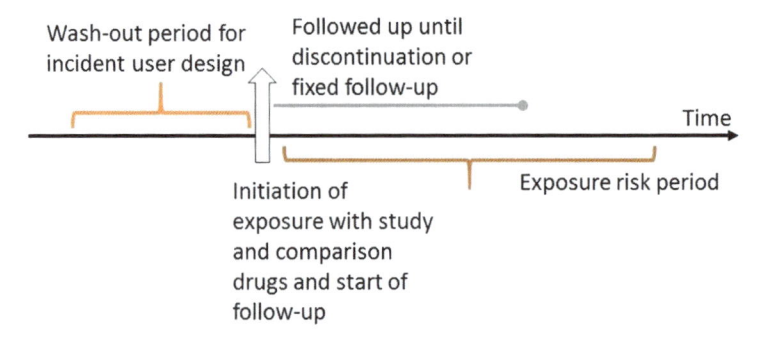

Fig. 11.2 Basic design of a pharmacoepidemiologic study

11.6 Defining Exposures and Outcomes

Drug exposures and outcomes in pharmacoepidemiological studies must be operationally defined considering the formulated research question and the data source to be used. Because administrative data are recorded for billing purposes and not for research, both systematic and random errors can occur in the identification of exposure and outcome. Importantly, data are only captured for individuals who seek care and whose care is obtained through the insurance payment system. Claims for prescription drugs are generally considered a valid measure of drug exposure (Strom et al. 1991). Claims for medical procedures and services have been found to have a high level of specificity, but substantial variability in sensitivity exists across diagnoses when compared with the gold standard of medical records (Wilchesky et al. 2004).

Prescription claims data provide a wealth of information on drug exposure including dispensing date, pharmacy identifier, and drug information (name, dose, duration, i.e., days supply). Drugs may be coded by established classification systems (e.g., World Health Organization's Anatomical Therapeutic Chemical system). Using details like date of dispensing and days supply, one can construct measures to assess medication adherence (discussed below). While EMR data capture whether the physician prescribed a medicine for a patient with information on the dose and intended regimen, they do not record whether the patient actually obtained the medication from the pharmacy. Again, a key limitation is that EMR data do not capture all medicines dispensed to patients.

Medical claims data provide information on final end points such as fractures, stroke, myocardial infarction, or death but are limited for outcomes that involve intermediate biomarkers or self-reported symptom scales and measures of patient functioning. Researchers may use a combination of diagnostic, procedures, or facility codes to develop proxy measures of intermediate outcomes. For instance, a study used diagnostic and inpatient hospital stays to classify severity of chronic obstructive pulmonary disease and found moderate accuracy to medical charts (McKnight et al. 2005). Recent years have seen an increasing use of laboratory results data linked to administrative claims data, but these data are not available on a large-scale across the globe.

Study cohorts are typically observed (followed) for a certain period of time after the start of treatment to assess the occurrence of outcomes—see Fig. 11.2. This is known as the exposure risk window. The exposure risk window is the time period during which the medicine puts individuals at risk for outcome(s) of interest. The choice of exposure risk period considers the duration of medicines use and the onset and persistence of drug toxicity. Typically, there is an extension after the drug is discontinued to account for the period when a drug is still biologically active in the body. The choice of exposure risk windows can influence the estimate of risks. Risk windows should be validated or sensitivity analysis should be conducted on the varying length of exposure risk window.

Table 11.2 Study designs for pharmacoepidemiology

Cohort studies follow one group that is exposed to an intervention and another group that is non-exposed to determine the occurrence of the outcome (estimating the relative risk). Cohort studies can examine multiple outcomes of a single exposure.
Case-control studies compare the proportion of cases with a specific exposure to the proportion of controls with the same exposure (estimating the odds ratio). Case-control studies can examine multiple factors that may be associated with the presence or absence of the outcome.
Within-subject methods: *The self-controlled case series method* assesses the association between a transient exposure and an outcome by estimating the relative incidence of specified events in a defined time period after the exposure. *Case-crossover design* estimates the odds of an outcome by comparing the probability of exposure between the exposure and control periods. *Case-time-control design* is case-crossover design with the addition of a traditional control group.
Cross-sectional studies are used to determine prevalence, that is, the number of cases in a population at a certain time and to examine the association between an exposure and an outcome. It cannot establish causality.
Ecological studies focus on the comparison of groups defined either geographically or temporally. They can be used to identify associations by comparing aggregate data on risk factors and disease prevalence from different population groups.
Quasi-experimental designs: *Interrupted time series design* involves a time series (repeated observations of a particular outcome) collected before and after the implementation of an intervention to evaluate its effects. It can be conducted without or with a time series from a comparison group (known as interrupted time series with comparison series). *Pre–post with/without comparison group design* involves one measurement of a particular outcome before and another measurement after the implementation of an intervention to evaluate its effects. Intervention effect is estimated by a difference-in-differences approach when there are also pre–post measurements from a comparison group. *Post-only with/without comparison group design* involves only measurements of a particular outcome after the implementation of an intervention to evaluate its effects.

11.7 Study Designs

Pharmacoepidemiological research typically uses epidemiological methods. This section introduces a range of study designs often used in pharmacoepidemiological studies; these are also summarized in Table 11.2.

11.7.1 Cohort Studies

Cohort design can be prospective or retrospective and has a number of applications, including the study of incidence, causes, and prognosis (Goldacre 2001; Rochon et al. 2005). In a retrospective cohort study, both the exposure and the outcome of interest have already occurred. A cohort study typically follows a group of people in which some have had or have an exposure of interest in order to determine the occurrence of outcome(s). In pharmacoepidemiology, the exposure is typically a drug or a medical intervention. The probability of developing the outcome in the exposed (intervention group) is compared with that in the unexposed group (control group); this is called the relative risk. Cohort studies measure exposure and outcome in temporal sequence, thereby avoiding the debate as to which comes first; thus, this design can demonstrate causal relationships. An advantage of the cohort design compared with the case-control approach is that one can examine a wide range of possible outcomes in one cohort study.

Cohort design is inefficient for studying the incidence of a latent or rare outcome (e.g., cancer) because individuals would need to be followed for many years. The major challenges of this design include: (1) selection bias occurs when there are systematic differences between the study groups in factors related to the outcome, (2) the inability to control all extraneous factors (confounders) that might be associated with the outcome and might differ between the study groups, and (3) bias by differential loss to follow-up due to migration, death, or dropouts (Rochon et al. 2005). Bias and confounding are discussed later in the chapter.

11.7.2 Case-Control Studies

Case-control studies are usually retrospective. An intervention group would include individuals who have the outcome of interest (i.e., cases) and they are matched with a control group who do not (i.e., controls or noncases). Same information on prior exposure is collected from both groups (Breslow 1982). The proportion of cases with a specific exposure is compared to the proportion of controls with the same exposure (the odds ratio) and, therefore, determines the relative importance of the exposure with respect to the presence or absence of the outcome.

As some of the subjects have been deliberately chosen because they have the outcome, case-control studies are more cost-efficient than cohort studies—that is, a smaller sample size is sufficient to generate adequate information because of a higher percentage of cases per study. Further, a large number of variables can be examined at one time but the outcome being studied is limited (i.e., presence or absence of the outcome). Case-control studies are commonly used for initial, inexpensive evaluation of risk factors and are particularly useful when there is a long period between an exposure and the outcome or when the outcome is rare. The main problems with case-control design are confounding, selection bias, and recall bias (when the study depends on data collected from subjects rather than administrative data because people with the outcome are more likely to remember certain antecedents or exaggerate or minimize what they consider to be risk factors).

11.7.3 Nested Case-Control Studies

A nested case-control study is comprised of subjects sampled from a cohort study. The case-control study is thus "nested" inside the cohort study (Etminan 2004). When the outcome of interest is rare, it is cost-efficient to construct a case-control study within the cohort once a sufficient number of cases have accumulated. If records of a specific exposure of the cases and a subset of noncases are available, one can examine an exposure not planned in advance. This relates to traditional cohort studies in which data on covariates must be collected from subjects; this is not relevant in studies using administrative or other secondary data where the marginal cost of data collection for covariates is minimal. Analysis methods appropriate for case-control studies are applicable to nested case-control studies with computation of an odds ratio.

11.7.4 Within-Subject Methods (Case-Only Designs)

Cohort and case-control studies are useful for examining cumulative effects of chronic exposures. However, to minimize a major challenge of these methods—confounding by indication (discussed below)—within-subject methods that use self-controls to address the potential bias due to unmeasured confounders have been developed. These include self-controlled case series method, case-crossover design, and case-time-control design (Maclure et al. 2012).

The self-controlled case series derives from the cohort (fixed exposure, random event) rather than case-control (fixed event, random exposure) logic (Farrington 2004). The self-controlled case series method was originally published by Farrington et al. (1995) to investigate the association between vaccination and acute potential adverse events and has also been used to examine effects of chronic exposures such as antidepressants (Hubbard et al. 2003). Using data on cases only, it is an alternative to cohort or case-control methods for assessing the association between a transient exposure and an outcome by estimating the relative incidence of specified events in a defined period after the exposure. Time within the observation period is classified as at risk or as control time in relation to the exposure. The key advantages are that it controls for individual-level confounders (measured and unmeasured) and allows for changes in the risk of exposure with time (Whitaker et al. 2006). Therefore, it provides valid inference about the incidence of events in risk periods relative to the control period and is suitable for studying recurrent outcomes.

Case-crossover studies are also less susceptible to confounding by indication because the exposure history of each case is used as his/her own control and thus eliminates between-person confounding (Maclure 1991). They are useful for examining effects of transient exposures (e.g., use of benzodiazepine) on acute events (e.g., car accidents) and the time relationship of immediate effects to the exposure.

It estimates the odds of an outcome by comparing the probability of exposure between the exposure and control periods. However, the underlying probability of exposure must be constant so that the exposure and control periods are comparable. Therefore, changes in prescribing over time or within-person confounding, including transient indication or changes in disease severity, may be problematic because they can influence the probability of exposure, that is, the case-crossover design may have time-trend bias (Schneeweiss et al. 1997).

Case-time-control design is an elaboration of the case-crossover design. This design uses data from a traditional control group to estimate and adjust for time-trend bias and control-time selection bias (Schneeweiss et al. 1997).

11.7.5 Cross-Sectional Studies

Cross-sectional studies are primarily used to determine prevalence, that is, the number of cases in a population at a certain time. Prevalence is important in pharmacy practice because it influences the chance of a particular diagnosis and the chance of treatment. This method is also used to examine the association between an exposure and an outcome (infer causation). The subjects are assessed at one point in time to determine whether they are exposed to an exposure and whether they have the outcome. A difference between cross-sectional studies and cohort and case-control designs is that some of the subjects will not have been exposed nor have the outcome of interest. The major advantage of cross-sectional studies is that they are generally quick to conduct and inexpensive because there is no follow-up. However, this method cannot differentiate between cause and effect or the sequence of events and is inefficient when the outcome is rare.

11.7.6 Ecological Studies

Ecological or correlational studies focus on the comparison of groups defined either geographically or temporally and are typically based on aggregate secondary data. The unit of analysis in an ecological study is an aggregate of individuals, and variables are often aggregate measures collected on this group. One can use ecological studies to identify associations by comparing aggregate data on risk factors and disease prevalence from different population groups. Because all data are aggregate at the group level, relationships between exposure and outcome at the individual level cannot be empirically determined but are inferred from the group level. An error of reasoning ('ecological fallacy') occurs when conclusions are drawn about individuals on the basis of group-level data, as relationships between variables observed for groups may not necessarily hold for individuals (Morgenstern 1995). Ecological studies provide relatively cheap and efficient source for generating or testing the plausibility of hypotheses for further investigation by case-control, cohort, or experimental studies to test whether the observations made on populations as a whole can be confirmed in individuals. Despite these practical advantages, there are major methodological problems that limit causal inference, including ecologic and cross-level bias, problems of confounding control, within-group misclassification, temporal ambiguity, collinearity, and migration across groups (Morgenstern 1995). Therefore, ecological studies should only be conducted when individual-level data are unavailable.

11.7.7 Quasi-experimental Study Designs

Quasi-experimental studies are those that evaluate interventions but do not use randomization. Similar to RCTs, quasi-experimental studies aim to demonstrate causality between an intervention and an outcome. For such studies, interventions of interest are often educational interventions, quality improvement initiatives, and health policies, rather than drug exposure in typical pharmacoepidemiological studies. The intervention often cannot be randomized; some reasons include: (1) ethical considerations, (2) not feasible to randomize patients, (3) not feasible to randomize locations, and (4) a need to intervene quickly.

An interrupted time series design is a strong quasi-experimental design. It consists of repeated measures of an outcome taken at regular intervals of time (e.g., monthly or quarterly) both before and after an intervention that occurs at a defined point in time. For example, studies may aim to assess the impact of a policy or regulatory actions on drug utilization and immediate outcomes (Lu et al. 2010, 2011, 2012, 2014; Adams et al. 2009). This method controls for most threats to internal validity (e.g., secular changes in prescribing, aging of the population) because it adjusts for baseline trends in study outcomes that are unrelated to the intervention. In an interrupted time series study, the post-intervention outcomes that might have occurred in the absence of the intervention are predicted based on patterns of historical data before the intervention of interest, so it is possible to get more valid and accurate measures of intervention effects. "Interrupted time series with comparison series design" is even stronger that includes a comparison time series from another region or group of providers or patients. Challenges include co-interventions (i.e., other events that may have occurred simultaneously at the time of intervention) and the typical need for relatively large effect sizes.

Quasi-experimental studies commonly use a pre–post with non-randomized comparison group design. This design examines a single measurement before and after an intervention in the intervention group as well as in a comparison group. The inclusion of a pretest provides some information about what the rates might have been had the intervention not occurred. In most cases, if the intervention achieves its expected impacts, the differences in effects observed between the groups should come from changes in the study group. It is, therefore, important to show that the intervention and comparison groups were similar on a variety of factors before the intervention takes place. Statistical methods (e.g., propensity scores) are sometimes used to adjust for differences in baseline characteristics between the groups. However, studies that depend on these types of statistical adjustment alone without strong study designs provide less convincing results.

Quasi-experimental studies can also use a "pre–post without comparison group" or "post-only" design. The former examines measurements in a single group before and after an intervention; the latter examines only measurements collected after an intervention has occurred. A pre–post study is a weak design; we cannot be confident that observed changes would have occurred anyway without the intervention due to previous trends or to external changes. A post-only study is also a weak design because we do not know anything about previous levels and trends of the measured effect; thus, we cannot be certain that observed effects are due to the intervention or to some other factor. Even if the study includes a comparison group ("post-only with comparison group"), there is no way to know whether the observed effects in study and comparison groups would have been different anyway without the intervention.

11.8 Common Measures for Medicines Use

This section introduces frequently used metrics to understand drug utilization and medication adherence, which are key study outcomes in pharmacoepidemiology and pharmacy practice research.

11.8.1 Drug Utilization Metrics

A commonly used measure of drug utilization is Defined Daily Doses (DDDs) per 1,000 inhabitants per day, the standard unit recommended by the World Health Organization (2009). This measure allows comparisons of medicines use independent of the country's population, the pack size, and dosage of the medication dispensed. The DDD is the assumed average maintenance dose per day for a drug used for its main indication in adults. The DDD is often a compromise based on a review of the available information about doses used in various countries. Sales, prescription, or dispensing data presented in DDD/1,000 inhabitants/day may provide a crude estimate of the proportion of the study population that may be treated daily with certain medicines. For example, 10 DDDs/1,000 inhabitants/day indicates that 1% of the population on average might get a certain drug or group of drugs every day. This estimate is most useful for chronically used drugs when there is good agreement between the average prescribed daily dose and the DDD.

The World Health Organization has recommended a number of quality indicators of medicines use (World Health Organisation 1993) that can be constructed from prescription or dispensing data. These aim to estimate the extent of appropriate use, overuse, underuse, or misuse of medicines. Indicators include:

- Average number of drugs per prescription (per encounter or per patient)
- Percentage of drugs prescribed by generic name
- Percentage of encounters with an antibiotic prescribed
- Percentage of encounters with an injection prescribed
- Percentage of drugs prescribed from essential drugs list or formulary
- Proportion of treatment according to standard treatment guidelines
- Average drug cost per encounter

Data on drug costs are important for policy design and development to manage drug supply, pricing, and use. Costs may be determined at government, health facility, hospital, health insurance plan, or other levels within the health sector. Costs are often broken down according to drug group or therapeutic area to determine, for example, the reason for an increase in drug costs. For instance, the introduction of new, expensive oncology therapies may be found to be driving the increase in drug costs in a hospital. Changes in drug costs can result from changes in prescription volumes, quantity per prescription, or in the average cost per prescription. Common cost metrics include: total drug costs; cost per prescription; cost per treatment day, month, or year; cost per DDD; cost as a proportion of total health costs; and cost as a proportion of average income (World Health Organisation 2003).

11.8.2 Medication Adherence Metrics

Medication adherence (also known as compliance) generally refers to whether a patient takes a medication according to schedule, while persistence generally indicates whether a patient continues with therapy or the time from initiation to discontinuation of therapy. The definitions and methods to determine adherence and persistence differ substantially in the published literature. Studies of medication adherence and persistence in large populations are important to understand factors related to low adherence (which will allow development of necessary interventions to improve adherence) and to assess clinical and economic outcomes related to low adherence and/or persistence. Medication adherence can be assessed by biochemical measures (e.g., levels of the drug or its metabolites in the blood or urine), patient interviews, pill counts, and clinician assessments. However, these are generally not practical to perform on large populations.

Administrative databases containing information on pharmacy claims are valuable sources for assessing medication adherence and persistence efficiently. Commonly used measures can be determined using days supply information in pharmacy claims and the duration between refills (Andrade et al. 2006). Medication possession ratio, which estimates the proportion (or percentage) of days supply obtained during a specified time period or over a period of refill intervals. Other related measures of medication availability include: proportion of days covered, adherence ratio, refill adherence, compliance rate, continuous multiple-refill-interval measure of medication availability, adherence index, compliance ratio, or total number of days supply dispensed during a specified time interval (Andrade et al. 2006). The adherence measure is often dichotomized or categorized so that patients are considered adherent if a specified threshold was attained. A value of 80 % or higher is generally considered adherent (Ho et al. 2009). One major limitation worth noting is that such measure cannot determine if the patient actually consumed the dispensed medication. Switching between drugs within a therapeutic class is defined as the dispensing of a different drug within the same class at some point during the study period (following the dispensing of the initial drug). Medication gaps related measures (continuous measure of medication gaps, cumulative gap ratio) are based on the number of days a patient is without medication. This allows calculation of proportion of days without medication during a specified time interval. Another metric is discontinuation and continuation rates, often known as persistence or the frequency of patients discontinuing/continuing medications. Discontinuation is the occurrence of a treatment gap of a defined period between one dispensing of the medicine and a subsequent dispensing, with continuous use based on the days supply of medication dispensed or a specified time period after each dispensing (e.g., days supply dispensed plus a grace period in days).

11.9 Challenges of Pharmacoepidemiological Studies

It is critical to minimize the effects of bias and confounding in pharmacoepidemiological studies in order to provide results that are credible and convincing. Bias and confounding are major threats to internal validity of a study and should always be considered as alternative explanations when interpreting the relationship between an exposure and the outcome. This section introduces major challenges in pharmacoepidemiological research: misclassification, selection bias, and confounding, which are also summarized in Table 11.3.

11.9.1 Misclassification

A major challenge using administrative data for defining exposure and outcome is misclassification (also known as information bias) (Vandenbroucke et al. 2007), that is, subjects may be classified as being exposed to a drug when they are not or not exposed when they are; similarly for the classification of outcome events. The likelihood of misclassification may differ between the exposed and non-exposed groups. The exposed group has a lower likelihood of outcome misclassification because they enter the health-care system, which increases the likelihood of

Table 11.3 Major challenges in pharmacoepidemiologic studies

Information bias[b] occurs when systematic differences in the completeness or the accuracy of data lead to differential misclassification of individuals regarding exposures or outcomes.
Selection bias[a]: Systematic error in creating intervention groups, such that they differ with respect to prognosis. That is, the groups differ in measured or unmeasured baseline characteristics because of the way participants were selected or assigned. Also used to mean that the participants are not representative of the population of all possible participants.
Confounding[a]: A situation in which the intervention effect is biased because of some difference between the comparison groups apart from the planned interventions, such as baseline characteristics, prognostic factors, or concomitant interventions. For a factor to be a confounder, it must differ between the comparison groups and predict the outcome of interest.

[a]Definitions by the CONSORT statement (Rochon et al. 2005)
[b]Definition by the STROBE statement (Vandenbroucke et al. 2007)

recording a diagnosis. In contrast, the non-exposed are more likely to be misclassified as not having the outcome, which is an artifact of not entering the health-care system.

With respect to drug exposure, misclassification may be due to the multiple channels by which subjects can receive their medications outside of the reimbursement system. Examples include physician samples, patient assistance programs, paying out-of-pocket, taking medications belonging to someone else, secondary insurance coverage, and low-cost generic programs offered by retail pharmacies. Misclassification of drug exposure can impact outcome measurement because an important choice in study design is the time-window during which patients are considered "exposed" and during which the risk of outcome is assessed (exposure risk window—see Fig. 11.2).

With respect to outcomes, misclassification of diagnostic or procedure codes may be due to payment arrangements. For instance, clinicians are less incentivized to submit claims documenting care under capitated payment systems. Coding practices also vary under fee for service systems (e.g., upcoding—billings deliberately exaggerated to obtain higher payments or undercoding—to avoid penalty). Ideally, researchers should use definitions that have been validated against medical chart reviews. When there are several approaches to define the outcome, sensitivity analysis should be conducted to understand the implications of the various definitions on the results.

11.9.2 Selection Bias

Selection bias is a systematic error due to design and execution errors in sampling, selection, or classification methods (Rochon et al. 2005). Factors that determined whether an individual received a drug could result in the intervention and comparison groups differing in particular factors that affect the outcome, either because people were preferentially selected to receive the drug or because of choices that they made (Rochon et al. 2005). To minimize, assess, and deal with selection bias, a recommended approach involves the selection of appropriate comparison groups, the identification and assessment of the comparability of potential confounders between the groups, and the use of appropriate statistical techniques in the analysis (Rochon et al. 2005). Confounding by indication (also known as channeling bias) is a form of selection bias, which occurs when treatments are preferentially prescribed to groups of patients based on their underlying risk profile (Psaty et al. 1999). Confounding by indication is one of the most important, frequent problems encountered in pharmacoepidemiological studies due to the natural presence of incomparability of prognosis between subjects receiving the drug and those who do not. Thus, selection of exposure is confounded with patient factors (clinical, nonclinical, or both) that are also related to the outcome.

11.9.3 Confounding

Selection bias can result in confounding. A factor can confound an association only if it differs between the intervention and comparison groups (Rochon et al. 2005). For a variable to confound an association, it must be associated with both the exposure and outcome, and its relation to the outcome should be independent of its association with the intervention(see Fig. 11.1). Confounding occurs when the differences in baseline characteristics between the study groups result in differences in the outcome between the groups apart from those related to the exposure of interest (Mamdani et al. 2005). Crude, unadjusted results of nonexperimental studies may lead to invalid inference regarding the effects of the intervention. Confounding can cause over- or underestimation of the true relationship and may even change the direction of the observed effect.

11.10 Common Analytical Techniques

Because pharmacoepidemiological studies typically use data that were originally collected for other purposes, not all the relevant information may have been available for analysis. Thus, there are unknown and/or unmeasured potential confounders. This section discusses methods that have been developed and adopted to improve the comparability of the intervention and control groups. Table 11.4 summarizes these strategies for controlling confounding.

In the design phase, methods to control for confounding include: (1) restriction—inclusion to the study is restricted to a certain category of a confounder (e.g., male). However, strict inclusion criteria can limit generalizability of results to other segments of the population; and (2) matching of controls to cases (frequency matching or one-to-one matching) to enhance equal representation of subjects

Table 11.4 Strategies to reduce confounding

Design phase
Restriction: inclusion to the study is restricted to a certain category of a confounder (e.g., male).

Matching of controls to cases to enhance equal representation of subjects with certain confounders among study groups.

Analytical phase
Stratification: the sample is divided into subgroups or strata on the basis of characteristics that are potentially confounding the analysis (e.g., age).

Statistical adjustments: regression—estimates the association of each independent variable with the dependent variable (the outcome) after adjusting for the effects of other variables.

Propensity score: a score that is the conditional probability of exposure to an intervention given a set of observed variables that may influence the likelihood of exposure. Propensity score may be used for matching, stratification, and regression.

Marginal structural models using inverse probability of treatment weighting (IPTW) have been developed to adjust for time-varying confounding.

Instrumental variables: a pseudo-randomization method that divides patients according to levels of a covariate that is associated with the exposure but not associated with the outcome.

with certain confounders among study groups. The effect of the variable used for restriction or matching cannot be assessed and is a disadvantage of these approaches.

In the data analysis phase, stratification can be used to control for confounding. The study sample is divided into subgroups or strata on the basis of characteristics that are potentially confounding the analysis (e.g., age). The effects of the intervention are measured within each subgroup (Normand et al. 2005). Disadvantages of stratification include reduced power of the study to detect effects because the number of participants in each stratum is smaller than the total study population and subgroups may not be balanced with respect to other characteristics. Significant heterogeneity between strata suggests the presence of effect-modification. In this case, stratum-specific estimates should be reported because effect-modification is a characteristic of the effect under study rather than a source of bias that needs to be eliminated. A pooled estimate that is substantially different from stratum-specific estimates indicates a possible presence of confounding.

Statistical adjustment for dissimilarities in characteristics between the study groups is a commonly used method in the data analysis phase to control for confounding. Regression (e.g., linear, logistic, proportional hazards regression) is the most common method for reducing confounding in observational studies (Normand et al. 2005). To capture and assess all the potential confounders, a thorough literature review should be conducted to identify variables that can influence treatment selection or the outcome. When using administrative data with limited clinical information, there are likely instances when the model cannot include known or suspected confounders, the regression estimates of treatment effect will be biased leading to omitted variable or residual confounding bias. Regression analyses estimate the association of each independent variable (i.e., measures of baseline characteristics and the intervention) with the dependent variable (the outcome) after adjusting for the effects of all the other variables. It is important to compare adjusted and unadjusted estimates of the effect. If these estimates differ greatly, it suggests that the differences in baseline characteristics were a source of confounding and have had a substantial effect on the outcome.

In the recent decade, major advances in methods to control for confounding include propensity score, marginal structural models, and instrumental variables, which are outlined below.

Propensity score, proposed by Rubin and Rosenbaum (Rosenbaum and Rubin 1984), is a statistical method increasingly used by researchers to control for confounding by indication, particularly when there are a large number of variables. This score is the conditional probability of exposure to an intervention (e.g., drug treatment), given a set of observed variables that may influence the likelihood of exposure. The propensity score can be derived from a multivariable logistic regression analysis including variables that are statistical significantly associated with the exposure. A higher score indicates a higher probability of receiving the exposure. The most critical issue of propensity scoring techniques is the appropriate selection of variables that are included to generate the propensity score. All factors that are related to the treatment selection and/or outcome should be carefully considered for inclusion (Brookhart et al. 2006a). There are three main applications of the propensity score: matching, stratification, and regression. Matching on the propensity score aims to find the nearest match of a treated (exposed) individual to comparison subject(s) based on the propensity score. When propensity scores are used with a matching technique, baseline characteristics of treated and untreated groups are comparable, often resembles those obtained from RCTs where measured covariates are nearly equally balanced across groups (McWilliams et al. 2007). However, balance between unmeasured covariates cannot be assumed across groups (i.e., there is residual confounding). Propensity scores can be used in stratified analyses by grouping treated and untreated subjects into quintiles, deciles, or some other stratification level based on the propensity score; the effects of treatment can be directly compared within each stratum. Also, covariate adjustment is another propensity score method. In this approach, the estimated propensity score is included as a covariate in the regression model.

Standard methods (matching, stratification, and regression adjustment) are not adequate to adjust for time-varying confounding and may be biased. In pharmacoepidemiological studies, drug treatment effects are often time dependent and affected by time-dependent confounders that are themselves affected by previous treatment (exposure). To solve this problem, marginal structural models using inverse probability of treatment weighting have been recently developed (Robins et al. 2000). An example is the effect of aspirin on the risk of myocardial infarction and cardiac death, and prior myocardial infarction is a time-dependent confounder affected by previous treatment (Cook et al. 2002). This is because prior myocardial infarction is associated with (subsequent) aspirin use and is associated with (subsequent) cardiac death; it is also associated with past aspirin use.

In recent years, the instrumental variable method, a technique originates from the field of econometrics, has been used more commonly in pharmacoepidemiological studies to overcome the potential lack of balance on unobserved prognostic factors (e.g., health behavior) (Greenland 2000). In brief, this pseudo-randomization method divides patients according to levels of a covariate that is associated with the exposure but not associated with the outcome. For example, Brookhart et al. (2006b) used the prescribing physician's preference to cyclooxygenase-2 inhibitors or nonselective, non-steroidal anti-inflammatory drugs as an instrumental variable to compare the risk of gastrointestinal complications associated with the use of these medicines. The instrumental variable method may lead to equal distribution of characteristics in both exposed and non-exposed people and thus, reduce potential confounding. However, finding good instrumental variables has demonstrated to be remarkably difficult. Researchers should focus efforts on reducing the sources of bias (e.g., measurement error, omitted variables) instead of wishing for a "magic bullet" from instrumental variables.

11.11 The Future of Pharmacoepidemiology

We have been fortunate to live in an era where large amounts of data are available for research. However, protection of the privacy and confidentiality of personal health information are issues of concern to all jurisdictions, database owners, and researchers. In particular, public, patient, and consumers are very sensitive about genetic information; higher privacy and confidentiality standards for such information than those for other medical information may be required. Genetic information in the field of medical care includes a person's genetic predisposition to disease (e.g., results of specific genetic tests), diagnosis of heritable medical conditions, or family history of disease with a known pattern of inheritance. Genetic testing may help to identify DNA variants that predict an individual's response to a drug, resulting in grouping the population in terms of treatment effectiveness and adverse effects. Many people have concerns about confidentiality and the inappropriate use of genetic information, for example, affecting employment or health insurance rights. To address these concerns, the International Declaration on Human Genetic Data was adopted in October 2003; this and the Universal Declaration on the Human Genome and Human Rights are the only international points of reference in the field of bioethics (Educational, Scientific and Cultural Organization 2003). Furthermore, in May 2007 member countries of Organization for Economic Cooperation and Development (OECD) adopted the Guidelines for Quality Assurance in Molecular Genetic Testing, which provide principles and best practice for the quality assurance of molecular genetic testing (OECD 2007). Based on OECD Privacy Guidelines, the protection of patient privacy has generally been safeguarded by laws in some countries including OECD member countries. Future pharmacoepidemiology will see increasing research involving genetic information. Researchers in the field should pay attention to legislations, policies, and guidelines for use of genetic information for research.

The availability of electronic health-care databases and advances in pharmacoepidemiological methods enable researchers to identify products in which effectiveness does not match efficacy(the efficacy-effectiveness gap) (Lu 2014). This will challenge the actions of all concerned—industry, regulators, payers, health-care providers, and patients. In recent years, European Medicines Agency and the US Food and Drug Administration have required risk management plans or risk evaluation and mitigation strategies as part of the drug approval process to help ensure that the benefits of a particular medicine outweigh its risks in the real-world setting. Observational studies are also increasingly requested by payers and other agencies to assess the value of medicines. Patients may also demand better systems to monitor effectiveness and safety of medicines. In fact, it is best practice to establish a systematic, comprehensive approach to monitor all marketed drugs post-launch, and abundant administrative health-care data present a unique opportunity. This monitoring may range from descriptive utilization statistics to sophisticated comparative effectiveness research, depending on the budget impact and level of uncertainty about the risk–benefit of the medicine at the time of marketing.

The data explosion in modern society will surely continue. As presented in this chapter, the nature of drug monitoring activities will be determined by the availability of data, advances in research methods and biostatistics, and competent pharmacoepidemiologists. Pharmacoepidemiology will also continue to be an area for collaboration between multiple stakeholders, including physicians, regulators, payers, manufacturers, patients, and the general public. Given the important contribution of pharmacoepidemiological studies, collaboration should also involve decision makers for drug formularies, health economists, and health policy researchers. Pharmacoepidemiology will likely continue to be one of the most dynamic and challenging research areas for the coming decades.

References

Adams AS, Zhang F, LeCates RF et al (2009) Prior authorization for antidepressants in Medicaid: effects among disabled dual enrollees. Arch Intern Med 169(8):750–756

Agency for Healthcare Research & Quality (2013) Linking data for health services research: a framework and guidance for researchers (a draft report)

Andrade SE, Kahler KH, Frech F, Chan KA (2006) Methods for evaluation of medication adherence and persistence using automated databases. Pharmacoepidemiol Drug Saf 15(8): 565–574, discussion 575–567

Austin PC, Mamdani MM, Juurlink DN, Hux JE (2006) Testing multiple statistical hypotheses resulted in spurious associations: a study of astrological signs and health. J Clin Epidemiol 59(9):964–969

Avorn J (2004) The role of pharmacoepidemiology and pharmacoeconomics in promoting access and stimulating innovation. Pharmacoeconomics 22(Suppl 2):81–86

Benson K, Hartz AJ (2000) A comparison of observational studies and randomized, controlled trials. N Engl J Med 342:1878–1886

Bertoldi AD, Barros AJ, Wagner A, Ross-Degnan D, Hallal PC (2008) A descriptive review of the methodologies used in household surveys on medicine utilization. BMC Health Serv Res 8:222

Breslow N (1982) Design and analysis of case-control studies. Annu Rev Public Health 3:29–54

Brookhart MA, Schneeweiss S, Rothman KJ, Glynn RJ, Avorn J, Sturmer T (2006a) Variable selection for propensity score models. Am J Epidemiol 163(12):1149–1156

Brookhart MA, Wang PS, Solomon DH, Schneeweiss S (2006b) Evaluating short-term drug effects using a physician-specific prescribing preference as an instrumental variable. Epidemiology 17:268–275

Brown JS, Holmes JH, Shah K, Hall K, Lazarus R, Platt R (2010) Distributed health data networks: a practical and preferred approach to multi-institutional evaluations of comparative effectiveness, safety, and quality of care. Med Care 48(6 Suppl):S45–S51

Brown JS, Kahn M, Toh S (2013) Data quality assessment for comparative effectiveness research in distributed data networks. Med Care 51(8 Suppl 3):S22–S29

Chung Y, Lu CY, Graham GG, Mant A, Day RO (2008) Utilization of allopurinol in the Australian community. Intern Med J 38(6):388–395

Concato J, Shah N, Horwitz RI (2000) Randomized, controlled trials, observational studies, and the hierarchy of research designs. N Engl J Med 342:1887–1892

Cook NR, Cole SR, Hennekens CH (2002) Use of a marginal structural model to determine the effect of aspirin on cardiovascular mortality in the Physicians' Health Study. Am J Epidemiol 155(11):1045–1053

Etminan M (2004) Pharmacoepidemiology II: the nested case-control study–a novel approach in pharmacoepidemiologic research. Pharmacotherapy 24:1105–1109

Farrington CP (2004) Re: "Risk analysis of aseptic meningitis after measles-mumps-rubella vaccination in Korean children by using a case-crossover design". Am J Epidemiol 159: 717–718, author reply 718–720

Farrington P, Pugh S, Colville A et al (1995) A new method for active surveillance of adverse events from diphtheria/tetanus/pertussis and measles/mumps/rubella vaccines. Lancet 345: 567–569

Glynn RJ, Knight EL, Levin R, Avorn J (2001) Paradoxical relations of drug treatment with mortality in older persons. Epidemiology 12(6):682–689

Goldacre M (2001) The role of cohort studies in medical research. Pharmacoepidemiol Drug Saf 10:5–11

Gram LE, Hallas J, Andersen M (2000) Pharmacovigilance based on prescription databases. Pharmacol Toxicol 86(Suppl 1):13–15

Greenland S (2000) An introduction to instrumental variables for epidemiologists. Int J Epidemiol 29:722–729

Ho PM, Bryson CL, Rumsfeld JS (2009) Medication adherence: its importance in cardiovascular outcomes. Circulation 119(23):3028–3035

Hubbard R, Farrington P, Smith C, Smeeth L, Tattersfield A (2003) Exposure to tricyclic and selective serotonin reuptake inhibitor antidepressants and the risk of hip fracture. Am J Epidemiol 158:77–84

Johnson ES, Bartman BA, Briesacher BA et al (2012) The incident user design in comparative effectiveness research. Effective Health Care Program Research Report No. 32. Agency for Healthcare Research and Quality, Rockville, MD

Kelly E, Lu CY, Albertini S, Vitry A (2014) Longitudinal trends in utilization of endocrine therapies for breast cancer: an international comparison. J Clin Pharm Ther. doi:10.1111/jcpt.12227

Kush RD, Helton E, Rockhold FW, Hardison CD (2008) Electronic health records, medical research, and the Tower of Babel. N Engl J Med 358(16):1738–1740

Lu CY (2009) Pharmacoepidemiologic research in Australia: challenges and opportunities for monitoring patients with rheumatic diseases. Clin Rheumatol 28(4):371–377

Lu CY, Williams KM, Day RO (2007a) Has the use of disease-modifying anti-rheumatic drugs changed as a consequence of controlled access to high-cost biological agents through the Pharmaceutical Benefits Scheme? Intern Med J 37(9):601–606

Lu CY, Williams KM, Day RO (2007b) The funding and use of high-cost medicines in Australia: the example of anti-rheumatic biological medicines. Aust New Zealand Health Policy 4:2

Lu CY, Soumerai SB, Ross-Degnan D, Zhang F, Adams AS (2010) Unintended impacts of a Medicaid prior authorization policy on access to medications for bipolar illness. Med Care 48(1):4–9

Lu CY, Law MR, Soumerai SB et al (2011) Impact of prior authorization on the use and costs of lipid-lowering medications among Michigan and Indiana dual enrollees in Medicaid and Medicare: results of a longitudinal, population-based study. Clin Ther 33(1):135–144

Lu CY, Srasuebkul P, Drew AK, Ward RL, Pearson SA (2012) Positive spillover effects of prescribing requirements: increased cardiac testing in patients treated with trastuzumab for HER2+ metastatic breast cancer. Intern Med J 42(11):1229–1235

Lu CY, Zhang F, Lakoma MD et al (2014) Changes in antidepressant use by young people and suicidal behavior after FDA warnings and media coverage: quasi-experimental study. BMJ 348:g3596

Lu CY (2014) Uncertainties in real-world decisions on medical technologies. Int J Clin Pract 68(8):936–940. doi:10.1111/ijcp.12434.

Maclure M (1991) The case-crossover design: a method for studying transient effects on the risk of acute events. Am J Epidemiol 133:144–153

Maclure M, Fireman B, Nelson JC et al (2012) When should case-only designs be used for safety monitoring of medical products? Pharmacoepidemiol Drug Saf 21(Suppl 1):50–61

Mamdani M, Sykora K, Li P et al (2005) Reader's guide to critical appraisal of cohort studies: 2. Assessing potential for confounding. BMJ 330:960–962

McKnight J, Scott A, Menzies D, Bourbeau J, Blais L, Lemiere C (2005) A cohort study showed that health insurance databases were accurate to distinguish chronic obstructive pulmonary disease from asthma and classify disease severity. J Clin Epidemiol 58(2):206–208

McWilliams JM, Meara E, Zaslavsky AM, Ayanian JZ (2007) Use of health services by previously uninsured Medicare beneficiaries. N Engl J Med 357(2):143–153

Morgenstern H (1995) Ecologic studies in epidemiology: concepts, principles, and methods. Annu Rev Public Health 16:61–81

Motheral BR, Fairman KA (1997) The use of claims databases for outcomes research: rationale, challenges, and strategies. Clin Ther 19(2):346–366

Normand SL, Sykora K, Li P, Mamdani M, Rochon PA, Anderson GM (2005) Readers guide to critical appraisal of cohort studies: 3. Analytical strategies to reduce confounding. BMJ 330:1021–1023

Organisation for Economic Cooperation and Development (2007) OECD guidelines for quality assurance in genetic testing. http://www.oecd.org/sti/biotech/oecdguidelinesforqualityassurance ingenetictesting.htm

Paniz VM, Fassa AG, Maia MF, Domingues MR, Bertoldi AD (2010) Measuring access to medicines: a review of quantitative methods used in household surveys. BMC Health Serv Res 10:146

Perrio M, Waller PC, Shakir SA (2007) An analysis of the exclusion criteria used in observational pharmacoepidemiological studies. Pharmacoepidemiol Drug Saf 16(3):329–336

Psaty BM, Koepsell TD, Lin D et al (1999) Assessment and control for confounding by indication in observational studies. J Am Geriatr Soc 47:749–754

Robins JM, Hernan MA, Brumback B (2000) Marginal structural models and causal inference in epidemiology. Epidemiology 11(5):550–560

Rochon PA, Gurwitz JH, Sykora K et al (2005) Reader's guide to critical appraisal of cohort studies: 1. Role and design. BMJ 330:895–897

Rosenbaum PR, Rubin DB (1984) Reducing bias in observational studies using subclassification on the propensity score. J Am Stat Assoc 79:516–524

Schneeweiss S (2007) Developments in post-marketing comparative effectiveness research. Clin Pharmacol Ther 82(2):143–156

Schneeweiss S, Sturmer T, Maclure M (1997) Case-crossover and case-time-control designs as alternatives in pharmacoepidemiologic research. Pharmacoepidemiol Drug Saf 6(Suppl 3): S51–S59

Schneeweiss S, Patrick AR, Sturmer T et al (2007) Increasing levels of restriction in pharmacoepidemiologic database studies of elderly and comparison with randomized trial results. Med Care 45(10 Suppl 2):S131–S142

Strom BL, Carson JL, Halpern AC et al (1991) Using a claims database to investigate drug-induced Stevens-Johnson syndrome. Stat Med 10(4):565–576

United Nations Educational, Scientific and Cultural Organization (2003) International declaration on human genetic data. http://www.unesco.org/new/en/social-and-human-sciences/themes/bioethics/human-genetic-data/

Vandenbroucke JP, von Elm E, Altman DG et al (2007) Strengthening the Reporting of Observational Studies in Epidemiology (STROBE): explanation and elaboration. Epidemiology 18(6):805–835

Vitry AI, Thai LP, Lu CY (2011) Time and geographical variations in utilization of endocrine therapy for breast cancer in Australia. Intern Med J 41(2):162–166

Wettermark B (2013) The intriguing future of pharmacoepidemiology. Eur J Clin Pharmacol 69(Suppl 1):43–51

Whitaker HJ, Farrington CP, Spiessens B, Musonda P (2006) Tutorial in biostatistics: the self-controlled case series method. Stat Med 25:1768–1797

Wilchesky M, Tamblyn RM, Huang A (2004) Validation of diagnostic codes within medical services claims. J Clin Epidemiol 57(2):131–141

World Health Organisation (1993) How to investigate drug use in health facilities: selected drug use indicators – EDM Research Series No. 007. World Health Organisation, Geneva

World Health Organisation (2003) Introduction to drug utilization research. World Health Organisation, Geneva

World Health Organization (2009) DDD – Definition and General Considerations. http://www.whocc.no/ddd/definition_and_general_considera/. Accessed 25 Feb 2014

Chapter 12
The Future of Pharmacy Practice Research

Zaheer-Ud-Din Babar and Anna Birna Almarsdottir

> *'Prediction is very difficult, especially if it's about the future'*
> *(Niels Bohr, Danish physicist, 1885–1962)*

Abstract The chapter starts by outlining the current and future scenario related to pharmacy practice research. This chapter then sets the scene by discussing issues that are pertinent for practice research. These issues are changes in population demographics; changes in technology, the role of the pharmacy as an institution and consumer behaviour; as well as changes in the pharmacy profession. It also outlines the major shifts in pharmacy practice research, which include interprofessional collaboration and teamwork with patients, describing and measuring outcomes of interventions as well as patients' cultural diversity. It concludes by drawing attention to methodologies that would be most commonly used in future pharmacy practice research. Some of the future methodological challenges could be the emergence of big and complex data sets, dealing with electronic health records and pharmacy practice researchers' adoption of a myriad of mixed methodologies.

It is estimated that 81 % of American adults take at least one medicine per week and one quarter of them take at least five (Slone Epidemiology Center 2005). Medicines continue to be the most common medical treatment offered to patients, and they contribute significantly to the healthcare budget (Babar and Susan 2014).

Around the globe, medicine use is changing with changing disease patterns and advances in technology and science (Kaplan et al. 2013). However, the less than optimal use of medicines commonly results in poor health outcomes and

---

Z.-U.-D. Babar (✉)
Faculty of Medical and Health Sciences, School of Pharmacy, University of Auckland, Private Mail Bag 92019, Auckland, New Zealand
e-mail: z.babar@auckland.ac.nz

A.B. Almarsdottir
Clinical Pharmacology, Institute of Public Health, University of Southern Denmark, 5000 Odense C, Denmark

Department of Clinical Chemistry and Pharmacology, Odense University Hospital, 5000 Odense C, Denmark
e-mail: abalmars@health.sdu.dk

unnecessary cost. The traditional roles of dispensing, distribution and administration fall under the umbrella of pharmacy practice, but so too does the optimal use of medicines and the activity associated with this. This chapter discusses the current state of pharmacy practice and the associated research in this field. In addition, there is a focus on the methodologies being used, the context and likely content of future practice research and the potential policy implications of such research.

The key drivers of change that will influence the field of pharmacy practice research include (1) population demographics, (2) technology (informatics and health/pharmaceutical/device technologies), (3) pharmacy as 'institution' and as 'profession', (4) consumers of healthcare services and (5) new research capabilities building on technological changes. These drivers of change for pharmacy practice research are considered here, and four plausible shifts that are likely to emerge in the coming decades are argued.

12.1 Population Demographics

According to official United Nations (UN) population estimates, the world population of 7.2 billion will increase to 8.1 billion in 2025 and will further increase to 9.6 billion in 2050 and 10.9 billion by the year 2100 (UNFPA 2013).

The additional 3.7 billion population increase between now and 2100 is expected to come from developing countries. The increase is projected to take place in high-fertility countries, mainly African countries, India, Indonesia, Pakistan, the Philippines and the USA. By contrast, the population of the more developed regions is expected to change minimally, increasing from 1.25 billion in 2013 to 1.28 billion in 2100. The net increase in these regions will be largely due to migration from developing to developed countries (UNFPA 2013).

Declining fertility and longer lives contribute to an older world, particularly in the developed world. Globally, the number of persons aged 60 or over is expected to more than triple by 2100, increasing from 841 million in 2013 to 2 billion in 2050 and close to 3 billion in 2100. Global demographic change encompasses far more than declining fertility and an ageing population. Social and human capital is far more mobile than it once was. Immigration has resulted in multicultural populations in most developed countries (Kymlicka 2010). For example, in the USA 321 different languages are spoken. By 2050, current racial and ethnic minorities will constitute 50 % of the total population of the USA (U.S. Census Bureau 2014).

Health disparities among these populations are of particular concern (Ling et al. 2008), and it will be important to think about how these demographic changes will affect medicine use, health, disease and public policy. This demographic change will be coupled with technological shifts alongside an ageing population living with long-term conditions. Together, these issues will have considerable influence on pharmacy practice activities and the optimal use of medicines (Babar et al. 2014). As such, a proactive research agenda that focuses on these challenges is warranted.

The process of globalisation has led to an increasingly interconnected world, with both benefits and costs to the health sector. The speed and ease of shared information, advancements to healthcare delivery and health policy and the increased pace of discovery through international research collaborations can all facilitate improvements to population health. At the same time, a significant increase in international travel forges the spread of communicable diseases; for example, the 2003 epidemic of severe acute respiratory syndrome (SARS) and the growth of antibiotic-resistant Pneumococcus species. Health priorities, for which the supply and use of medicines is often central, must increasingly be viewed from a global perspective (Murdan et al. 2014).

12.2 Technology

The traditional model of community pharmacy is being challenged, and technology is driving change in pharmacy practice. The increased use of technology includes automation at community pharmacies, e-prescribing and e-communication, as well as pharmacists' access to integrated patient records. These technological advances impact on how patients and consumers are accessing and using pharmacy services and medicines (Smith et al. 2013). Robotics and electronic prescribing are reshaping the dispensing of medicines, and this has the potential to release pharmacists to undertake more patient-centred care (Smith et al. 2013). However, the pace of technological development varies among countries. For example, dispensing with robots has become widespread within hospital pharmacy, and in community pharmacy in some countries such as the Netherlands when compared with UK.

Increasing use of medical diagnostics means that consumers are now in a position to be more aware of their health status. Companies like Google and Apple are working to develop new applications, tools and devices whereby consumers will be much more aware of their health status and will be able to store their electronic health record (EHR). This technological development will mean that consumers will be much more aware of disease states and medications, and as a result pharmacists will need to remain current with skill sets and knowledge.

Use of the internet to supply pharmaceuticals is also becoming more common; for example, through established networks such as Amazon. Advances in science will allow innovative new drugs to treat specific populations based on their genetic makeup. In the next 5–10 years, it is expected that the pharmaceutical industry will deliver drugs to people based on their preferences and will tailor specific treatment regimens supporting their lifestyles and behaviours (The Future of Pharmaceuticals 2001). It has been mooted that 3D printing will play its part in the generation of pharmaceuticals, where users would go to an online drugstore with their digital prescription, buy the 'blueprint' and the chemical 'ink' they need and then print the drug at home with software and a 3D molecular printer. In this manner, the chemicals and dosages can be tailored to the specific needs of the individual (Gayomali 2013).

Developments such as these are expected to significantly change the face of healthcare and pharmacy practice and the research underpinning it. With this in mind, the future research agenda must align with addressing some of these influences and challenges.

12.3 Role of Pharmacy as 'Institution' and 'Profession'

12.3.1 Community Pharmacy as 'Institution'

With over 40,000 registered pharmacists in England alone, pharmacy is the third largest health profession after medicine and nursing. Internationally, health systems are increasingly recognising the role of pharmaceutical care and community pharmacy (Scottish Government 2013; Pharmaceutical Care 2012). As many health systems are under pressure due to shortages of funding and manpower, community pharmacy has a window of opportunity in many countries where they are the most accessible type of care.

In England community pharmacy is under pressure, as NHS funding for dispensing and other services is constrained, reimbursement of drug costs is diminishing, non-pharmaceutical sales are falling and the oversupply of pharmacies and pharmacists also contributes to this pressure (Health and Social Care Information Centre 2012). Internationally, this will only be reversed if pharmacies are able to create new extended roles based on patient-centred care and persuade funders to purchase services as part of wider programmes of public health, treatment of common ailments, care for people with long-term conditions and so forth (Smith et al. 2013).

However, much has been written about the role of pharmacy as an institution in society, the state of play—'where it is' and 'where it should be going' community pharmacy seems to be marginalised in the health and social care system at local and national levels. Pharmacy is seen by others as an insular profession, busy with its own concerns and missing out on debates and decisions that other health and social care organisations are engaging with in the wider world of health policy (Smith et al. 2013; Lewis et al. 2014).

It is not clear to healthcare and social professionals, policy-makers, patients and the population at large what is meant by the terms 'pharmaceutical care' and 'medicines optimisation'. Whilst hotly debated within pharmacy circles, the terms are not well understood and there is no consensus even among informed health policy and management experts. Consumers also have misconceptions about the role of pharmacists. A 2008 consumer survey in the UK found that 43 % of people would consider consulting a pharmacist for tests related to their long-term condition, but that only 6 % had actually done so (Which 2008). This raises very important questions about the actual availability and services that pharmacists can provide for patients, in comparison with the assertions often made about the potential of pharmacy to deliver such care (Smith et al. 2013).

The global picture of the 'place' of community pharmacy as an institution is also rather varied. In some parts of the world, pharmacy has been gaining a foothold, as is seen in the USA (Lewis et al. 2014). Conversely, relatively strong professional systems have been dismantled and restructured where pharmacy has moved to a more commercial identity, such as in some Nordic countries (Almarsdóttir and Traulsen 2009). The question could be raised as to whether community pharmacies in their current form may disappear if only seen as commercial sellers of medicines and be replaced by mail order, robot technology and automatic delivery of medications.

12.3.2 The Pharmacy Profession

In line with the developments of pharmacy as 'institution', earlier research focused on the dual role of the community pharmacist as a business person, which was juxtaposed to that of a healthcare professional (Kronus 1975; Hindle and Cutting 2002). In this focus, their education, job content and satisfaction have been of interest. Deprofessionalisation and loss of autonomy to business has been an important topic within this research. Researchers in Canada and Australia have suggested that despite increased efforts and important policy initiatives (Canadian Pharmacists Association 2008; The Fifth Community Pharmacy Agreement 2010), the majority of pharmacists still prefer the status quo, with dispensing as their main professional activity (Rosenthal et al. 2010; Mak et al. 2011). Each year, 84 % of adults in England visit a pharmacy at least once, 78 % of these attendances being for health-related reasons. Whilst medicine use reviews (MUR) and new medicine services for chronic illnesses are now widely available in pharmacies, some pharmacies are still not taking advantage of the opportunities afforded by these programmes to provide, screening, diagnosis, advice, medicines support and public health services. There needs to be a significant change in this area, as the low preparedness of pharmacists indicates that research on pharmacists and how the world views them is not the most promising way forward.

It is fair to say that hospital pharmacists have not been split according to a business versus professional clinical image. This sector of the profession has largely developed a role as clinical pharmacists, increasingly focusing on patient care in addition to pharmacy's traditional distribution and compounding role in the hospital setting. In a sense, one can view this as a different type of duality of roles (sourcing vs advice) which has manifested differently around the globe.

Internationally, healthcare systems are under pressure from changing population demographics and service demand, coupled with relatively decreasing resources (Ling et al. 2008). As such, health funders, planners and policy-makers have been keen to explore new practice models that will fulfil political objectives. This means that pharmacists will have to continue adjusting to an environment of shifting boundaries and new clinical roles as healthcare professionals. There is fertile ground with many innovative ideas, but these are usually localised and have not been taken to a wider context (Smith et al. 2013). A few notable exceptions are, for example, the Medicaid Medication Therapy Management Program (2014) and the Australian Home Medication Review (HMR) (Australian Government Department of Health and Ageing 2010).

In the last instance, HMRs were kept as community pharmacy provided services until 2012, where this was widened to include independent pharmacist consultants. Another example of a proactive pharmacy is Bromley-by-Bow in London; an NHS walk-in centre is co-located with a green-light pharmacy, and the walk-in centre pharmacists triage people who do not need to see a doctor or nurse to the pharmacy for advice and self-care (Smith et al. 2013; Thomas and Plimley 2012).

12.4 Role and Expectations of Consumers

The lay public is becoming more literate and better educated with more resources at their disposal than was the case 20–30 years ago. The literature dealing with trends in consumerism of healthcare defines the 'new consumer' as having the following characteristics: being information strong, information seeking, non-authoritarian and increasingly demanding (Winkler 1987; Herzlinger 1997; Traulsen and Noerreslet 2004).

One very important phenomenon is the baby boomers coming into retirement age (Barr 2014). As noted above, this demographic shift will put pressure on healthcare systems and speed up the requirement for development of new models of care which are cost-effective, integrated and team based. The boomer's political prowess and sheer numbers will force pharmacy to adapt to this through monitoring carefully what this group wants from pharmacy and the wider healthcare sector and how the cohort might influence the healthcare agenda.

12.5 New Horizons for Pharmacy Practice Research

As the institution and profession of pharmacy develops within the realm of rapidly changing healthcare technology, healthcare systems and patient populations, it faces future challenges and has to respond to these. This will mean four types of major shifts for research within pharmacy practice. Some of these shifts are well under way in many countries.

12.5.1 *From Uniform Pharmacy Practice/Pharmacist Implemented Interventions to Cross-Disciplinary or Interprofessional Collaboration and Team Work with Patients*

The opinion has been voiced that pharmacy practice research all too often has been aimed at evaluating narrowly focused pharmacy services and the world view of these (Almarsdottir et al. 2013). In addition, the challenges faced by healthcare systems are forcing providers and professionals to implement more large-scale team-based healthcare services. This is an opportunity for pharmacists to get involved and/or build on models of care that have been generated internationally. Smaller projects started by enthusiastic 'trail blazers' within pharmacy have often been successful, since these pioneer pharmacists have high motivation and sound connections within the community they work in. Making their models transferrable to a larger scale and different settings is the challenge facing both practitioners and researchers.

The researchers can play an important role, with their knowledge of pharmaceutical policy analysis and implementation research. Research activity can be implemented within a framework coined by Useem (2002) as 'leading up'. This approach recognises that an organisation's best efforts are accomplished when leaders move forward strategically, but also earnestly look back to the rank and file and listen and act upon the thoughts and insights shared by those who follow. The successes within pharmacy practice have illustrated that 'leading up' requires researchers to find out what the rank and file ('leader followers') think and are willing to do, to react to the changes ahead.

Pharmacy sometimes gets forgotten in collaborative schemes to improve quality in healthcare, and researchers and pharmacy professional organisations need to monitor closely developments within the wider framework of healthcare (Scahill 2011). This leads to further pressure when undertaking programme evaluation and implementation research and making it known what pharmacists can contribute to patient care within the cross-disciplinary framework. Pharmacy practice researchers will have to prepare themselves to communicate with funders to become recognised as integral members of healthcare teams. They can then push forth pharmacy practitioners within the framework. When planning projects are centred on interprofessional collaboration, pharmacy professional bodies need to be aware of the benefits that pharmacy practice researchers bring to the table.

12.5.2 From Describing and Measuring Outcomes of Interventions Towards Systematising and Understanding Implementation of Large-Scale Initiatives

Policy-makers and administrators commission healthcare services and purchase specific clinical interventions. It will not suffice to plan an intervention without being able to demonstrate its value to purchasers, based on theoretical and empirical merits. Questions that need to be answered include:

- What does the intervention entail?
- Why are individual components of the intervention chosen?
- What is the long-term cost for the organisation?
- And what impact will interventions have on the way the organisation works?

There has been enough research into effects and outcomes carried out (Smith et al. 2013). What is required is a shift to focus on implementation research and how decision-makers can be influenced to incorporate pharmacy in large-scale health services planning. Researchers will also need to follow the trend towards increased team work within healthcare and refrain from studying interventions undertaken by pharmacy in a vacuum.

Placing the patient at the centre of the system has been a weakness of pharmacy practice research which is focused on itself as a subject of study. Future pharmacy practice research will have to shift towards studying collaborative models, identifying problem areas and reaching consensus on systematised approaches. It will be even more important to listen to professions that pharmacists will collaborate with and to social and organisational scientists in order to avoid the programmes' failure due to unobserved negative attitudes. Clinical pharmacology is one of the most important disciplines to ally with in this respect (Burckart 2012). Similarly, healthcare authorities and their administrators may want to impress by implementing new services such as medication reviews, but may omit setting up real outcomes goals and institute process indicators that will not improve process. For example, an outcome measure of how many interventions the pharmacists suggest to GPs may actually be counterproductive and lead to both lower quality and alienation of doctors from the project. Researching successful collaborative approaches will be one of the most important strands in pharmacy practice in the future (see for example Snyder et al. 2010).

12.5.3 Patients Are Increasingly Culturally Diverse and Active Analyzers and Decision-Makers Who Use IT to Their Advantage

With the baby boomers ageing, there will be a domineering group of people expecting healthy ageing who involve many different approaches to prevention and life enhancement. They are more health literate, critical and information seeking than the generations before them, and they have a stronger voice in healthcare politics (Barr 2014). This will impact all of healthcare research. On the pharmacy practice front, this will go hand in hand with demand for evidence for practising in a certain way. Why pharmacists do as they do will be questioned, just as for other healthcare professionals. This will mean that interventions need to be interpreted and founded not only in professional but in patient rationalities.

The trends reviewed regarding the ageing of the population constituting the baby boomers, coupled with fast-evolving IT decision support systems for patients and healthcare professionals, will mean that they have more (evidence-based) information about health and medicines ready at their fingertips which they are able to use due to their high level of health literacy and will show little or no submissiveness to authority, rather looking at health professionals as partners in their decisions about healthcare and life style. This will make physicians, pharmacists and other healthcare professionals into 'guides/facilitators/advocates' and not all-knowing experts.

Practising pharmacists and their pharmacy researcher colleagues will have to adapt to this new reality by studying how they use the informatics available, and how this information/informatics influences them. It will become even more imperative for pharmacists to maintain patient-centredness, since the baby boomers will require pharmacists to have a holistic view of them and be guides in their quest for good health.

Cultural differences—especially within countries with significant immigration—make for a burgeoning field of research within the pharmacy practice sector. This trend will be escalated as the baby boomers are primarily a phenomenon of the inhabitants of industrialised developed countries. There will also be large minority groups within this part of the world who have recently immigrated and will need a totally different healthcare approach.

12.5.4 Blurring of Boundaries Between What Has Been Termed Pharmacy Practice Research and Related Fields

Many researchers who classify themselves pharmacy practice researchers also work in departments that define their work as part of drug utilisation research (DUR), clinical pharmacy, pharmaceutical policy, health services research, health economics or social pharmacy. Some pharmacy practice researchers can even relate to having one or more of these as areas of expertise. As pressure increases to participate in large multidisciplinary consortia, the relationship between those working in the fields of DUR, pharmacoepidemiology, social science theories and clinical pharmacy research will be expected to intensify and develop a common front towards the public. Other research areas such as pharmacogenetics and drug formulation—which have not traditionally been integrally connected with pharmacy practice research—may also increasingly be invited to 'enter this space' or may be a competence of many who define themselves as pharmacy practice researchers.

12.6 Methodologies in the Future of Pharmacy Practice Research

As demonstrated within previous chapters of this book, there are a wide variety of methods in use within pharmacy practice research. Historically, the research area has been characterised by being more inclusive of qualitative methods than related pharmaceutical subjects such as pharmacoepidemiology and drug utilisation research (DUR). One of the reasons for this has been noted as the inclusion of the patient/user perspective in pharmacy practice research. This is currently more fluid and changing, as being outlined in the chapter on pharmacoepidemiological methods in the book. These related fields are moving towards more breadth in methodological and design choices.

Another important development is the increased availability of 'big data' in many countries around the globe. Big data in healthcare refers to electronic health data sets so large and complex that they are difficult (or impossible) to manage with traditional software and/or hardware; nor can they be easily managed with traditional or common data management tools and methods (Raghupathi and Raghupathi 2014). This development will increase the pressure on pharmacy practice researchers to be knowledgeable about the use of extensive data sets in understanding the patient/user perspective and in evaluating pharmacy practice-related healthcare initiatives. More breadth will be required of researchers within the field, although those involved in qualitative methodologies may also have to become savvier in using big secondary qualitative data.

Due to the expansion of techniques available and challenges faced, researchers will have to be able to use a larger palate of methods and be ready to use mixed methods. They will have to be even more knowledgeable about various designs and methods when working in teams of researchers who do not have the same educational background. Pharmacy practice researchers need to be clearer about who they are, where they sit on the epistemological spectrum and what special competences they bring to large-scale interprofessional projects.

Funders of research have views of what they want to achieve and how this should be evaluated. As key stakeholders, they are likely to require a broad healthcare services focus and be less likely to fund pharmacy-focused research. These projects are then often led and administered by social science trained persons who make crucial decisions on funding. Therefore, pharmacy practice researchers will have to closely follow developments in methods and theories within the social sciences.

Future research could focus on medicines optimisation and on improving safety and effectiveness of medicines. With active engagement of pharmacists in local primary care networks and their access to integrated patient records, they will be in a better position to conduct this type of research. Other uses of integrated patient records data could include pharmacists undertaking predictive risk analysis of local populations of patients. This could also help to identify and target patients considered at risk of developing complications in conditions like asthma or when taking high-risk medicines.

12.7 Summary

The chapter has outlined the changes in pharmacy practice research. The key drivers of change to influence pharmacy practice research are population parameters, changes in technology, consumers of healthcare services and new research capabilities building on technological changes. As the institution and profession of pharmacy develops within the realm of rapidly changing healthcare technology, it faces future challenges and has to respond to these. The growing focus on pharmacy practice research would include interprofessional collaboration and teamwork with patients, describing and measuring the outcomes of interventions as well as cultural diversity of patients. The future methodological development in pharmacy practice research would be the emergence of big data and dealing with large and complex electronic health records. Due to the expansion of techniques available and challenges faced, researchers will have to be able to use a larger palate of methods and be ready to use mixed methods. Also, as most research projects are often led and administered by social science researchers, pharmacy practice researchers will have to closely follow developments in methods and theories within the social sciences.

References

Almarsdóttir AB, Traulsen JM (2009) Multimethod research into policy changes in the pharmacy sector – the Nordic case. Res Social Adm Pharm 5(1):82–90

Almarsdottir AB, Kaae S, Traulsen JM (2013) Opportunities and challenges in social pharmacy and pharmacy practice research. Res Social Adm Pharm 10(1):252–255

Australian Government Department of Health and Ageing (2010) Home medicines review program qualitative research project final report. Campbell Research and Consulting, Australia

Babar Z-U-D, Susan F (2014) Identifying priority medicines policy issues for New Zealand. BMJ Open 4(5):e004415

Babar ZU, Gray A, Kiani A, Vogler S, Ballantyne P, Scahill S (2014) The future of medicines use and access research: using the *Journal of Pharmaceutical Policy and Practice* as a platform for change. J Pharm Policy Pract 7:8. http://www.joppp.org/content/7/1/8

Barr P (2014) The boomer challenge. Trustee February:13–16

Burckart GJ (2012) Clinical pharmacology and clinical pharmacy: a marriage of necessity. Eur J Hosp Pharm 19:19–21

Canadian Pharmacists Association (2008) Blueprint for pharmacy: designing the future together. Canadian Pharmacists Association, Ottawa, ON. http://blueprintforpharmacy.ca/docs/pdfs/2011/05/11/BlueprintVision.pdf. Accessed 11 November 2014

Gayomali C (2013) Can you 3D print drugs? *The Week*, 26 June. http://theweek.com/article/index/246091/can-you-3d-print-drugs

Health and Social Care Information Centre (2012) General pharmaceutical services in England: 2002–03 to 2011–12. www.hscic.gov.uk/searchcatalogue?productid=9731&q=title%3a%22general+pharmaceutical+services%22&sort=relevance&size=10&page=1#top

Herzlinger RE (1997) Market-driven health care: who wins, who loses in the transformation of America's largest service industry. Addison–Wesley, New York, NY

Hindle K, Cutting N (2002) Can applied entrepreneurial education enhance job satisfaction and financial performance? An empirical investigation in the Australian Pharmacy Profession. J Small Bus Manag 40:162–167

Kaplan W, Wirtz VJ, Mantel-Teeuwisse A, Stolk P, Duthey B, Laing R (2013) Priority medicines for Europe and the World: 2013 update. World Health Organization, Geneva

Kronus CL (1975) Occupational values, role orientations and work settings: the case of pharmacy. Socio Q 16:171–183

Kymlicka W (2010) The current state of multiculturalism in Canada and research themes on Canadian multiculturalism 2008–2010. http://www.cic.gc.ca/english/pdf/pub/multi-state.pdf

Lewis NJW, Shimp LA, Rockafellow S, Tingen JM, Choe HM, Marcelino MA (2014) The role of the pharmacist in patient-centered medical home practices: current perspectives. Integr Pharm Res Pract 3:29–38

Ling AM, Panno NJ, Shader ME, Sobinsky RM, Whitehead HN, Hale KM (2008) The evolving scope of pharmacy practice: perspectives from future pharmacists. http://www.pharmacy.ohio-state.edu/forms/outreach/intro-to-pharmacy/Evolving_Scope_of_Pharmacy_Practice.pdf

Mak VSL, Clark A, Poulsen JH et al (2011) Pharmacists' awareness of Australia's health care reforms and their beliefs and attitudes about their current and future roles. Int J Pharm Pract 20 (1):33–40

Medication Therapy Management (2014) Centers for Medicaid and Medicare services. http://www.cms.gov/Medicare/Prescription-Drug-Coverage/PrescriptionDrugCovContra/MTM.html

Murdan S, Blum N, Francis SA, Slater E, Alem N, Munday M, Taylor J, Smith F (2014) The global pharmacist. http://www.ioe.ac.uk/Global_Pharmacist_-_FINAL.PDF, UCL School of Pharmacy

Pharmaceutical Care (2012) Policies and practices for a safer, more responsible and cost-effective health system. European Directorate for the Quality of Medicines & HealthCare, EDQM. www.edqm.eu/en/pharmaceutical-care-1517.html

Raghupathi W, Raghupathi V (2014) Big data analytics in healthcare: promise and potential. Health Inform Sci Syst 2:3

Rosenthal M, Austin Z, Tsuyuki RT (2010) Are pharmacists the ultimate barrier to pharmacy practice change? CPJ 143(1):37–42

Scottish Government (2013) Prescription for excellence: a vision and action plan for the right pharmaceutical care through integrated partnerships and innovation. Scottish Government, Edinburgh. www.scotland.gov.uk/publications/2013/09/3025

Scahill SL (2011) Community pharmacy doesn't appear as part of the collaboration discourse within New Zealand primary care. J Prim Healthcare 3(3):244–247

Slone Epidemiology Center at Boston University (2005) Patterns of medication use in the United States 2005: a report from the Slone Survey. http://www.bu.edu/slone/SloneSurvey/AnnualRpt/SloneSurveyWeb.Report2005.pdf. Accessed 23 June 2008

Smith J, Picton C, Dayan M (2013) Now or never: shaping pharmacy for the future, the report of the Commission on future models of care delivered through pharmacy November 2013. Royal Pharmaceutical Society of Great Britain, London UK. http://www.rpharms.com/promoting-pharmacy-pdfs/moc-report-full.pdf

Snyder ME, Zillich AJ, Primack BA, Rice KR, McGivney MAS, Pringle JL, Smith RB (2010) Exploring successful community pharmacist-physician collaborative working relationships using mixed methods. Res Social Adm Pharm 6(4):307–323

The Fifth Community Pharmacy Agreement between the Commonwealth of Australia and the Pharmacy Guild of Australia (2010) http://www.guild.org.au/docs/default-source/public-documents/tab---the-guild/Community-Pharmacy-Agreements/fifth-community-pharmacy-agreement.pdf. Accessed 11 November 2014

The Future of Pharmaceuticals (2001) Healthcare Horizons, Institute for the Future. http://www.iftf.org/uploads/media/SR-756_Future_of_Pharmaceuticals.pdf

Thomas M, Plimley J (2012) The future of community pharmacy in England. AT Kearney, London. www.atkearney.com/documents/10192/649132/the+future+of+community+pharmacy.pdf/1838dede-b95a-4989-8600-6b435bd00171

Traulsen JM, Noerreslet M (2004) The new consumer of medicine – the pharmacy technicians' perspective. Pharm World Sci 26:203–207

U.S. Census Bureau (2014) Population projections, U.S. interim projections by age, sex, race, and Hispanic origin: 2000–2050. http://www.census.gov/ipc/www/usinterimproj/

United Nations Fund Population Fund (2013) Linking population, poverty and development. http://www.unfpa.org/pds/trends.htm

Useem M (2002) Leading up. Center for Leadership & Change. http://leadership.wharton.upenn.edu/l_change/up_lead/Exec_Excellence.shtml. Accessed 11 November 2014

Which (2008) A test of your own medicine. October, pp 12–15

Winkler F (1987) Consumerism in health care: beyond the supermarket model. Policy Polit 15(1):1–8

Chapter 13
Pharmacists' Attitudes Towards Pharmacy Practice Research: A Review

Ahmed Awaisu, Nadir Kheir, Noor Alsalimy, and Zaheer-Ud-Din Babar

Abstract Despite an increase in pharmacy practice research, literature addressing the attitudes and involvement of pharmacists is limited. Our own observations as pharmacy practitioners and educators lead us to believe that, so far, pharmacists are reluctant to participate in research at any level and indicate some barriers to research. In this chapter, we review the literature and gauge the views and attitudes of pharmacists with regard to their involvement in research. We also identify the barriers as well as outline the enablers to conducting such research. The chapter highlights pharmacists' attitudes and trends towards pharmacy practice research over the past three decades. We mainly utilised MEDLINE, PubMed, EBSCO, ScienceDirect, ProQuest and Google Scholar to identify published studies surrounding this issue.

13.1 Evolution of Pharmacy Practice as a Catalyst for Research

The pharmacy profession has undergone tremendous changes, and the scope of pharmacy professional practice has expanded in the past few decades (Bond 2006; Holland and Nimmo 1999; Van Mil and Fernandez-Llimos 2013). This is further supported by the evolution of the concept and practice of pharmaceutical care in the 1990s (Hepler and Strand 1990; Holland and Nimmo 1999; Penna 1990). Pharmacists have extended their roles beyond the traditional services of medicinal products preparation and distribution to ensuring that optimal therapeutic outcomes are

---

A. Awaisu (✉) • N. Kheir
College of Pharmacy, Qatar University, Doha, Qatar
e-mail: aawaisu@qu.edu.qa; nadirk@qu.edu.qa

N. Alsalimy
Al-Rumailah Hospital, Hamad Medical Corporation, Doha, Qatar

Z.-U.-D. Babar
Faculty of Medical and Health Sciences, School of Pharmacy, University of Auckland, Auckland, New Zealand

© Springer International Publishing Switzerland 2015
Z.-U.-D. Babar (ed.), *Pharmacy Practice Research Methods*,
DOI 10.1007/978-3-319-14672-0_13

achieved through patient-centred cognitive services (Holland and Nimmo 1999; Tsuyuki and Schindel 2008). These cognitive functions include, but are not limited to, patient education and counselling, providing drug information, monitoring drug therapy, health promotion and disease prevention, disease state management, clinical pharmacokinetic consultations and clinical recommendations to other members of the healthcare team. This new paradigm in pharmacy practice has resulted from several factors such as increased prevalence of drug-related morbidity and mortality (Johnson and Bootman 1997), escalating costs of healthcare delivery due to demographic changes in the population and technological advancements (Bond 2006) and patients' increased demands, preferences and expectations. The changing roles for pharmacy are also attributed to the ease with which the public accesses pharmacy services as well as changes in pharmacy curricula that led to increased expertise in therapeutics.

13.2 Why Be Interested in Pharmacists' Attitudes Towards Practice-Based Research?

According to the Canadian Pharmacists Association, "pharmacy practice research" is defined as a component of health services research that focuses on the assessment and evaluation of pharmacy practice (Bakker 1996). The new roles for pharmacists evolve in parallel with evidence-based practice, which is a new paradigm in health services delivery (Sackett et al. 1996). As new professional services and practices evolve, there is a need to demonstrate evidence of their benefit and cost-effectiveness (Bond 2006; Kritikos et al. 2013; Roberts and Kennington 2010b, c; Schommer et al. 2010; Anderson et al. 2008).

Some US-based studies have reviewed the literature on the evidence of benefit of clinical pharmacy services (Hatoum and Akhras 1993; Hatoum et al. 1986; Schumock et al. 1996, 2003). However, often local evidence is needed that could demonstrate the need for a new service or different method of service delivery (Bond 2006; Peterson et al. 2009; Roberts and Kennington 2010a, b, c). Such evidence can be provided through pharmacy practice and clinical research that can inform policy and confirm the value or feasibility of the potential new roles and services (Bond 2006; Kritikos et al. 2013; Roberts and Kennington 2010b; Ambler and Sheldrake 2009; Schommer et al. 2010). This places pharmacy practice in a central role for establishing new pharmacy services by justifying the need, effectiveness and the value of these services (Ambler and Sheldrake 2009; Bond 2006; Roberts and Kennington 2010b). Moreover, pharmacy practice research serves as the cornerstone for evidence-based pharmacy practice and is an essential component in the advancement of the pharmacy profession (Roberts and Kennington 2010b, c; Bond 2006; Ambler and Sheldrake 2009; Schommer et al. 2010).

Despite the increased awareness, published literature addressing the attitudes and involvement of pharmacists in practice research indicates limited involvement and reluctance among pharmacists for participating in such research-based activities. Understanding pharmacists' attitudes and perception about practice-based research is critical in developing a critical mass of pharmacy professionals who are actively involved in advancing practice through high-quality research and innovation. It is also instrumental in raising awareness, cultivating a culture change, inculcating a positive attitude and strengthening research support, as well as improving the building of research capacity (Kritikos et al. 2013; Awaisu et al. 2014).

13.3 What Does the Literature Report About Pharmacists and Research?

To explore how pharmacists understand issues around pharmacy-related research and to gain an insight into their attitude towards research, we conducted a systematic search. The aim of this review was to identifying published studies that report pharmacists' attitudes and involvement in research as well as perceived enablers and barriers. Our inclusion criteria were studies that included either specialised or unspecialised community, hospital, primary healthcare or industrial pharmacists and studies that utilised surveys/questionnaires, focus groups or interviews. We used a systematic search for original studies published or indexed in MEDLINE, PubMed, EBSCO, ScienceDirect, ProQuest and Google Scholar. Sixteen articles that looked at pharmacists' attitudes towards pharmacy practice-based research were reviewed according to the criteria described. Most of these studies were conducted in community pharmacies in the UK, Australia, and Canada.

These studies reported that pharmacists had positive attitudes in relation to willingness and interest in participating in pharmacy practice research. However, the extent of interest in participation in research varied widely and ranged from 28 % to 83 % of all the surveyed pharmacists. Several motivational factors to participation in research were reported by most of the studies and could be categorised into the following: personal interest in a particular research project, a belief regarding the perceived importance of research, the research's impact on patients' health, and the desire to improve the profession of pharmacy. Between 6 % and 54 % of the surveyed pharmacists reported previous involvement in research; this was observed more in hospital than in community settings. A general trend of establishing pharmacy practice-based research networks (PBRNs) started and greatly increased after the year 2000. The evolution of PBRNs could be attributed to the popularity of the pharmaceutical care concept among pharmacies in the last decades. Barriers to research participation were highlighted in all the reviewed studies, and lack of time, support and training were identified as the most common barriers.

Due to the impact of the philosophy and practice of pharmaceutical care introduced in the early 1990s, it is logical to analyse and view pharmacists' involvement in research using a decade-wise approach starting from the 1990s.

Before the 1990s During this era, pharmacists in most parts of the world had a minimal involvement in research. Based on our personal reflection, we know pharmacists generally did not have much interest in research, did not see it as a professional mandate or a way to advance practice, and were rarely involved in practice research activities. Prior to 1990, and since the early 1960s and 1970s, pharmacists have strived to move away from the traditional pharmacy practice that was dominated by inventory control, drug supply and dispensing to something new and different. This was a dissatisfaction with old practice, and it was increasingly expected that the health professionals should have updated knowledge of the therapeutic use of drugs (Miller 1981). The clinical pharmacy movement began at the University of Michigan in the early 1960s, with some beginnings that could be traced back to the latter part of the 1960s. Up to the late 1980s, pharmacy-related research was mostly limited to research associated with postgraduate studies (Masters and Doctorate in Pharmacy). Many pharmacists did their postgraduate degrees in pharmacology and pharmaceutical sciences, and they were rarely exposed to pharmacy practice. However, even in those years, when compared with community pharmacists, hospital pharmacists showed higher motivational levels to participate in research activities. On the other hand, it would appear that pharmacists working for pharmaceutical companies were involved much more in research than other pharmacists, for reasons associated with trials involving drugs. For example, pharmaceutical companies conducted 393 trials in Norway, of which over 55 % of staff involved in these controlled drug trials were pharmacists (Eriksen and Andrew 1986). Furthermore, 94 % of these clinical trials staff reported previous attendance in external workshops related to clinical drug trials methodology, compared to 41 % of hospital pharmacists who reported some knowledge through attendance of continuing pharmacy education courses.

1990–1999 In general, there was an increasing awareness, interest and willingness to be involved in future practice research among pharmacists. Only a minority of UK pharmacists were reported to be involved in practice-based research, although there was an increasing trend in pharmacists' opinion regarding the importance of it (Krska et al. 1998; Liddell 1996). It has actually been observed that the majority of the pharmacists considered that practice-based research was important (Krska et al. 1998; Liddell 1996). It was obvious, therefore, that there was a trend of an increase in the positive attitude towards research with time. Supporting service development, preregistration requirement and personal interest were among the most commonly reported reasons for initiating research projects. For example, there was a general agreement among pharmacists on the need for practice research training programmes.

2000–2009 There was a paradigm shift towards increased recognition of the value of research among community pharmacists. Studies during this period indicated increased awareness and positive attitude towards research among pharmacists, mostly in the community setting (Rosenbloom et al. 2000; Simpson et al. 2001; Saini et al. 2006; Armour et al. 2007; Peterson et al. 2009). Future development of community pharmacy practice and new practice models could be among the motivational factors for this trend. Previous experience with research seems to be a factor affecting pharmacists' willingness to participate in future research. Saini et al. suggested that willingness to participate in practice research varied between those who had prior experience in research and those who had not. Only 34 % of research-naïve pharmacists showed interest in involvement in research, compared to over 75 % of those with previous research experience (Saini et al. 2006). Other investigators linked the willingness of pharmacists to participate in research with their perception of the benefit of research findings (Peterson et al. 2009). It was observed that the pharmacists with this opinion were most likely to be interested in participating in research when they perceived, or expected, clear benefit in terms of improving patient care.

2010–2014 During the period 2010–2014, pharmacists seem to be more aware of the importance of research and also to participate in the professional development. Many pharmacists recognise the need to be involved in research and strive to document the value of new services through drug audits and by conducting research. There is a general consensus that lack of dedicated time, shortage of research funding and support and lack of adequate knowledge and training are significant barriers for pharmacists' involvement in practice-based research.

However, the positive factors noted to promote a culture of research were continuing professional development, changes in pharmacy education including mandatory research projects, licensing requirements, competition for job opportunities and accreditation requirements. Up to 50 % or more of the surveyed hospital and intensive care unit pharmacists reported previous involvement in pharmacy practice research. The interest of pharmacists in participating in research was relatively high and ranged between 40 and 84 % (Carr et al. 2011; Perreault et al. 2012; Kanjanarach et al. 2012; Hébert et al. 2013; Elkassem et al. 2013; Awaisu et al. 2014). Overall, pharmacists agreed on the importance of conducting practice-based research and shared their beliefs that research is part of their professional responsibility and is a critical tool for improving patients' care. Motivational factors, however, varied widely between pharmacists. The motivational factors include impact of research on clinical practice, having access to continuing education programmes and the development of clinical tools.

In recent years, an evolving initiative in practice-based research environments is the development of practice-based research networks (PBRNs), a form of collaborative learning organisations. The Agency for Healthcare Research and Quality (AHRQ) defines a primary care PBRN as a group of ambulatory practices devoted principally to primary care patients. The aim of this initiative is to investigate questions related to community-based practice and to improve the quality of primary care (Agency for Healthcare Research and Quality 2012). These networks have been envisioned as places of learning where clinicians are engaged in reflective practice inquiries and where clinicians and academic researchers can collaborate to develop new ways to improve delivery of primary care. These collaborative learning networks are becoming a commonplace in pharmacy, whereby many pharmacy practice-based research networks are evolving (Farland et al. 2012; Goode et al. 2008; Lipowski 2008; Marinac and Kuo 2010).

13.4 Pharmacists' Attitudes Towards Practice-Based Research: An Interpretation of the Literature

The area of pharmacy practice research is rapidly evolving and falls under the umbrella of "health services research" (Bond 2006). This area emerged in the 1990s with the evolution of patient-centred pharmacy practice. There appears to be clear evidence that pharmacists continue to recognise the value of practice-based research in advancing evidence-based pharmacy practice and express a high level of interest in being involved in such research. In general, pharmacists expressed positive attitudes towards research, and there was an increasing trend over time in the proportion of pharmacists who indicated interest as well as involvement. Pharmacy practice research is becoming essential to generate new knowledge for improving therapeutic use of medicines, as well as to improve healthcare outcomes (Bond 2006; Kritikos et al. 2013; Peterson et al. 2009). Research is needed in order to advance education and evidence-based pharmacy practice and to improve rational clinical decision-making. Therefore, having pharmacists who are competent in the delivery of pharmaceutical care and possess the skills for conducting research is critical, because their role in direct patient care is rapidly advancing (Bond 2006; Dowling et al. 2009; Hepler and Strand 1990; Holland and Nimmo 1999; Poloyac et al. 2011; Schumock et al. 2003; Schwartz 1986; Smith et al. 2009).

Although a large proportion of pharmacists in various settings (hospital, community, industry) had expressed interest in pharmacy practice and health-related research, in reality studies have reported pharmacists' reluctance and limited involvement in research activities (Armour et al. 2007; Bond 2006; Ellerby et al. 1993; Liddell 1996; Peterson et al. 2009; Rosenbloom et al. 2000; Saini et al. 2006). The research is not regarded as a mandate for pharmacists or a requirement for preregistration training in many countries, and this partly contributes to pharmacists' limited involvement. There is a clear need for concerted efforts to educate pharmacists and pharmacy students that existing pharmacy services are an end product and outcome of research, and if new services are to be developed, then more practice-based research is needed.

By involvement in practice-based research, pharmacists can improve the quality of existing cognitive services and develop new services through research evidence. They can also contribute to other health services research in collaboration with other healthcare professionals. In some parts of the world, hospital pharmacists, especially those with clinical training and affiliations, are increasingly becoming involved in collaborative research (Fagan et al. 2006; Knapp et al. 2011; Smith et al. 2009).

Pharmacists in many studies admitted the lack of competence in research methodologies including research design, implementation and dissemination of research findings. This is in spite of the fact that many of the pharmacists had experience and have had some aspects of previous research training. However, it was observed that the content, depth, structure and mode of delivery of such training programmes would determine whether the pharmacists have gained sufficient exposure to the core competencies to undertake such research. The methods for training individuals in skills to conduct pharmacy practice as well as clinical and translational research have been extensively discussed in the literature (Blouin et al. 2007; Dowling et al. 2009; Knapp et al. 2011; Poloyac et al. 2011; Smith et al. 2009). Most pharmacists in community and hospital practices have limited exposure to clinical and practice research (Awaisu et al. 2014; Elkassem et al. 2013; Simpson et al. 2001). These inadequacies call for intervention. These interventions should be targeted to practising pharmacists and pharmacy students, who should be given adequate training to conduct research and scholarly activities (Armour et al. 2007; Kritikos et al. 2013).

Professional pharmacy organisations across the world including North America, UK, Europe and Australia have developed research training and support for practice-based research (Bakker 1996; Lipowski 2008; Marinac and Kuo 2010; Smith 1999). We believe that it will be useful to include elements of research training for community and hospital pharmacists as part of their continuing professional development. Furthermore, it is imperative to establish pharmacy practice research networks (PBRNs) between the academia and other pharmacy practice settings. These academic interactions and practice experiences would promote research culture. This would also facilitate mentoring and would be a key component in training and development of new researchers (Bakker 1996; Farland et al. 2012; Kritikos et al. 2013; Peterson et al. 2009). In this context, PBRNs in pharmacy are increasingly been recognised (Farland et al. 2012; Goode et al. 2008; Lipowski 2008; Marinac and Kuo 2010).

PBRNs often link practising clinicians with investigators experienced in clinical and health services research while enhancing the research skills of the network members (Agency for Healthcare Research and Quality, 2012). There is evidence that these research networks will increasingly augment pharmacists' active participation in practice-based research (Carr et al. 2011; Hébert et al. 2013; Peterson et al. 2009; Rosenbloom et al. 2000). Furthermore, studies have investigated pharmacists' attitudes and willingness to participate in PBRNs (Carr et al. 2011; Hébert et al. 2013; Rosenbloom et al. 2000) and others have discussed the importance of PBRNs (Peterson et al. 2009; Rosenbloom et al. 2000; Simpson et al. 2001). Up to 84 % of pharmacists in three studies expressed interest in participating in PBRNs. In addition, such networks can foster community engagement and create links between academia and practitioners for broader scope of health services research. The networks can also strengthen the robustness of research and can facilitate research capacity building and mentoring (Carr et al. 2011; Peterson et al. 2009; Simpson et al. 2001). It also offers researchers the opportunity for greater input to generate research questions. This could also be a forum in which seasoned researchers can offer mentoring to less experienced members (Farland et al. 2012).

Key facilitators to research participation reported by the studies were recognition of the value of research to the advancement of pharmacy profession, the desire to improve the profession, incentives as well as personal interest in research. Conversely, the literature reported a lack of skills and knowledge, financial support or funding, lack of dedicated time to conduct research and workload and lack of awareness of opportunities as the greatest barriers to participation in research. These factors could negatively impact participation in practice-based research. Given the significant role pharmacy practice research plays in evidence-based healthcare and advancing practice, it is imperative to employ measures that will address these barriers encountered in practice. Research should be viewed as a mandate for pharmacy practitioners because it is a means of documenting and sharing evidence in the interest of improved healthcare and the evolving roles of pharmacy (Bond 2006; Elkassem et al. 2013; Peterson et al. 2009; Roberts and Kennington 2010a, b).

It is evident from the current study that the studies evaluating pharmacists' attitudes towards practice research utilised questionnaire surveys, focus groups, interviews or a combination of these (mixed methods). Though most of the studies reported in the literature have utilised quantitative research methods, with few on qualitative research, the trend to use qualitative methods is, however, on the rise. We strongly believe that it is pertinent to use mixed-method, as it will be helpful to gain a deeper insight of pharmacists' attitudes towards practice-based research. This could be further strengthened with triangulation of qualitative and quantitative data and integration of findings within or across different stages of research (Dougherty and Conway 2008; Koshman 2011; Smith 1999).

13.5 Conclusion

There is ample evidence that pharmacists recognise the importance of research in advancing evidence-based practice. Moreover, pharmacists have expressed a high level of interest and willingness to be involved in independent and collaborative research. However, lack of time, unawareness of opportunities, lack of funding and lack of training and support were identified as the major barriers to participating in practice-based research. There is a need to promote the development of PBRNs. Other strategies to promote pharmacy practice-based research could include offering informal research training programmes for pharmacists, increased research funding, creating protected time for pharmacy researchers and support from pharmacy leaders.

Acknowledgement Reprinted from Research in Social & Administrative Pharmacy, doi: 10.1016/j.sapharm.2014.12.008., Awaisu A and Alsalimy N, Pharmacists' involvement in and attitudes towards pharmacy practice research: a systematic review of the literature, 2014, with permission from Elsevier.

References

Agency for Healthcare Research and Quality (2012) Primary care practice-based research networks: An AHRQ initiative. Agency for Healthcare Research and Quality, Rockville, MD. http://www.ahrq.gov/research/findings/factsheets/primary/pbrn/index.html

Ambler S, Sheldrake L (2009) Pharmacy practice research: challenges and opportunities. Prim Health Care Res Dev 10:4–6. doi: 10.1017/S1463423608000935

Anderson C, Blenkinsopp A, Armstrong M (2008) The contribution of community pharmacy to improving the public's health: literature review update 2004–07. PHLink, London

Armour C, Brillant M, Krass I (2007) Pharmacists' views on involvement in pharmacy practice research: strategies for facilitating participation. Pharm Pract 5(2):59–66

Awaisu A, Bakdach D, Elajez RH, Zaidan M (2014) Hospital pharmacists' self-evaluation of their competence and confidence in conducting pharmacy practice research. SPJ doi: 10.1016/j.jsps.2014.10.002

Bakker A (1996) Pharmacy-practice research: a challenge for academia and practicing pharmacists. Pharmaceutica Acta Helvetiae 71(5):373–379. doi:10.1016/S0031-6865(96)00036-2

Blouin RA, Bergstrom RF, Ellingrod VL, Fletcher CV, Leff RD, Morris A, Okita RT, Roberts JC, Tracy TS, Sagraves R, Miller KW (2007) Report of the AACP Educating Clinical Scientists Task Force. Am J Pharm Educ 71(4):S05

Bond C (2006) The need for pharmacy practice research. Int J Pharm Pract 14(1):1–2. doi:10.1211/ijpp.14.1.0001

Carr MB, Divine H, Hanna C, Freeman PR, Blumenschein K (2011) Independent community pharmacist interest in participating in community pharmacy research networks. J Am Pharm Assoc 51(6):727–733

Dougherty D, Conway PH (2008) The "3 T's" road map to transform US health care: the "how" of high-quality care. JAMA 299(19):2319–2321. doi:10.1001/jama.299.19.2319

Dowling TC, Murphy JE, Kalus JS et al (2009) Recommended education for pharmacists as competitive clinical scientists. Pharmacotherapy 29(2):236–244. doi:10.1592/phco.29.2.236

Elkassem W, Pallivalapila A, Al Hail M, McHattie L, Diack L, Stewart D (2013) Advancing the pharmacy practice research agenda: views and experiences of pharmacists in Qatar. Int J Clin Pharm 35(5):692–696. doi:10.1007/s11096-013-9802-z

Ellerby DA, Williams A, Winfield AJ (1993) The level of interest in pharmacy practice research among community pharmacists. Pharm J 251:321–322

Eriksen IL, Andrew E (1986) Pharmacist involvement in Norwegian clinical drug trials: a questionnaire study. Drug Intell Clin Pharm 20(5):391–395

Fagan SC, Touchette D, Smith JA, Sowinski KM, Dolovich L, Olson KL, Cheang KI, Kolesar JM, Crismon ML (2006) The state of science and research in clinical pharmacy. Pharmacotherapy 26(7):1027–1040. doi:10.1592/phco.26.7.1027

Farland MZ, Franks AS, Byrd DC, Thomas JL, Suda KJ (2012) Development of a primary care pharmacist practice-based research network. Curr Pharm Teach Learn 4(2):150–154

Goode JV, Mott DA, Chater R (2008) Collaborations to facilitate success of community pharmacy practice-based research networks. J Am Pharm Assoc 48:153–162

Hatoum HT, Akhras K (1993) A 32-year literature review on the value and acceptance of ambulatory care provided by clinical pharmacists. Ann Pharmacother 27(9):1108–1119

Hatoum HT, Catizone C, Hutchinson RA, Purohit A (1986) An eleven-year review of the pharmacy literature: documentation of the value and acceptance of clinical pharmacy. Drug Intell Clin Pharm 20(1):33–48

Hébert J, Laliberté M-C, Berbiche D, Martin E, Lalonde L (2013) The willingness of community pharmacists to participate in a practice-based research network. Can Pharm J 146(1):47–54

Hepler CD, Strand LM (1990) Opportunities and responsibilities in pharmaceutical care. Am J Hosp Pharm 47(3):533–543

Holland RW, Nimmo CM (1999) Transitions in pharmacy practice, part 1: beyond pharmaceutical care. Am J Health Syst Pharm 56(17):1758–1764

Johnson JA, Bootman JL (1997) Drug-related morbidity and mortality and the economic impact of pharmaceutical care. Am J Health Syst Pharm 54(5):554–558

Kanjanarach T, Numchaitosapol S, Jaisa-ard R (2012) Thai pharmacists' attitudes and experiences of research. Res Soc Admin Pharm 8(6):e58–e59

Knapp KK, Manolakis M, Webster AA, Olsen KM (2011) Projected growth in pharmacy education and research, 2010 to 2015. Am J Pharm Educ 75(6):108. doi:10.5688/ajpe756108

Koshman SL (2011) What is pharmacy research? Can J Hosp Pharm 64(2):154–155

Kritikos VS, Carter S, Moles RJ, Krass I (2013) Undergraduate pharmacy students' perceptions of research in general and attitudes towards pharmacy practice research. Int J Pharm Pract 21 (3):192–201. doi:10.1111/j.2042-7174.2012.00241.x

Krska J, Kennedy EJ, Hansford D, John DN (1998) Pharmacists' opinions on their involvement in a community pharmacy based practice research study. Pharm J 261:R54

Liddell H (1996) Attitudes of community pharmacists regarding involvement in practice research. Pharm J 256:905–907

Lipowski EE (2008) Pharmacy practice-based research networks: why, what, who, and how. J Am Pharm Assoc 48(2):142–152

Marinac JS, Kuo GM (2010) Characterizing the American College of Clinical Pharmacy practice-based research network. Pharmacotherapy 30(8):865

Miller RR (1981) History of clinical pharmacy and clinical pharmacology. J Clin Pharmacol 21 (4):195–197

Penna RP (1990) Pharmaceutical care: pharmacy's mission for the 1990s. Am J Health Syst Pharm 47(3):543–549

Perreault MM, Thiboutot Z, Burry LD et al (2012) Canadian survey of critical care pharmacists' views and involvement in clinical research. Ann Pharmacother 46(9):1167–1173

Peterson GM, Jackson SL, Fitzmaurice KD, Gee PR (2009) Attitudes of Australian pharmacists towards practice-based research. J Clin Pharm Ther 34(4):397–405. doi:10.1111/j.1365-2710. 2008.01020.x

Poloyac SM, Empey KM, Rohan LC et al (2011) Core competencies for research training in the clinical pharmaceutical sciences. Am J Pharm Educ 75(2):27

Roberts R, Kennington E (2010a) Pharmacy practice research has an impact on each and every pharmacist. Pharm J 284:267–268

Roberts R, Kennington E (2010b) What are the benefits for pharmacists of engaging in practice research? Pharm J 284:291–292

Roberts R, Kennington E (2010c) Getting involved in pharmacy research. Pharm J 284:365–367

Rosenbloom K, Taylor K, Harding G (2000) Community pharmacists' attitudes towards research. Int J Pharm Pract 8(2):103–110. doi:10.1111/j.2042-7174.2000.tb00994.x

Sackett DL, Rosenberg WM, Gray JA, Haynes RB, Richardson WS (1996) Evidence based medicine: what it is and what it isn't. Br Med J 312(7023):71–72

Saini B, Brillant M, Filipovska J, Gelgor L, Mitchell B, Rose G, Smith L (2006) Factors influencing Australian community pharmacists' willingness to participate in research projects — an exploratory study. Int J Pharm Pract 14(3):179–188. doi:10.1211/ijpp.14.3.0004

Schumock GT, Butler MG, Meek PD, Vermeulen LC, Arondekar BV, Bauman JL (2003) Evidence of the economic benefit of clinical pharmacy services: 1996–2000. Pharmacotherapy 23(1):113–132

Schumock GT, Meek PD, Ploetz PA, Vermeulen LC (1996) Economic evaluations of clinical pharmacy services: 1988–1995. Pharmacotherapy 16(6):1188–1208

Schommer JC, Brown LM, Doucette WR, Goode J-V, Oliveira DRd (2010) Innovations in pharmacy through practice-based research. Innov Pharm 1(1): Article 9

Schwartz MA (1986) Academic pharmacy 1986: are clinical pharmacists meeting the clinical scientist role? Am J Pharm Educ 50:462–464

Simpson SH, Johnson JA, Biggs C, Biggs RS, Kuntz A, Semchuk W, Tsuyuki RT (2001) Practice-based research: lessons from community pharmacist participants. Pharmacotherapy 21(6):731–739

Smith F (1999) Health services research methods in pharmacy: triangulation. Int J Pharm Pract 7(1):60–68. doi:10.1111/j.2042-7174.1999.tb00949.x

Smith JA, Olson KL, Sowinski KM (2009) Pharmacy practice research careers. Pharmacotherapy 29(8):1007–1011

Tsuyuki RT, Schindel TJ (2008) Changing pharmacy practice: the leadership challenge. Can Pharm J 141(3):174–180

Van Mil J, Fernandez-Llimos F (2013) What is 'pharmaceutical care' in 2013? Int J Clin Pharm 35:1–2

Printed by Printforce, the Netherlands